COMPLEX INTERVENTIONS
IN HEALTH

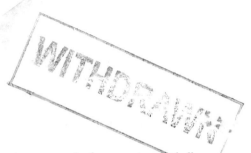

Health and human services currently face a series of challenges – such as ageing populations, chronic diseases and new endemics – that require highly complex responses, and take place in multiple care environments including acute medicine, chronic care facilities and the community. Accordingly, most modern health care interventions are now seen as 'complex interventions' – activities that contain a number of component parts with the potential for interactions between them which, when applied to the intended target population, produce a range of possible and variable outcomes. This in turn requires methodological developments that also take into account changing values and attitudes related to the situation of patients receiving health care.

The first book to place complex interventions within a coherent system of research enquiry, this work is designed to help researchers understand the research processes involved at each stage of developing, testing, evaluating and implementing complex interventions, and assist them to integrate methodological activities to produce secure, evidence-based health care interventions. It begins with conceptual chapters which set out the complex interventions framework, discuss the interrelation between knowledge development and evidence, and explore how mixed-methods research contributes to improved health. Structured around the influential UK Medical Research Council guidance for use of complex interventions, four sections, each comprised of bite-sized chapters written by multidisciplinary experts in the area, focus on:

- Developing complex interventions
- Assessing the feasibility of complex interventions and piloting them
- Evaluating complex interventions
- Implementing complex interventions.

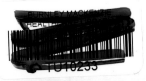

Accessible to students and researchers grappling with complex interventions, each substantive chapter includes an introduction, bulleted learning objectives, clinical examples, a summary and further reading. The perspectives of various stakeholders, including patients, families and professionals, are discussed throughout as are the economic and ethical implications of methods.

A vital companion for health research, this book is suitable for readers from health and social care disciplines such as medical, nursing, public health, health services research, human services and allied health care backgrounds.

David A. Richards is Professor of Mental Health Services Research at the University of Exeter Medical School. For many years he has been at the forefront of national and international efforts to improve access to treatment for those suffering from high-prevalence mental health problems such as depression. A nurse by professional background, he is a UK National Institute of Health Research Senior Investigator, President of the European Academy of Nursing Science and chair of the European Science Foundation REFLECTION Research Network Programme, an interdisciplinary European faculty of researchers, equipped to design, plan and implement programmatic, mixed-methods and complex interventions research. Like Ingalill, he has frequently challenged the research community to reduce waste in their work by refocusing their research activity towards clinically relevant programmes, driven by the uncertainties of clinical practice and the real concerns of the public, patients and clinicians.

Ingalill Rahm Hallberg is Professor in Health Care Science at Lund University, Sweden. She has been the pro-dean of the Medical Faculty, the assistant vice-chancellor and pro vice-chancellor of Lund University. She is a nurse by professional background. Her research has been on ageing, care and services for older people and living with severe diseases, an area in which she has been at the forefront nationally and internationally. Her frequent involvement in reviewing research proposals, research at universities, and research by national and international groups inspired her to initiate a debate on how research was very often scattered, lacking coherent programmes and dominated by descriptive studies with no impact on health care. As the previous president of the European Academy of Nursing Science she was, together with David, a driving force to change the unwelcome preponderance of small-scale, descriptive projects.

COMPLEX INTERVENTIONS IN HEALTH

An overview of research methods

*Edited by David A. Richards and
Ingalill Rahm Hallberg*

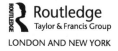

Routledge
Taylor & Francis Group

LONDON AND NEW YORK

First published 2015
by Routledge
2 Park Square, Milton Park, Abingdon, Oxon OX14 4RN

and by Routledge
711 Third Avenue, New York, NY 10017

Routledge is an imprint of the Taylor & Francis Group, an informa business

British Library Cataloguing in Publication Data
A catalogue record for this book is available from the British Library

Library of Congress Cataloguing in Publication data
Richards, David A., author.
  Complex interventions in health: an overview of research methods / David A. Richards and Ingalill Rahm Hallberg.
      p.   cm.
  Includes bibliographical references.
  I. Hallberg, Ingalill, author.   II. Title.
  [DNLM: 1. Comparative Effectiveness Research–methods.   2. Research Design. W 84.3]
  R850
  610.72–dc23
  2014031766

ISBN: 978-0-415-70314-7 (hbk)
ISBN: 978-0-415-70316-1 (pbk)
ISBN: 978-0-203-79498-2 (ebk)

Typeset in Bembo
by Out of House Publishing

CONTENTS

Section 2: Investigating feasibility and undertaking pilot testing of complex interventions 121

FIGURES

TABLES

BOXES

CONTRIBUTING AUTHORS

Charles Abraham DPhil, BA, CPsychol
Professor of Psychology Applied to Health
University of Exeter Medical School
United Kingdom

Michael Allen PhD, BSc
Senior Modeller
University of Exeter Medical School
United Kingdom

Douglas G. Altman DSc
Professor of Statistics in Medicine
Centre for Statistics in Medicine
University of Oxford
United Kingdom

Salla Atkins PhD, MA, BSocSci (Hons), BA
Postdoctoral Researcher
Department of Public Health Sciences
Karolinska Institutet
Sweden

Suzanne Audrey PhD, MSc
Research Fellow
DECIPHer UKCRC Public Health Research Centre of Excellence
School of Social and Community Medicine
University of Bristol
United Kingdom

Janis Baird PhD, MBBS
Senior Lecturer in Public Health
MRC Lifecourse Epidemiology Unit
University of Southampton
United Kingdom

Mary Barker PhD, MSc
Senior Lecturer in Psychology
MRC Lifecourse Epidemiology Unit
University of Southampton
United Kingdom

Lyndal Bond PhD, MA, BA (Hons)
Principal Research Officer
Centre of Excellence in Intervention and Prevention Science, Melbourne
Australia

Chris Bonell PhD, MSc, MA
Professor of Sociology and Social Policy
Department of Childhood, Families and Health
Institute of Education
University of London
United Kingdom

Gunilla Borglin PhD, MSc, BSc, RN
Associate Professor and Senior Lecturer in Nursing Science
Faculty of Health and Society
Department of Care Science
Malmö University
Sweden

Susanne Buhse MSc, RN
Research Fellow
University of Hamburg
Germany

Christopher R. Burton DPhil, PGCert, BN, RGN
Senior Research Fellow
School of Healthcare Sciences
Bangor University
United Kingdom

Jackie Chandler MSc, RN
Methods Coordinator
Cochrane Collaboration
Oxford
United Kingdom

Sylvie Cossette PhD, RN
Professor
Montreal Heart Institute Research Center
University of Montreal
Canada

Peter Craig PhD, MSc
Senior Research Fellow
MRC/CSO Social and Public Health Sciences Unit
Institute of Health and Wellbeing
University of Glasgow
United Kingdom

Nicky Cullum DBE, PhD, BSc, RGN
Professor of Nursing
The University of Manchester
United Kingdom

Sarah Dean PhD, MSc, BSc, CPsychol
Senior Lecturer in Psychology Applied to Health
University of Exeter Medical School
United Kingdom

Sarah Denford PhD, MSc, BSc
Research Fellow in Psychology Applied to Health
University of Exeter Medical School
United Kingdom

Elizabeth J. Dogherty PhD, MSc, RN
Postdoctoral Research Fellow
Faculty of Nursing
University of Alberta
Canada

Jo Dumville PhD, MSc
Senior Lecturer in Applied Health Research
The University of Manchester
United Kingdom

Carole A. Estabrooks PhD, RN
Professor and Canada Research Chair in Knowledge Translation
University of Alberta
Canada

Paul Ewings PhD, MSc, BSc
Professor
Director of NIHR Research Design Service South West
National Institute for Health Research
United Kingdom

Nancy Feeley PhD, MSc, BSc
Associate Professor
Ingram School of Nursing
McGill University
Canada

Lora M. Giangregorio PhD
Associate Professor
Department of Kinesiology
University of Waterloo
Canada

Colin Greaves PhD, CPsychol, BSc, BEng
Associate Professor in Psychology Applied to Health
University of Exeter Medical School
United Kingdom

Karin Hannes PhD, MSc
Assistant Professor
Methodology of Educational Sciences Research Group
KU Leuven
Belgium

Wendy Hardeman PhD, MSc
Senior Research Associate in Behavioural Science
Primary Care Unit, Department of Public Health and Primary Care
University of Cambridge
United Kingdom

Karin Harms-Ringdahl PhD, RPT
Professor of Physiotherapy
Department of Neurobiology, Care Sciences and Society
Karolinska Institutet, and Karolinska University Hospital, Stockholm
Sweden

Henna Hasson PhD, MSc
Associate Professor
Medical Management Centre
Karolinska Institutet, Stockholm
Sweden

Sascha Köpke PhD, RN
Professor of Nursing Research
University of Lübeck
Germany

Sallie Lamb DPhil, MSc, MCSP
Professor
Oxford Clinical Trials Research Unit
University of Oxford
United Kingdom

Natalie Leon PhD, MA, MClinPsych
Senior Resarcher
South African Medical Research Council, Cape Town
South Africa

Simon Lewin PhD, MBChB
Senior Researcher
Global Health Unit, Norwegian Knowledge Centre for the Health Services,
Norway and
Health Systems Research Unit, Medical Research Council of South Africa,
South Africa

Jenny Lloyd PhD, MSc, BA (Ed) Hons
Senior Research Fellow in Child Health
University of Exeter Medical School
United Kingdom

Elizabeth Lutge PhD, FCPHM, MSc (Epidemiology), MPH, MBChB
Manager: Epidemiology, Health Research and Knowledge Management
KwaZulu-Natal Department of Health
South Africa

Brendan McCormack DPhil (Oxon), BSc (Hons), PGCEA, RGN, RMN
Professor of Nursing and Head of the Division of Nursing
Queen Margaret University, Edinburgh
United Kingdom

Carl May PhD, BScEcon
Professor of Healthcare Innovation
University of Southampton
United Kingdom

Gabriele Meyer PhD, RN
Professor
Medical Faculty, Institute for Health and Nursing Science
Martin-Luther-Universität Halle-Wittenberg
Germany

Thomas Monks PhD, MSc, BSc (Hons)
Senior Research Fellow
Faculty of Health Sciences
University of Southampton
United Kingdom

Graham Moore PhD, MSc, BSc
Research Fellow
DECIPHer UKCRC Public Health Research Centre of Excellence
School of Social Sciences
Cardiff University
United Kingdom

Laurence Moore PhD, MSc
Professor
Director, MRC/CSO Social and Public Health Sciences Unit
University of Glasgow
United Kingdom

Ingrid Mühlhauser PhD, MD
Specialist in Internal Medicine, Endocrinology and Diabetology
Professor of Health Sciences
University of Hamburg
Germany

Lena Nilsson-Wikmar PhD, RPT
Associate Professor in Physiotherapy
Department of Neurobiology, Care sciences and Society
Division of Physiotherapy
Karolinska Institutet, Stockholm
Sweden

Jane Noyes DPhil, RN
Professor of Health and Social Services Research and Child Health and Co-Chair
Cochrane Methods Executive,
Bangor University
United Kingdom

Alicia O'Cathain, PhD, MA, MSc, BSc
Professor of Health Services Research
School of Health and Related Research
University of Sheffield
United Kingdom

Willem Odendaal MA
Senior Scientist
South African Medical Research Council
South Africa

Katherine Payne PhD, MSc, DipClinPharm, BPharm, MRPharmS
Professor of Health Economics
Manchester Centre for Health Economics
University of Manchester
United Kingdom

Martin Pitt EngD, MSc, BSc
Associate Professor of Healthcare Modelling and Simulation
University of Exeter Medical School
United Kingdom

Ingalill Rahm Hallberg PhD, BSc (Hons), RN
Professor of Health Sciences
Lund University
Sweden

David A. Richards PhD, BSc (Hons), RN
Professor of Mental Health Services Research
University of Exeter Medical School
United Kingdom

Jo Rycroft-Malone PhD, MSc, BSc (Hons), RN
Professor of Implementation Research
Bangor University
United Kingdom

Anne E. Sales PhD, MSN, RN, BA
Professor
School of Nursing
University of Michigan
USA

Walter Sermeus PhD, MSc, RN
Professor of Healthcare Management
KU Leuven
Belgium

Ted A. Skolarus MD, MPH
Assistant Professor of Urology
University of Michigan
VA Ann Arbor Healthcare System
USA

Jane R. Smith PhD, PGCert, PGDip, BSc (Hons)
Research Fellow in Psychology Applied to Health
University of Exeter Medical School
United Kingdom

Mark Tarrant PhD, BA (Hons)
Senior Lecturer in Psychology Applied to Health
University of Exeter Medical School
United Kingdom

Rod S. Taylor PhD, MSc, PGCert, BSc
Professor of Health Services Research
University of Exeter Medical School
United Kingdom

Lehana Thabane PhD, MSc, BSc
Professor of Clinical Epidemiology and Biostatistics
Departments of Anesthesia/Pediatrics
McMaster University
Canada

Alexander J. Thompson MSc
Research Associate in Health Economics
The University of Manchester
United Kingdom

Tannaze Tinati PhD, MSc, BSc
Research Fellow
MRC Lifecourse Epidemiology Unit
University of Southampton
United Kingdom

Shaun Treweek PhD, BSc (Hons)
Professor of Health Services Research
Health Services Research Unit
University of Aberdeen
United Kingdom

Obioha C. Ukoumunne PhD, MSc, BSc
Senior Lecturer in Medical Statistics
University of Exeter Medical School
United Kingdom

Theo van Achterberg PhD, MSc
Professor of Quality Care
Centre for Health Services and Nursing Research
KU Leuven
Belgium

Louise von Essen PhD, MSc
Professor of Health Care Sciences
Uppsala University
Sweden

Fiona C. Warren PhD, MSc
Lecturer in Medical Statistics
University of Exeter Medical School
United Kingdom

Mathew P. White PhD, MSc, BSc (Hons)
Lecturer in Psychology Applied to Health and the Environment
University of Exeter Medical School
United Kingdom

Daniel E. Wight PhD, MA (Hons)
Professor
MRC/CSO Social and Public Health Sciences Unit
University of Glasgow
United Kingdom

Katrina Wyatt PhD, BSc (Hons)
Associate Professor
University of Exeter Medical School
United Kingdom

Yan Hu PhD, MSN, RN
Professor
School of Nursing
Fudan University
P.R.China

FOREWORD

Peter Craig

Recent reports on avoidable waste in the conduct and reporting of research have re-emphasized the need for guidance to help researchers, and others involved in the research process, such as funders and publishers, to make appropriate methodological and practical choices (Chalmers and Glasziou, 2009; Chalmers *et al.*, 2014; Chan *et al.*, 2014; Glasziou *et al.*, 2014; Ioannidis *et al.*, 2014; Macleod *et al.*, 2014; Salman *et al.*, 2014). Some of the sources of waste identified in those reports, such as over-regulation of low-risk research and the imbalance of investment in basic and applied research, are outside the scope of guidance aimed at the conduct of specific studies. Others, such as inefficient priority-setting, failure to take account of what is already known, poor design and incomplete reporting, are matters that all researchers should take seriously.

The 2008 MRC guidance on the development and evaluation of complex interventions (Medical Research Council, 2008) was motivated by the need to take stock of the rapid evolution of the field since the first edition of the guidance was published in 2000 (Campbell *et al.*, 2000) and to address issues that had been overlooked first time round. A workshop involving the original authors of the guidance, and others directly involved in research on complex health care and public health interventions, raised four key concerns with the 2000 guidance: a lack of evidence for some of the recommendations, too little attention to the early and later phases of the research process, such as pilot and implementation studies, and a failure to recognize the importance of context, or the need to take account of systematic reviews in both the planning and reporting of complex intervention studies. There were also concerns about adopting a model based on the phases of drug development and testing, and the relative lack of attention to non-randomized designs.

Following the workshop, a small writing group was convened. We resolved to base our recommendations on practical examples and to avoid suggesting approaches that, however appealing in principle, had not been successfully implemented at least once in practice. The first draft of the new document, in an attempt to avoid being too prescriptive, adopted a question-and-answer format. This was dropped in the light of feedback from workshop participants and others, in favour of a more conventional approach to presenting the key recommendations in terms of what we saw as the key phases of the development and evaluation process.

While both editions of the guidance have been found useful by researchers, and are widely cited in the evaluation literature, the 2008 guidance is equally liable to the charge of neglecting or dealing superficially with important issues. Such is the interest in complex interventions nowadays, that many of these gaps are rapidly being filled with more detailed and specific guidance. The MRC's Population Health Sciences Research Network, which sponsored the revision of the complex interventions guidance, has since supported work on natural experimental approaches (Craig et al., 2012) and on process evaluation (Moore et al., 2014).

There are several other areas where the 2008 guidance could usefully be supplemented by further work. One is research priority-setting. The guidance stressed the need to consider implementation issues at the outset, rather than deferring them to the end of the research process, to undertake a systematic review, unless there is an up-to-date review already available, and to involve users at all stages in the research process. This is consistent with Chalmers and colleagues' emphasis on identifying questions that are important to patients and practitioners, and basing new research on a systematic and comprehensive understanding of what is already known (Chalmers et al., 2014). But these approaches should be supplemented by a systematic appraisal of whether the important questions can be answered at reasonable cost. So-called 'value of information' methods have been applied to health care research priority-setting but they have not been extensively used to prioritize complex intervention studies (Fenwick et al., 2008). Whether or not such methods do turn out to have wider applicability, the value of pre-trial modelling, using existing evidence and emerging findings from pilot and feasibility studies to optimize design and to take an informed decision on whether to proceed, should be evident from reports of the high proportion of funded trials that produce inconclusive results (Raftery and Powell, 2013).

The 2008 guidance emphasized the need for careful development, feasibility and pilot work before embarking on a full-scale evaluation, but did not distinguish sufficiently clearly between the questions appropriate to feasibility and pilot studies. This blurring of the distinction between pilot and feasibility studies has since been shown to be a widespread flaw in the reporting of research (Arain et al., 2010). Guidance for applicants provided by the National Evaluation Trials and Studies Co-ordinating Centre, which manages many important UK funding streams, usefully distinguishes between feasibility studies, which look at specific aspects of the design of the proposed full study, and pilot studies, which seek to test whether the entire set of procedures of the full study work together. It follows that while randomization may not be needed in a feasibility study, unless for example there is uncertainty about its acceptability among the target population, it would be required in a pilot for a randomized trial. Another key aspect of pilot and feasibility studies insufficiently emphasized in the 2008 guidance is the need for clear criteria for progression. Findings such as low recruitment or high attrition rates should be taken seriously as an indication of problems that need to be addressed in the design of the full study, or of the need for further feasibility or pilot work.

One important aspect of the reporting of complex intervention studies where good progress is being made is the systematic description of interventions. This has been a weakness in the past, leading to difficulties in synthesizing and implementing evidence about complex interventions, and incorporating that evidence into the design of future research (Glasziou *et al.*, 2008, Michie *et al.*, 2009). Michie and colleagues are developing methods for classifying behaviour change techniques systematically (Michie *et al.*, 2011, 2013). Their taxonomy should enable improvements in intervention design, by helping researchers to identify appropriate techniques, and reporting, by helping researchers to systematically describe interventions in terms of their component techniques. Publication of the TIDieR template for reporting health care interventions (Hoffmann *et al.*, 2014), and the development of an extension of the CONSORT checklist to cover social and psychological interventions (Mayo-Wilson *et al.*, 2013), should help to consolidate progress.

In publishing the 2008 guidance we did not expect to have the last word on how to develop and test complex interventions, and we explicitly drew attention to the ongoing methodological debates. We were also aware that in places we were dealing with some complex issues in just a few sentences. This book, which expands on the guidance, draws on many more examples, and a wider range of expertise, is therefore very welcome.

ACKNOWLEDGEMENTS

We would like to thank all the contributors to this volume for their expert contributions and insights, and the European Science Foundation for funding the REFLECTION research network programme, out of which the idea for this book was born. We would also like to thank our friends and colleagues on the REFLECTION Steering Committee, in universities, health services and organizations across Europe and the world who have provided support and insights. Particular thanks go to members of the European Academy of Nursing Science for providing multiple opportunities for discussion about complex interventions research methods. Final thanks to Marte Lavender for administrative support to us during the writing and editing of the book

1

THE COMPLEX INTERVENTIONS FRAMEWORK

David A. Richards

In the year 2000, the Medical Research Council (MRC) in the United Kingdom (UK) published a document that aimed to guide researchers on how to investigate the effects of health care interventions that could be regarded as complex (Medical Research Council, 2000). Whilst this document was found extremely useful by many researchers internationally, it was superseded in 2008 by a revision that has arguably led to an even larger impact (Medical Research Council, 2008). As noted by Peter Craig in the foreword to this book, the second edition arose as a consequence of methodological and theoretical developments in health services research together with a desire to focus on aspects of the topic that had been omitted from the first guidance. This introductory chapter will provide an overview of complex interventions and research methods. It will examine the MRC framework for complex interventions research methods and set the scene for the subsequent sections and chapters, each of which will describe in depth elements of research methods necessary for developing, testing, evaluating and implementing complex interventions in health care and public health.

Learning objectives

- Understand the nature of complexity in health care interventions.
- Consider the need for guidance on complex interventions research methods.
- Be familiar with an overview of the complex interventions research framework.

Given that we as book editors and chapter contributors are focused on 'complex interventions', it would be reasonable to define what a complex intervention actually is. It is a relatively simple process to define what we mean by an intervention.

Most dictionaries include the idea of an intervention as an action taken for medical purposes. In this book we have extended this definition to mean any action taken by health care workers (including people working in social care and public health situations) with the aim of improving the well-being of people with health and/or social care needs. These actions might also be taken by informal carers, or by people and patients themselves in the form of self-care interventions directed at, for example, better glycaemic self-control by people with diabetes. When we use the term 'intervention', therefore, we subsume terms such as 'activities' or 'actions' often used to describe the work of nurses or other people labouring in health and social care.

Unfortunately, when we turn our attention to our second definitional concept of 'complex' the task is not as easy as one might at first assume. What, after all, is a 'simple' intervention? It might be assumed that an oral antibiotic agent prescribed by a doctor and taken by a patient in order to reduce an infection is a good example of this simplicity. However, if one takes a moment to consider this proposition, it quickly breaks down.

At the biological level, different people absorb active drug reagents at different rates and amounts. People metabolize the same drug in different ways or even not at all. Gut motility varies. At a psychological level, individual people are motivated differently, have different recall and different views about medication. As a consequence, the drug may be taken exactly as prescribed, sporadically, at an insufficient daily dose and for varying durations, often being terminated before the full course has been taken. Interpersonally, the relationship between the medical practitioner and the patient may influence 'compliance' as may the individual's view of the competency of the doctor. The doctor may have a preference for one drug type over others, and may prescribe according to preference or manufacturer marketing techniques, rather than through evidence. The patient may have an allergy to one type of drug. Even before the medical encounter happens, an individual's perception of himself or herself as a 'candidate' for treatment varies from person to person. This is in itself influenced by both the dominant cultural values of society and the many groups within society to which an individual identifies.

All this, for just a short-term dose of an antibiotic. Pharmacological interventions for mental health conditions, long-term physical conditions and multi-morbidity create additional levels of complexity. On close examination it would seem that there is barely any intervention that we should not consider as 'complex'. Simple interventions might be merely our desire for simple solutions to the problems of the human condition. Beguiling as it may seem, simplicity is probably a chimera.

Given the above reservations, the current fascination in research circles for the idea of a separate notion of 'complex interventions' is slightly puzzling. Indeed, one of the original authors of the MRC framework (Medical Research Council, 2008) has made the suggestion that definitions of simple and complex should not begin with the intervention itself but with the questions being asked in research projects (Petticrew, 2011). He makes the point that if most interventions are inherently complex then it might not be the intervention that determines the most appropriate research strategy, but the questions being posed. 'Does it (the intervention) work?' is a very different question to 'How does it work?' or 'What would work in this situation?' or even 'How can we optimize it?' independent of the actual complexity of the intervention itself. Notwithstanding this, registers of randomized controlled trials suggest that almost 50 per cent of entries could refer to trials of interventions regarded by their investigators as complex (http://www.clinicaltrials.gov/ct2/resources/trends; http://www.controlled-trials.com/news/statistics).

Although this sophisticated understanding of interventions and research methods is helpful, it is still necessary to understand what we mean when we talk about the complexity of an intervention. Throughout this book, our contributors return again and again to several important concerns. Of these, perhaps the major one is that of implementation. Whilst we have a full section on implementation, many people believe that it is foolish to develop, test and evaluate an intervention without considering its sustainability and the likelihood it can be routinely adopted by clinical services. The MRC framework describes development, testing, evaluation and implementation as separate, albeit non-linear, steps with important feedback loops to previous and subsequent stages. However, this is really for convenience sake.

As Ingalill Rahm Hallberg notes in Chapter 2 on knowledge generation, although there is a direction of travel through discovery, evaluation and implementation, the route often requires frequent stops, doubling back and retracing of steps. Whilst every journey might start with a single step, most people have an idea where they expect to end up. Complex intervention research methods have been developed to maximize the likelihood that knowledge generated will be ultimately of benefit to humanity. The idea is to be able to develop something useful, demonstrate its effect beyond the vagaries of chance and then embed it in situations where it will bring most benefit. The complex interventions researcher always has an eye on this prize. However, the more complex an intervention, the more difficult it can be to make it a routine part of health care.

Three definitions of complexity are presented in Table 1.1. The MRC definition (Medical Research Council, 2000, 2008) focuses mainly, though not exclusively, on characteristics of the intervention itself and the importance of specifying the individual components, the way in which these components might interact and the amount of flexibility in intervention delivery. It asks researchers to consider the way in which an intervention might be designed to address itself to different groups or organizational targets and to further consider the possible range of different outcomes sought. Latterly, some authors have categorized complexity beyond components of the intervention (Anderson et al., 2013) and have also considered implementation complexity (how an intervention might vary as it is implemented), context (the varied situations in which an intervention is implemented) and participants (the variation in participants receiving the intervention). The final definition cited in Table 1.1 was developed empirically by content analysing authors, descriptions of complex interventions in 207 journal articles (Datta and Petticrew, 2013). This thematic analysis discovered that researchers publishing about complex

TABLE 1.1 Three published examples describing components of intervention complexity

Source	Type of complexity	Sub-themes
Medical Research Council, 2000, 2008	Behaviours	Number of different behaviours
		Parameters of behaviours
		Methods of organizing and delivering behaviours
		Interactions between behaviours
		Difficulty of these behaviours for clinicians and recipients
	Outcomes	Number and variability
	Delivery	Degree of flexibility and tailoring
Anderson *et al.*, 2013	Intervention	Anticipated effects may be modified by intervention characteristics
	Implementation	Anticipated effects may be modified by implementation process
	Context	Anticipated effects may be modified by context where interventions are implemented
	Participant response	Anticipated effects may be modified by participant characteristics
Datta and Petticrew, 2013	Design	Theoretical understanding
		Standardization and treatment fidelity
	Implementation	Staffing issues
		Patient issues
	Context	
	Outcomes	Multidimensional measures
		Assessment methods
	Evaluation	Formative and process

interventions described them in terms of intervention design, implementation, context, outcomes and evaluation challenges.

It is apparent, therefore, that later definitions have been extended to pay more attention to issues of context and implementation, notwithstanding the fact that the original MRC definition did indeed note their importance. We now think of a complex intervention as much more than the sum of its component parts. Its effects are likely to be modified by both the site and process of implementation. It is likely to have more than one target for change. It is also likely that the more components of complexity present within and between the different elements, the more complex an intervention will be, although one might also argue that some elements (for example the number and variety of intervention components) will have a greater impact on the level of complexity. Crucially, complex interventions present considerable evaluation challenges as they progress along the knowledge development pipeline.

Principles for researching complex interventions

Vast amounts of time and resource are expended in research into human health and well-being, amounting to around US$240 billion annually (Rottingen et al., 2013). From basic scientists aiming to discover underlying disease mechanisms to applied researchers wishing to translate these insights into new therapeutic compounds and regimens, efforts to prolong life and reduce distress preoccupy individuals and societies worldwide. Although tremendous progress has been made, the return on investment is much less than one might expect, referred to by some authors as 'research waste' (Chalmers and Glasziou, 2009). This waste arises when the health care research community asks the wrong questions, uses unnecessary or poor-quality research methods, fails to publish research promptly or not at all, and reports research findings in a biased or unusable manner (Chalmers and Glasziou, 2009). In the field of nursing, Rahm Hallberg made a similar observation three years before Chalmers and Glasziou, in that only 15 per cent of papers published in two international nursing science journals in 2005 were addressing 'research that may carry strong evidence for practice' (Rahm Hallberg, 2006: 924). Recent reviews have suggested that experimental work comprises no more than 5–10 per cent of research into nursing (Yarcheski et al., 2012; Richards et al., 2014). Given that nursing represents an exemplar of an applied (and complex) science (Richards and Borglin, 2011), these are serious allegations.

Conversely, one of the other reasons behind the efforts to improve research methods, cited in the MRC framework guidance itself (Medical Research Council, 2008), was that promising interventions might be rejected as inefficacious because insufficient effort had been made to develop and pilot test the intervention, or identify and select the right outcome(s) and measures before proceeding to a full clinical trial. Alternatively, many trials fail because of over-optimistic assessments of trial procedures, for example failing to recruit sufficient participants and thereby producing inconclusive results. The most serious problem, however, is in the area of implementation or 'normalization' (May and Finch, 2009) of new interventions, a problem that has so bedevilled health sciences that a whole new field of 'implementation science' has grown up to address it. Researchers and clinicians can appear to be at loggerheads as the researchers wonder why apparently effective interventions are not widely adopted while clinicians often refer to the unsuitability of carefully controlled, research-based interventions when applied to their own unique clinical context. In some fields many researchers have rejected the idea of experimental trials at all, in favour of observational research, often with a unique qualitative focus. Ironically, therefore, while some health scientists are concerned with preventing badly planned clinical trials of poorly conceptualized interventions from proceeding, others want to see more trials of interventions in areas where traditions have developed that question the validity of clinical trials at all (Richards and Hamers, 2009; Melnyk, 2012).

The MRC complex interventions framework, together with the growing popularity of mixed methods, described by Borglin in Chapter 3 of this book, promised to usher in a new integrative world from that where previous opponents of alternative paradigms would argue vociferously against each other's positions. The guidance recognized that insights gained from qualitative and descriptive research could provide important contextual information when either developing interventions or understanding how they are received and delivered. The use of alternative evaluative designs was suggested, particularly where randomization might be impossible, difficult or extremely costly. Process evaluations, natural experiments, 'n of 1' studies, the importance of feasibility and piloting, and attention to context and implementation issues throughout the knowledge development process were all considered in the guidance. The guidance opened up the world of clinical trials to alternative or additive methods and allowed those suspicious of the usefulness of clinical trials to consider that there might be merit in such endeavours after all.

Central to research methods in complex interventions is that research should be programmatic. The original guidance was also programmatic, but was considered by many to be too linear, apparently based too closely on the process of new drug development. The 2008 guidance retained the idea that interventions can only be taken from 'bench to bedside' or 'campus to clinic' if a programme of research is sequential and builds upon itself. However, as noted earlier (Anderson *et al.*, 2013) this must not be at the expense of ignoring new, perhaps unexpected, feedback loops from the clinical practice context into the development and testing process itself. McCormack's Chapter 31 in this book describes one research method that explicitly uses this feature of complex interventions to embed them in practice through researcher and clinician co-production of the intervention itself.

A framework for researching complex interventions

The remainder of this chapter will now devote itself to briefly describing the suggested components of the MRC's complex interventions framework as contained in the guidance (Medical Research Council, 2008). This is helpfully (albeit rather simplistically) summarized as a four-stage process of 'develop–test–evaluate–implement'. At all stages in this process, researchers aim to address the key uncertainties in their intervention, their research design and their procedural strategies before moving on to reporting the effects of their intervention and working to embed it into routine health care. What follows is, therefore, a short introduction. All four elements of the framework are covered thoroughly and comprehensively, each as a separate section of this book, within which are multiple chapters. Readers will find that our contributing authors cite many relevant and varied clinical examples in their chapters and we advise that the following section of this chapter be regarded as merely the appetizer for the full menu to follow.

Developing complex interventions

Although much guidance on complex interventions does exhort the research community to consider how non-randomized or alternatively randomized (such as cluster randomized) clinical trial designs can be used where the situation dictates, much of the guidance concentrated on what could be done to improve the performance of complex interventions before taking them to trial. The development stage of the framework is best seen as the design stage in the research endeavour. It is here that researchers construct a model of their intervention. This model will be based on two major components – existing data on similar or comparable interventions, and a coherent idea of the theory behind the proposed intervention.

In order to provide a secure starting point for the proposed intervention, it is best to systematically assess existing data, ideally by locating a systematic review of the intervention itself, to provide a clear answer to the question of likely intervention effect. One might ask that if a review does exist, and that it indicates the proposed intervention is effective, then why conduct further research. Indeed, this might be the result after searching for and locating a review. If the evidence were clear, then further research would only contribute to more research waste. However, the review might indicate that results are uncertain; perhaps the meta-analysis of results from the combined studies might be heterogeneous. The researchers might be left not knowing whether intervention outcomes in their context would be at the positive or less encouraging end of the distribution of results from the combined studies. There may even be the possibility that certain intervention components appear to be present in studies with better outcomes but not in those with poorer results, but that no studies have constructed an intervention with all these factors in combination. New methods of qualitative evidence synthesis might provide insights from multiple studies of qualitative data from patients or health professionals, alerting us to intervention characteristics that could be better tailored to their needs.

All the scenarios above are very common. Even more common is that either no review exists, or that existing reviews are of poor quality or have not addressed the specific intervention being designed. One of the first steps in developing a complex intervention is more often than not, therefore, to conduct a systematic review oneself. We devote several chapters in this book to review methods. What we might now regard as 'traditional' systematic reviews of effectiveness such as those that follow methods pioneered by the Cochrane collaboration (http://www.cochrane.org/), the Centre for Reviews and Dissemination (http://www.york.ac.uk/inst/crd) or the Joanna Briggs Institute (http://joannabriggs.org/) have been joined by review methods that address the synthesis of qualitative data, data from mixed-methods studies and the synthesis of data using alternative orientations such as realistic evaluation (Pawson and Tilley, 1997). A number of complementary reviews might be needed, therefore, in order to address questions of known effectiveness, contextual variation, intervention acceptability, feasibility and mechanisms of action.

The question of mechanisms of action is also addressed through the identification and development of the theory that underpins the proposed intervention. Indeed, there might be more than one theory, perhaps a biological one, to explain the physical impact of the proposed intervention (exercise or diet, for example) and a psychological one to explain how the intervention will act to change behaviour (the theory of planned behaviour, for example). If the intervention being designed were to be an educational one, a theory about learning would be appropriate to underpin what the health care professional and their patient partner would be doing. Just as in the previous section about identifying and reviewing the existing evidence base, researchers may find out that there is no theory that satisfactorily explains their intervention's proposed mechanism of action and they may have to develop their own theoretical ideas. Once again, some empirical work may be required, often of a qualitative or possibly survey nature, to propose how the deliverers and recipients of the proposed intervention may behave in order to construct a specific theory of behaviour change appropriate for the planned intervention. Abraham *et al.* in Chapter 11 address this process.

There is also a need to model the intervention before testing it. Modelling is a complex process that can be approached from many different standpoints, as Sermeus amply demonstrates in Chapter 12 and Pitt and colleagues describe in detail in their contribution to this book (Chapter 32). Essentially, researchers can undertake a paper-based exercise to visualize the pathways that patients will take through their intervention components, using the model to answer questions about who will deliver the intervention, how long it will take to deliver and what each partner (professionals, patients, carers, etc.) will actually do as part of the intervention.

Finally, as discussed earlier in this chapter, the issue of final implementation should be addressed during the intervention development phase. It is becoming increasingly apparent that thinking about the process of routine implementation during initial intervention design could be critical for eventual widespread adoption should the intervention prove effective. This type of thinking can be quite difficult for researchers who are also obliged to think about high-quality experimental methods. On the one hand, researchers need to produce an intervention that can be shown to have good 'internal validity' (i.e. any results can be properly attributed to the intervention) in an experimental evaluation, whereas they also need to demonstrate 'external validity' (i.e. the intervention and its effects can generalize to situations outside those of a carefully controlled experiment). This second criterion is an important element of assessing the implementation potential of any new complex intervention. There is simply no point in developing something that is so specialized it has no chance of being taken up by health services or people for whom it was designed. In order to avoid this further example of research waste, researchers need to consider the setting in which they expect their intervention to be placed, to conduct primary research to assess the likely chance of it being embedded in routine practice and to consult with health care providers, patients, policy-makers and other stakeholders before embarking on an expensive evaluation. As noted earlier, there are implementation science models such as Normalization Process Theory (May and Finch, 2009) that can help researchers with this task.

At the end of the development phase of the complex interventions research framework, therefore, researchers should be clear about the theoretical basis of their proposed intervention, they should have a firm grasp of the existing evidence for their intervention, should be able to describe very clearly who will do what, have modelled the way the intervention will be operationalized in practice, and will be sufficiently convinced that their intervention, should it prove effective, will be taken up by those for whom it is intended. Only at this stage should they then go on to conduct an evaluation. However, there may be further uncertainties that need to be addressed and for this, feasibility and pilot work may be required.

Feasibility and piloting

As indicated above, the development stage may leave a number of uncertainties remaining, uncertainties that would potentially undermine the conduct of a thorough evaluation of the planned intervention. These uncertainties often concern the feasibility or even the selection of the appropriate research method. They may also concern how acceptable the intervention will be to those for whom it is intended or may have to deliver it, and finally, there may be uncertainties around the practical research procedures to be adopted.

Opinion tends to be divided in the field between those who make a sharp distinction between feasibility trials and pilot studies and those who regard the terms as interchangeable, plus all positions in between (Lancaster *et al.*, 2004; Arain *et al.*, 2010; Thabane *et al.*, 2010). The MRC guidance does not make a clear distinction (Medical Research Council, 2008) whilst others distinguish feasibility studies as independent pieces of work around specific uncertainties to determine whether a future study can be done at all, and pilot studies as a small-scale test of how all the components of a planned study that closely follows the proposed main study procedures will function together (http://www.ccf.nihr.ac.uk/RfPB/Pages/FAQ.aspx). Giangregorio and Thabane discuss this further in this book (Chapter 13). Whether these distinctions are applicable or not, settling uncertainties before embarking on a large-scale evaluation can only be a sensible course of action for researchers interested in testing their interventions.

The primary methodological uncertainty will lie in the selection of the research design. It is good practice to undertake as unbiased a 'fair test' of the new intervention as possible. This usually involves some kind of comparison. As investigators attempt to design rigorous studies, they strive to select a design that minimizes the potential for biasing the results in favour of one comparator group over another. Systematic bias (Shadish *et al.*, 2002) can occur in terms of: the groups being compared (selection bias); differences between the way care is provided to comparison groups apart from the intervention being tested (performance bias); the rates of withdrawals from the study (attrition bias); and the way in which outcomes are assessed (detection bias).

Although the gold standard in terms of experimental comparison is the randomized controlled trial because of its ability to control for unknown selection biases and the way in which known confounders can be controlled for in the process of randomization, there are many situations where it may not be possible to exert this degree of control. In the feasibility and piloting phase of researching complex interventions one aim may be to investigate the feasibility of conducting a randomized trial. It may not be necessary to actually pilot randomization but to assess whether people would be prepared to be randomized into such a trial, work that can be done through survey or simulation methods. If a randomized trial is deemed possible and particularly desirable, the feasibility and piloting stage may be used to determine the most appropriate unit of comparison (individual or cluster, for example) or the type of trial being proposed (superiority or non-inferiority, for example). It might be possible to address these uncertainties through non-randomized feasibility studies, but it is equally possible to test them out in small-scale randomized pilots that closely approximate to the intended evaluation.

Moving on to the use of feasibility or pilot trials to assess intervention uncertainties, it is here that notions of intervention delivery and acceptability are most prominent in researchers' minds. Having designed an intervention from a clear theoretical base, developed on an existing evidence base and with a clear implementation plan, there is no guarantee that the intended providers of the intervention will be prepared, able or sufficiently skilled to deliver the intervention as designed. Nor will the recipients of the intended intervention be necessarily prepared to accept the intervention or undertake activities associated with it. The main question to be addressed here is whether researchers have evidence that their intervention can be delivered as they intend it to be, and whether those for whom it is designed to help will accept it. Much of this work can be undertaken in stand-alone feasibility studies, often drawing on qualitative research methods to gather data. It is certainly not necessary to undertake a pilot randomized controlled trial to answer the question, 'Will the intervention be accepted by trial participants?' Furthermore, uncontrolled data could be used to deduce the likely magnitude of effect of the proposed intervention, data that can then be used to help inform sample size calculations for the planned evaluation. Once again, these data can be gathered in an uncontrolled manner or as part of a pilot randomized trial that closely mimics the proposed trial procedures.

The third set of uncertainties that can be addressed in this stage of the complex interventions research framework are procedural. For example, investigators need to know whether their population of interest is big enough to recruit sufficient participants for their study. They need to know whether people would be prepared to be in such a study, and how they might be identified and approached. Issues of poor recruitment lead to very many trials failing, discussed at length by Shaun Treweek in Chapter 16. Likewise, the feasibility and pilot stage can be used to test the likely participant attrition rates for both intervention adherence and study follow-up procedures. These factors will be required for determining the sample size for a subsequent evaluation.

In summary, therefore, the feasibility and pilot stage of the complex interventions framework allows researchers to identify the methodological, clinical and procedural uncertainties, formulate questions to be answered and conduct one or more preparatory studies to address them. Each study should have clear criteria by which researchers will know whether the proposed study is 'feasible'. At the end of this stage, researchers should be ready to move to the main evaluation stage with reasonable certainty that their intervention can be delivered as intended, is acceptable to providers and recipients and that they have the required methodological and procedural information to ensure that the proposed study can be undertaken successfully.

Evaluation of complex interventions

As discussed in the previous section, choosing the most rigorous evaluation design is absolutely critical. The main aim of any evaluation of an intervention, complex or not, is to establish *causality*, i.e. the link between the intervention and the effect. The choice of design strategy will be one crucial factor for determining the ability of the evaluation to show the effects of the intervention at as good an approximation of the 'real' effect as possible. For the reasons cited earlier, controlling selection bias and the resulting confounders is one of the most important elements in a fair test of the planned intervention and is usually best achieved through randomization.

Nonetheless, there are many circumstances where randomization may not be possible, for example when large-scale policy changes are made throughout a health system or where patients and professionals will not accept a randomized design. In these circumstances, researchers must consider how best they can establish that causality exists beyond reasonable doubt. One of the pioneers of health services research, Austin Bradford-Hill, proposed criteria by which this assessment can be arrived at (Hill, 1965). Although the Evidence Based Medicine movement has supplanted this thinking by placing the randomized controlled trial (RCT) at the top of a hierarchy of evidence-generating research methods (Sackett et al., 1996), recently several thinkers have suggested that a broader look at causality, based on Bradford-Hill's thinking, could be more helpful (Howick et al., 2009). For example, some causality–effect links are so obvious that they do not need to be tested in RCTs (these authors use the Heimlich manoeuvre as one such example). They adapt Bradford-Hill's criteria for establishing causality and categorize them into sources from direct evidence (such as: clear evidence that effects are not due to confounding; there is a link in time between the intervention and the effect; there is a dose response), mechanistic evidence (there is an established mechanism by which the effect can be caused by the intervention) and parallel evidence (the proposed causal link is coherent in terms of current scientific knowledge; can be replicated elsewhere; is similar across populations and settings) (Howick et al., 2009).

Whilst direct evidence can be obtained from traditional evaluations – such as RCTs of the intervention when applied to the population in question to achieve the desired outcome in comparison to an alternative intervention – mechanistic and parallel evidence can be gathered in different ways. It follows, therefore, that the choice of evaluation method should establish as fairly as possible whether the intervention has the effect intended, and where RCTs are not feasible observational, case control, 'n of 1' studies can all be considered. These designs are covered in depth in later chapters of this book.

Running within evaluation methods designed to measure clinical effects, current guidance recommends two other types of investigation within the evaluation phase of the complex interventions research framework – process and economic evaluations (Medical Research Council, 2008). A process evaluation is designed to understand the mechanisms by which the intervention exerts its effects, getting into the 'black box' of the intervention. It can be used to evaluate the theory of action upon which the intervention has been developed. Process evaluations can also investigate intervention fidelity (the extent to which it was delivered as intended), can ask questions about patient buy-in to the intervention and can explore the contexts in which the intervention was delivered, including how this might be related to variations in the measured outcomes. For example, in a study of a psychological therapy, differences in outcomes might be partially explained by patients receiving treatment from different therapists or in different study sites, or indeed by different levels of engagement with elements of the therapy.

Process evaluations can be conducted in many different ways, depending on the question being asked. Some require monitoring of intervention delivery, others measurement of potential mediators of effect and others qualitative interviews with participants and professionals. An evaluation without a process evaluation component is at the very least a waste of an opportunity to understand what is happening and at worst will leave the results of the trial as uncertain as ever. Consequently, there is much interest and theorizing about process evaluations underway and work to develop guidance (Moore *et al.*, 2014) and frameworks by which process evaluations can be designed and reported (Grant *et al.*, 2013). (See this volume, Chapter 23.)

Equally, it is now almost mandatory to conduct an economic evaluation in parallel with the main evaluation. There are a number of standard approaches to health economic evaluation, explained in detail by Payne and Thompson's Chapter 26 in this book, but the importance of undertaking a well-designed economic evaluation cannot be overestimated. All health care systems exist only within the economic life of a culture or country. Understanding the effect of an intervention is of little use if we cannot also determine the cost of its benefit compared to alternative approaches or doing nothing. Decision-makers and policy-makers will be balancing funding priorities and need to understand these relationships, not just the clinical effects. Health economists have developed generic ways of estimating the value of treatments to individuals so that the benefits and costs of different interventions can be compared using the same metric, allowing policy-makers to make decisions about which interventions should be supported, and which of these are affordable to a society. Quality-adjusted life years or disability days are two examples.

Complex interventions present some additional challenges regarding economic evaluation. As noted by Payne and Thompson later (Chapter 26), a key aim of the economic evaluative framework for complex interventions is to be clear about the number of intervention- and condition-specific patient pathways, and then the relevant use of health care resources. However, all evaluations of complex interventions should endeavour to include an economic evaluation where costs of the intervention are collected, estimated or modelled and the benefits clearly measured in a way that policy-makers can use.

Implementation

The issue of implementation or 'implementability' has been referred to throughout this chapter. The days when researchers can expect that their responsibility ends once they have published the results of their work in peer-reviewed academic journals have long passed. We should differentiate here between dissemination – the communication of information to others – and implementation – the embedding of the new intervention into routine health or social care systems and activities. Dissemination, even if it is comprehensive and repeated, is not the same as implementation. Implementation requires attention to multiple factors and is a highly active process involving 'the use of strategies to adopt and integrate evidence-based health interventions and change practice patterns within specific settings' (http://www.fic.nih.gov/News/Events/implementation-science/Pages/faqs.aspx).

Richard Grol and colleagues in the Netherlands (Grol et al., 2005) were pioneers in the development of what is now called 'Implementation Science'. A number of academic journals have been set up to publish research on *how* rather than *what* to implement into clinical practice. The classic case of implementation failure is Antman and colleagues' 1992 analysis of the routine use of thrombolytic drugs in the treatment of myocardial infarction (Antman et al., 1992) which demonstrated a 13-year lag between the establishment of the clinically significant and positive therapeutic effect of these drugs and their routine recommendation in guidelines and textbooks. There are many other such examples.

Given that traditional dissemination is insufficient for implementation, what should researchers do to ensure any positive results from their trials are taken up and implemented in practice? Clearly, as noted earlier, designing and feasibility testing a complex intervention with implementation in mind at the very start is likely to improve the chances of embedding the new intervention into routine practice. Likewise, involving patients and members of the public throughout the complex interventions research process can only help, discussed in depth in Chapter 4. Dissemination of results beyond traditional journals so that they are read by relevant stakeholders is vital – policy-makers, patient pressure groups, professional and managerial organizations, politicians – all are important people who will influence the likely uptake of your intervention.

However, probably the key to ensuring that implementation proceeds rapidly is to undertake a strategic and systematic approach to the problem, an approach that examines both the positive factors that would facilitate intervention adoption and the barriers to embedding the intervention routinely. The final section of our book details these approaches in some detail. Essentially, diagnostic methods are used to understand the resistance points and the openings for implementation, and a plan of action is arrived at based on strategies to increase the positive pressure and decrease the barriers.

The strategies one might adopt are extremely varied and like interventions themselves, some are more effective than others. Common strategies include audit and feedback, computerized decision support and enrolling opinion leaders to influence intervention adoption. Alternatively, compulsory methods such as legislation – often used for major public health concerns such as smoking, the wearing of seat belts in vehicles – are also options as are financial incentives to care providers or even patients.

Researchers are now taking a scientific approach to implementation itself, in effect regarding implementation strategies to embed clinical interventions into practice as interventions in their own right. This can lead to confusion when using terms and in this book we have tried to make a distinction between clinical *interventions* and implementation *strategies*. However, this by no means suggests that we regard the evaluation of implementation strategies as unimportant. Research into models and techniques for successful implementation of effective interventions is one of the most important health care challenges of our times. As with studies into interventions themselves, more than one study of specific implementation strategies will be needed before we can be sure that a particular approach is more or less effective than alternatives.

As an example of this scientific approach, there are a number of systematic reviews of implementation strategy effectiveness. Indeed, the Cochrane collaboration has had a specific group looking at this topic for many years, the Effective Practice and Organization of Care group (EPOC http://epoc.cochrane.org/). There is now evidence from these reviews, summarized in an overview of reviews in this area, that multicomponent interventions appear to perform better than single-strand approaches, albeit even these achieving only moderate effect sizes at best (Boaz *et al.*, 2011). There are a number of potential models to embed these strategies into a coherent action plan, for example Intervention Mapping (Bartholomew *et al.*, 1998) and Normalization Process Theory (May and Finch, 2009).

One further issue in implementation is that of surveillance, monitoring and long-term outcomes. Many research outcomes are relatively short-term. It is in the nature of research funding and commercial pressures that studies do not collect data far into the future. At this point it is often health services themselves that must be relied upon in order to collect, extract and analyse routine data. Nonetheless, observational prospective cohort studies can be set up to detect long-term outcomes and particularly rare but significant adverse events that might be detected only by routine monitoring of large numbers of intervention recipients in health systems.

Indeed, despite the difficulties in capturing data from disparate health providers and organizations, discovering how a new intervention is performing in routine health care is essentially the acid test of any researcher's work.

Conclusion

This chapter has set the scene for what follows. The remainder of the book will take the issue of complexity in treatments and place it in a detailed framework of research methods and knowledge generation. This introduction has outlined just how pervasive complexity is in almost all health and social care interventions and how important it is to consider the final goal of implementation from the very beginning of intervention development. Several factors will assist researchers in their work, not least the involvement of members of the public, patients, informal carers and professionals in designing and testing new interventions, and a programmatic approach to development, feasibility, piloting, evaluation and final implementation. That this endeavour will involve a plethora of different methods and study designs seems axiomatic. The following pages will open up these topics for further elaboration.

Further reading

Evans, I., Thornton, H., Chalmers, I. and Glasziou, P. 2011. *Testing Treatments: Better Research for Better Healthcare*, 2nd edn. London: Pinter & Martin.

Goldacre, B. 2009. *Bad Science*. London: HarperCollins.

Macleod, M. R., Michie, S., Roberts, I., Dirnagl, U., Chalmers, I., Ioannidis, J. P., Al-Shahi Salman, R., Chan, A. W. and Glasziou, P. 2014. Biomedical research: increasing value, reducing waste. *The Lancet*, 383: 101–4.

Medical Research Council. 2008. *Developing and Evaluating Complex Interventions: New Guidance*. London: Medical Research Council.

2

KNOWLEDGE FOR HEALTH CARE PRACTICE

Ingalill Rahm Hallberg

Introduction

Evaluating or establishing the effect of complex interventions in terms of effects, causes and consequences is just one step in the process of developing knowledge that can be applied and used in health care practice. Several studies have to be conducted before arriving at the stage where an intervention study can be developed, as well as additional subsequent studies related to implementation of the new knowledge. This process of developing knowledge for practice normally draws on various designs in preparation for the phase where a complex intervention can be planned and carried out successfully. Even after the intervention has yielded successful results, additional studies are needed to confirm or reject the results regarding their usefulness for practice. Thus developing knowledge is more than simply producing evidence. From a research perspective this means constructing research programmes rather than isolated projects and formulating theories that can explain how a phenomenon operates and how to intervene. From a health care practitioner's perspective it means understanding how science and experience contribute to knowledge that can be used in a more sophisticated manner when health care providers are faced with novel situations. This chapter will address how the research framework is both encapsulated within and is subservient to the theoretical knowledge framework.

Learning objectives

The learning objectives of this chapter are to understand

- The process of developing knowledge that can be applied and used in practice.
- How to construct a research programme.

- The kinds of knowledge that different research designs produce.
- The process of developing and testing theory.
- Requirements that should be fulfilled when applying research findings in practice.

Knowledge development

The real meaning of the term knowledge is still debated. Commonly knowledge is thought of as a collection of facts, information or descriptions of a phenomenon or a thing. From a health care perspective, knowledge to be applied in practice is expected to be scientifically scrutinized so as to prevent harm being done the patient, maximize the outcome of the care and treatment and ensure the best use of the organization's resources. Some knowledge is supposed to remain stable over time, or at least a longer time, e.g. that the Earth is round, whilst other knowledge is more ephemeral, e.g. the surgical procedure for prostatic cancer. Knowledge is also imbued with the societal values that change perhaps faster than other ideas. Not so long ago homosexuality was believed to be a disease with a biological background. Nowadays the predominant view is that it is a normal sexual variation among human beings as well as most other beings. Thus a challenge for the health care system is to remove practices that are founded on old knowledge, regardless of whether they are rooted in societal attitudes or in empirical science that did not lay bare the problem thoroughly. Another difficulty for the health care system is to assess the current level of knowledge and, if it is found usable, implement it in practice (see Section 4).

From the health care researcher's perspective the task is to develop knowledge that can be used in practice. Arriving at the stage of presenting knowledge that can be applied in practice is a process and commonly means going back and forth over the ground many times before being able to successfully manipulate a phenomenon and establish an outcome that is better than if nature had taken its course. It also means integrating results developed by other researchers regarding the research questions, designs and methods used. The process of knowledge development is often presented in terms of three phases: of discovery, of evaluation and finally of implementation. It may appear to be a linear process but this is not the case. The researcher moves in particular between discovery and evaluation and, once effect and effectiveness have been proved, to implementation. These phases in turn give rise to new questions and hypotheses to be tested in new studies and thus the researcher may have to turn back to discovery or evaluation.

Discovery is commonly understood as the phase where we become aware that there is a problem, or a resource, or something that interferes with a phenomenon of interest. For example quite a lot of research presents findings that social resources, social networks or variables such as education or income are related to the outcome of a treatment or a health care intervention. This has been shown in many studies, particularly in epidemiological studies and in cross-sectional studies exploring determinants of quality of life (Durst *et al.*, 2013). Thus it seems fair to state that research has discovered a phenomenon that is of great importance for successful treatment or care outcome; let us call this phenomenon people's social resources. However, this phenomenon is not yet fully understood. Is there a conglomerate of variables or just one or two variables that are pivotal for a successful outcome? Is it culturally stable in that it is the same in all societies or is there variation related to context/culture? Does it operate only under some circumstances, early in a disease process or throughout the process? Is it possible that genetic or epigenetic factors determine how a person develops his/her social network and thus strength when in difficult life situations? What are the causes and what are the consequences? Thus the discovery phase regarding this phenomenon is not yet complete since we have not reached the level of knowledge required to explain how aspects of social networks develop and function or how this can be manipulated in the best interests of people. More work is needed before this very important phenomenon can be fully understood and applied in practice.

In order to make full use of the knowledge about people's social resources, or even more importantly how to intervene in instances of poor social resources, in a health care treatment process it is necessary to enter the next phase of knowledge development, that of *evaluation*. This is the phase where the researcher tries to manipulate/intervene in the phenomenon in order to improve the outcome or reduce negative effects that may interfere with a positive outcome. To the best of my knowledge there is very little research in health care concerning understanding how strong or weak social resources can be used to improve the outcome of a health care process. A tentative theoretical model about how social resources operate and how to improve or make use of their positive effects is needed in order to set up an intervention study. Since it is obviously a complex phenomenon, any intervention study will probably be complex, as described in the MRC guidelines for complex interventions (Medical Research Council, 2008). Such an intervention study will probably also cast new light on the mechanisms of social resources and thereby also lead to new discoveries. The conclusion right now would be that our knowledge about social resources is not yet at a stage where it can be used in practice. To take it to the next level, the effectiveness of various interventions needs to be evaluated. Testing the effect of an intervention may lead to new questions that need to be addressed, not in an intervention but perhaps in personal interviews or surveys that lead to new discoveries.

Once we know for certain how to manipulate/intervene in health care practice, the next phase is that of *implementation* in the health care system. This can certainly not be done based on successful results from one intervention study only. The findings need to be confirmed and refined in the same or other contexts. Many challenges in terms of aspects that may hinder or facilitate implementation such as attitudes, organizational or personal barriers, power distribution, etc. are carried forward into the implementation phase (see Section 4). From a knowledge development perspective this is the phase where it can be established whether the intervention really works in a natural environment, not controlled by researchers' directives, whether it works over time or whether it works in some but not in other contexts. Thus, during this phase new questions arise that may return the researcher to the evaluation or the discovery phase. Knowledge development from the researcher's perspective is therefore an ongoing process, a movement back and forth until the knowledge is solid and can inform practice. From the practitioner's perspective, while it may be interesting to know more about the results obtained during the discovery phase, the results from the evaluation and implementation phases may be the most useful in terms of applicability in practice. This reduces the burden of scientific reading. A study by Mantzoukas (2009) showed that only 13 per cent of the top ten nursing journals reported results from intervention studies. The study did not evaluate the quality of the studies but taking that aspect into account would have reduced the percentage even more. Another study by Richards *et al.* (2014) focusing on European nursing research showed a similar figure for experimental studies. They also reported that methodological description was poor or absent and thus difficult to build further research on. These studies showed that much of the knowledge was not ready for implementation in practice, but remained in the discovery phase. The published research may well be useful in terms of adding to discovery/understanding of a phenomenon but not for practice in terms of implementation since how to successfully intervene has not been tested. In essence, the phases of discovery, evaluation and implementation call for researchers to have a programme for their work rather than pursuing isolated projects if they are to be successful in providing knowledge for practice.

Constructing a research programme

It is characteristic of a research programme that it deals with a problem in a more general sense. Such a programme may be concerned with understanding how social resources, social capital or related concepts operate to protect the individual from poor outcomes, quality of life or traumatic stress disorder when confronted with a life-threatening situation, perhaps even how to improve survival and how to manipulate the phenomenon. Thus a programme addresses an area rather than a specific question and to solve the problem the researcher needs to go back and forth and move between discovery and evaluation many times until the knowledge of how to use this phenomenon effectively in practice has been gained. The programme description is a living document in that it changes from time to time depending on what has been done or found and the new questions that have arisen from the findings. This description covers, apart from the research area, a description of what has already been done, what is currently going on and what can be foreseen as needing to be done. In a back-and-forth process, the programme is broken down into projects and a more sophisticated plan defining a specific research question, the design, sample and methods employed, is developed and the research is geared to implementation in practice. Such a project could be to explore in depth the relationship between different variables related to socio-economic factors, social networks or social capital over time in a population that is in a challenging health situation, perhaps to understand their interrelationship, their relationship to quality of life or even their relationship to bio-molecular variables. Another approach would be to go and explore in depth, to reveal the meaning of the factors from the perspective of the person affected. By going back and forth between samples and questions and by using the literature already available, the researcher may come up with a preliminary theory to explain how the phenomenon of social resources operates to protect or to hinder a positive outcome, how to identify those with poor social resources compared with those with strong social resources and how to manipulate these resources to improve their protective power in those where social resources are weaker. This means constructing a theory about how social resources operate and how they can be used in practice to obtain better outcomes than if it were left to nature. It is well known from testing psychosocial interventions that if the intervention is applied to everyone the outcome will be diluted; there will be no positive effect simply because some people did not need the intervention (Cook and Campbell, 1979). Thus one challenge is to differentiate between those who need the intervention and those who do not. The problem of determining who would benefit from an intervention and who would not may be a study in its own right.

According to the guidelines for developing and evaluating complex interventions in health care (Medical Research Council, 2008), although best placed in the phase of evaluation, the actual task to be carried out is in itself an example of a research programme or at least a large part of a research programme. The guidelines clearly demonstrate that the evaluation phase is a complex research activity and entails tasks that may be regarded more as discoveries than evaluation. The guidelines are described in terms of development and modelling which means assembling the research already done and making sense of it in terms of the modelling. It entails descriptive work and theoretical development and some of the results will be new discoveries. Feasibility and pilot studies help to test whether the ideas based on the development and modelling are applicable and make sense, and new ideas will be developed. This work needs to be done before entering into a major study on the effect and effectiveness of the intervention to be tested. Thus the guidelines clearly show that there is a lot of work to be done before arriving at the stage where a new intervention can be studied for its effectiveness and before a successful outcome can be implemented in practice. The guidelines cover the research work that needs to be done when the researcher is at the stage of wanting to manipulate a situation and achieve an outcome that is better than that already achieved or better than if nature runs its course. Before that stage the researcher has probably carried out several studies to discover aspects of the phenomenon, epidemiological studies, qualitative studies, cross-sectional studies or the like, studies that help the researcher to understand the phenomenon more deeply and start to develop ideas about how to manipulate it.

Constructing research programmes does not mean that the idea of project plans has to be discarded. The programme is made up of projects highlighting specific research questions. It is normally the project plan that is used when applying for grants but the specific plan is embedded in a larger programme. It strengthens the application for funding if the project is embedded in a long-term commitment to solve a specific problem, demonstrating that the researcher has worked on the problem for some time, is moving the understanding of the problem forward and is conversant with the current knowledge base.

Working with research programmes rather than jumping from one project to another with no plan or overarching aim also highlights the question of working in solitude or with a group of researchers. The research programme approach requires a variety of competences depending on the specific question in focus. However, it also requires a group of people who remain in the group. Ideally there is a core of researchers with different scientific competences working together for a longer time augmented by other researchers who come and go depending on the question in focus. In the best of worlds there would a group of people at senior and junior levels as well as doctoral candidates working together to solve the problem. Multidisciplinary research groups may have difficulty in using a common language and understanding each other, but on the other hand they bring necessary tension or critical reflection into the group simply by being trained in different scientific cultures.

In summary, setting up and carrying out a complex intervention is only just one step of the way in constructing solid knowledge useful for practice. The researcher may find all the knowledge and inspiration needed simply by reading what has already been done and reported in scientific journals. However, constructing knowledge for practice requires the researcher to be involved in the entire process of knowledge development, discovery, evaluation and implementation.

Types of knowledge derived from different designs

Planning and carrying out research using a programme approach also means that the researcher needs to be flexible in terms of using various designs and applying a variety of methods related to the research question. Once a researcher decides on an approach to a research question, the kinds of knowledge the research design produces are also determined, and the knowledge obtained is more or less positioned as discovery, evaluation or implementation. Thus the researcher should think twice about the research question and the kind of knowledge that is to be produced. The outcome of a research study delivers a specific kind of knowledge. The inductive approach (Creswell, 2007) is supposed to present the problem or phenomenon per se; as it is and not as the researcher thinks it is. This can be done using quantitative as well as qualitative methods. However, it is not entirely true that the inductive approach tells the researcher about the phenomenon itself since the methods chosen determine what the researcher recognizes, identifies or selects as being of interest, and is in fact determined by the researcher's expectations and ideas although they may perhaps not be verbalized or conscious. The deductive approach is driven by an explicit idea, i.e. by hypotheses, theories or more-or-less developed ideas about the research question. The selection of methods is also driven by a specific idea concerning the area of research. Research about quality of life is often based on measures tapping into negative aspects of life, such as those connected with depression, neglecting the fact that there may be positive aspects that balance the negative aspects and make them less difficult, which in turn can convey ideas for interventions.

The hierarchy of evidence is built on the belief that different designs produce different levels of evidence (see GRADE – The Grading of Recommendations Assessment, Development and Evaluation; http://www.gradeworkinggroup.org). The concept of evidence (Sackett et al., 1996) has been criticized since there is no clear definition of what is meant by evidence (Worrall, 2002; Cartwright et al., 2007). Given that a study is of high quality, it may produce knowledge that can be regarded as evidence, even if it is not an intervention study. Epidemiological studies may produce evidence applicable in practice even though they may be best at producing knowledge about relationships. They do not generally disclose how to manipulate a certain aspect or situation and demonstrate the outcome. Almost every design may produce new ideas and in that sense serve discovery. Systematic reviews of different kinds – cross-sectional, correlational, epidemiological studies, etc. – are very good at producing new ideas. This is also true of qualitative studies, whether purely descriptive or interpretative. The designs mentioned are very good at revealing relationships between variables, providing ideas for new hypotheses that can be tested in other designs and helping to develop theories that can be tested. A hypothesis can be more or less complex or more or less developed. These designs are, however, not as good at saying anything about effect or causality or how to manipulate a situation to obtain a desired result. The quantitative approach gives a surface overview of a certain problem, phenomenon, etc. whilst the qualitative approach gives a deeper understanding of the area of research.

In order to establish effect or effectiveness or causality, designs other than the merely descriptive or cross-sectional are required. In terms of systematic reviews, meta-analysis may produce this knowledge, depending on the quality of the studies already reported and the results they indicate. Longitudinal studies or controlled cohort studies may also produce knowledge about effect or effectiveness. Natural experiments, for instance a sudden change in situations or behaviour or the like, may tell us about effect (Morgan, 2013). For instance, a law enforcing the mandatory use of safety belts in cars or of a helmet when bicycling speaks to the protective effect of wearing a helmet and the outcome can be studied through examining statistics for brain damage, for instance. The most common designs used in answering questions about effect, effectiveness or causality are those where there is manipulation (intervention, experimenting) of the variable in focus and the outcome of this manipulation is investigated. There are several types of intervention study (Section 3) and they need to be controlled in one way or another to make sure that the outcome is not determined by some irrelevant process or accidental intervention. There is a difference between establishing effect or effectiveness in a natural environment like health care as opposed to a laboratory situation, where all confounding variables can be kept under control. The complexity may be connected with the context or with the applied interventions (see Chapter 1). It may be argued that all interventions are complex. However, there is a big difference between testing an intervention in a laboratory-like context and in a natural context like everyday health care. There is also a big difference in terms of establishing the outcome between an intervention with a single aspect, such as the effect of a drug, and one with a systems approach, such as employing a multi-professional team in depression treatment (Richards *et al.*, 2013).

Establishing effect means explaining the variation in the dependent variable in relation to the intervention and possible explanatory variables; these could be sex, age, health or the like (Cook and Campbell, 1979). Such a study tells us not only about the effect of a certain intervention but also about the circumstances under which it is most effective. It may be more effective for women than for men, for example. Establishing causality on the other hand is about demonstrating that a certain factor causes a specific effect. Strictly speaking this means that the effective component in the intervention can be linked to both the outcome and the dose–response. In order to establish that level of causality, all other variables (explanatory) need to be under control. As such a situation does not mimic real life, establishing causality is often related to low external validity. Research about new drugs is an example of when external validity may be, and perhaps should be, questioned due to the fact that the participants do not mimic those likely to use the drug, for instance the elderly and children. The closer the intervention study is to real life the more difficult it is to establish exactly what caused the effect. However, external validity may be much stronger. Kerry *et al.* (2012) suggested a less strict definition of causality. This may, however, cause confusion as to the meaning of causality. Using a multi-method approach may increase the possibility of establishing effect and also of understanding the mechanisms involved in the outcome of the intervention. Effectiveness is connected with how much intervention is needed to obtain a certain level of effect, and the level of effect should make a difference in terms of the patient's experience or health outcome.

Much more remains to be done in developing designs for intervention studies and also in eradicating the idea that the only method that should be used is the traditional randomized controlled study, preferably blind (Worrall, 2010). This approach is applicable to some situations but certainly not always to others, particularly not to testing the effect of interventions addressing individuals, organizations or systems for delivering health care, all of which require complex interventions. Combining different methods in the same study, so-called multi-method or mixed-methods designs (Creswell and Plano Clark, 2011), provides richer results than using only one method (see Chapter 3). The value of constructing research programmes and combining methods indicates that researchers should be flexible and open-minded when setting up studies rather than repeatedly applying the same method in different contexts.

An intriguing challenge for health care is to understand by and for whom, when and under what circumstances effective support for people in difficult health situations can and should be provided, be it for stroke, depression or cancer or any other demanding disease. There are several research studies showing that some people have a better outcome than others which cannot be explained purely by disease severity or treatment burden. The findings are revealed by including measures to assess, for example, resilience (Yu and Xhang, 2007), sense of coherence (Antonovsky, 1993), hardiness or self-efficacy. These concepts are generally well developed from a theoretical perspective and translated into measures. Quite a lot of the available studies show that these factors, as assessed by the measures above, interfere in some way with the disease process and with the outcome in terms of adaptation and quality of life. This is also seemingly a cross-cultural phenomenon. For instance, Ding *et al.* (2013) reported that sense of coherence was significantly related to quality of life in women with early-stage cervical cancer but not in later phases of the disease. In order to take this kind of knowledge forward, intervention studies are needed. It may be that resilience or sense of coherence or similar phenomena cannot be manipulated but they may be useful when selecting people for an intervention that buffers the strain caused by the disease or the treatment. Much research is still needed both at the level of understanding the phenomenon and also in making it useful in practice. Thus the knowledge base is not yet at the implementation phase.

Developing and testing theory

Constructing knowledge in a sense is about developing and testing theories and thus is an important part of a research programme and an ongoing process. The entire model of the MRC guidelines for developing and testing complex interventions, although it does not explicitly refer to theoretical development, covers such work, in particular the part about development and modelling but also feasibility and pilot studies. Whether researchers like it or not, whenever they approach a research question they have some ideas in their heads, implicitly or explicitly. The ideas can be more or less complex and the researcher may be more or less aware of the idea driving the research design and the methods applied. This idea may be the embryo of a theory or a more developed theory. It is risky when the theories or ideas are implicitly hidden in the way the study is set up or the way in which methods are selected or discarded. For instance, most of the time the impact of informal care-giving for older people is researched using methods that tap burden, strain, demands, costs, challenges, etc. (Ekwall and Rahm Hallberg, 2007). This means that the researcher constructs the study on the assumption that it is a burden to provide care for a next of kin and, since that is what the measures used or the interviews carried out focus on, the researcher cannot report anything else. Thus useful knowledge showing that informal care-giving may include joy, contribute to the feeling of performing meaningful actions, give meaning to life or is just a natural self-evident action occurring between human beings who care for each other is lost. Research that takes such a perspective for granted distorts the knowledge base in that it only describes one perspective. Thus it is important to recognize that any research study is imbued more or less with the researcher's understanding of the world. This needs to be recognized and dealt with explicitly, meaning that the researcher has to be clear about the assumptions behind the setting up of a study and this is even more important when studying complex interventions. This does not necessarily mean that a method or an approach cannot be understood differently from what the inventor had in mind. Section 1 addresses developing theories for investigating the effect of complex interventions. Such theory development is needed for the intervention per se as well as for the design and methods used to study the outcome of a certain intervention.

Ideas, assumptions or more or less developed propositions about how things hang together in a sense precede or occupy an early stage of a theory. A theory is commonly thought of as a set of assumptions that explains something (Meleis, 2004). The assumptions are linked to each other more or less loosely and they may also determine a certain outcome. The theory may be more or less general and more or less scientifically scrutinized. A general theory as to how humans react to a severe crisis may originally have been developed in a very specific situation such as a fire in a night-club that claimed many lives (Lindemann, 1944; Sleiku, 1990). A theory can be stronger or weaker in explaining a situation or phenomenon. It is strong when it can show how the assumptions connect together, their order and their effect and also how to manipulate the situation to achieve an effect (Meleis, 2004). A weaker theory may be exemplified by that of social capital (Bolin et al., 2003; Nieminen et al., 2013) which states that social capital, through social networks and communities, impacts on a person's ability to handle stressful situations such as cancer. It does not reveal, however, how social capital is related to socio-economic or personality factors and which of the factors are more important to the outcome, or how social capital can be manipulated or what should be focused on in practice to improve the situation of those with less social capital than others. Attempts to implement social capital in practice may be under way (Putland et al., 2013). In summary, a theory is an explanatory framework, more or less complex, more or less empirically well-grounded and as such it is helpful in developing hypotheses. The theory in part or in whole also has to be tested empirically. In research that aims to discover new perspectives on a certain situation or phenomenon or evaluate the effect of any intervention, tentative or early-stage theories are needed to avoid getting lost in myriad possible measures. The research helps to support the tentative idea or the discarding of it if it is not supported. Unfortunately medical as well as nursing research has been criticized for its lack of theories.

Requirements before applying findings in practice

It is often stated that it takes far too long for new research findings to be used in practice and that the evidence–practice gap is too large (Bryant et al., 2014). That may well be true but the opposite may also be a problem in health care, where staff may introduce ideas based on weak research results not yet ready to be applied in practice. The idea or the findings may be close to their heart but have weak or no scientific underpinnings. The risk of introducing findings from research that is not yet proven to improve practice may be higher in research-intensive settings. This may be due to the researchers who are carrying out research – doing intervention studies, developing new self-reported or laboratory methods, etc. – and are convinced that a specific method is effective even if it has not been tested sufficiently to be able to state that it is good enough to be implemented. There is also pressure from scientific journals which expect or demand that authors add a section stating the implications of the findings for practice. There is also a tendency to include such a paragraph in applications for research funds. These demands do not take into account the research process where the programme has not yet reached a stage where implementation or implication can be either reliably stated or discussed. Thinking in terms of knowledge that needs to be constructed through taking various perspectives, various designs, various research methods and samples means that in the process of developing knowledge for practice some very important studies do not produce knowledge ready to be introduced in practice. A groundbreaking experimental study by Norberg and colleagues (1986, reprinted 2003) demonstrates this. The research group worked on testing the idea that people in a severe stage of dementia reacted to stimuli of various kinds (touch, music and objects). The predominant attitude to people in this stage of dementia was that they were no longer reachable. The study was small, with only four participants, but showed that the patients reacted to stimuli. The findings at that stage could not easily be implemented. However, it opened the way for psychosocial interventions in dementia care and also for the understanding that care quality and the care environment played a vital role in the patients' behaviour. These findings, together with those from several other studies, changed attitudes to people with dementia. Thus the study, together with others, contributed to effecting a change in attitudes and also in the long run to the ways in which nursing care, medical treatment and support for informal care-givers are provided. To achieve this change, much more research had to be carried out to inform practice about how to use the knowledge that people with dementia are not beyond contact and not indifferent to what goes on around them.

Requirements that need to be taken into account before implementing research findings in practice should include that the effect of an intervention is in fact established and in addition its effectiveness, its safety and also perhaps when and where to implement it. Effect concerns the intervention actually having the expected effect, being capable of producing the desired result. Thus an intervention deemed to be effective has the intended and expected outcome. This is not enough; its effectiveness also needs to be established. Effect is different from the effectiveness of an intervention which concerns establishing the extent, the effort involved or whether the costs of the intervention are justified. Thus it is not enough to establish that an intervention works, it also has to be established that the outcome of the intervention is feasible, that it is strong enough in terms of producing clinically significant effect, and is cost-effective in that the resources needed are reasonable and afford-able in terms of the time needed for the implementation, the general cost or other resources. There is a risk that the term effectiveness will be used interchangeably with effect. It says nothing about how big the effect is or what is required to obtain a reasonable effect, an effect that is clinically meaningful. Statistical significance may be misleading as it concerns only a significant effect. This effect, however, may not be clinically significant or it may be so costly that it is simply not feasible. This has been expressed in terms of minimally clinically important difference (Richards et al., 2013). The effectiveness should tell us about costs and the outcomes expressed in numerical terms, allowing health care providers to make decisions about whether implementing the new interventions or methods is worthwhile.

The health care provider also needs to consider the safety of the new method and ensure that it does not involve risks that are hazardous to the patient or staff. In addition the provider needs to consider what this new method is replacing as well as under what circumstances and when the new method should be used. For instance psychosocial interventions are needed to support processing and adap-tation to the fact that a person has got cancer and needs some serious treatment, but is given no promises for the future. No one is disputing this. The problem is really when in the process of receiving the diagnosis, starting the treatment, getting treatment and finally leaving treatment is it most effective to apply a psychosocial intervention. Furthermore, in a population of people with cancer there is great variation in terms of the severity of the disease, of the person's strength to cope with a life crisis of this kind and of social resources available to them to handle the new situation. Thus the challenge is to obtain the knowledge that will inform practice in terms of who should receive the intervention, who could perhaps be left to deal with it with a minimum of support and who should have the biggest 'dose' of psychosocial support. Providing the same intervention to all, irrespective of the severity of the disease, personal and social resources seems to be a waste of resources. In terms of prioritization it means that some patients who are more in need of the intervention, perhaps not because of the cancer, may not get the help to handle the challenges that confront them, simply because resources are limited. Before implementing new research findings in practice some important questions have to be answered. How to introduce new findings is another story dealt with in Section 4. That is the story about implementation. However, implementation cannot be considered on the basis of one study showing effectiveness; more work and repeated studies are needed to ensure that the results were not achieved due to other circumstances.

Summary

Developing knowledge for practice is an ongoing process and the problem or ques-tion in focus needs to be studied from several perspectives before entering the stage where a complex intervention can be considered. When the researcher feels ready to develop and evaluate a complex intervention, she or he is entering into a new stage of developing the intervention, as described in the MRC guidelines. The process of developing knowledge for practice and of developing a complex intervention includes theoretical work; in essence all research is about theorizing. Thus, applying a programme approach to an area of interest is more effective in terms of costs and manpower than moving from one project to another, without being systematically connected. With the programme approach, the research will probably be more successful in providing knowledge that can be implemented in practice.

3

THE VALUE OF MIXED METHODS FOR RESEARCHING COMPLEX INTERVENTIONS

Gunilla Borglin

Introduction

In the twenty-first century, it is more obvious than ever before that health services research and its practitioners exist in an extremely complex contextual environment. Consequently, at the heart of understanding how to develop interventions in a setting characterized by multifaceted health care demands, is the realization that no one research method in isolation will suffice. In this chapter an overview of mixed methods and their potential contribution in undertaking research on complex interventions (Medical Research Council, 2008) will be provided.

Learning objectives

- To appreciate the philosophical background to the development of mixed methods as a research paradigm.
- To understand the potential contribution of mixed methods to researching complex interventions.
- To be able to recognize the principles and structure of common mixed-methods designs.
- To appraise the place of mixed methods in modern health services research.

Background

In comparison with quantitative and qualitative methods, mixed methods are a relatively 'new' idea for those researching the acceptability, delivery, effectiveness, economics and organization of patient care in health and social care, often referred to as 'health services research' (Lohr and Steinwachs, 2002). Mixed methods as a distinct concept is increasingly gaining ground even if its methods and methodology can still be considered to be in their infancy. Published health services research studies classified as mixed methods have increased from about 17 per cent in the latter part of the twentieth century to about 30 per cent in the early twenty-first century (O'Cathain, 2009). Methodologically, mixed methods are substantially more than an *ad hoc* combination of numerical data (quantitative) and textual data (qualitative). About ten years ago, research designs, which these days are referred to as mixed methods, started to appear more frequently in scientific literature within medicine, nursing, education and sociology but under different names such as integrative research, multi-method and triangulation research (Polit and Tatano Beck, 2012). Those looking for guidance in how and what the *method* (procedure to collect, analyse and interpret data) and the *methodology* (strategy, plan, design of the research study) could entail, did not receive much guidance in comparison with the greater number of text and methods books published more recently. Among the leading authors in the field are Creswell and Plano Clark (2011) and Teddlie and Tashakkori (2009). Despite an increased access to literature in the topic it is important to remember that even though the methodology is not new, it is still considered a research paradigm under development (Collins and O'Cathain, 2009; Johnson *et al.*, 2007). Consequently, the foundations for different potential designs are not set in stone, and the research community has not yet reached consensus about what mixed methods can entail or how to define it. This means that taking on a mixed-methods design can be a challenge for researchers, as few explicit clinical examples are available for guidance. Furthermore, published papers and textbooks introduce different definitions, which tend to contrast with each other by only including methodology (Teddlie and Tashakkori, 2009), or including method and/or philosophy (Creswell and Plano Clark, 2011). In this chapter, mixed methods will be discussed principally from the perspective of Creswell and Plano Clark's (2007: 5) definition:

> A research design with philosophical assumptions as well as methods of inquiry. As a methodology, it involves philosophical assumptions that guide the direction of the collection and analysis of data and the mixture of qualitative and quantitative approaches in many phases in the research process. As a method, it focuses on collecting, analysing and mixing both quantitative and qualitative data in a single or series of studies. Its central premise is that the use of quantitative and qualitative approaches in combination provides a better understanding of research problems than either approach alone.

As the definition reveals, mixed methods are characterized by the integration of a qualitative and quantitative approach. The integration of the two different methods can take place at any point in the research process, i.e. during data collection, data analysis or the interpretative phase. The main aim of mixed methods is to achieve the optimum answer to the research question(s). It is important to note that utilizing quantitative and qualitative methods within the same frame of a single study is not a new idea. This 'technique' has been around for at least 20 years. Indeed, two decades ago, Morgan (1998) suggested that health service researchers' interest in combining methods came down to 'the complexity of the many different factors that influence health' (1998: 362). However, this insight appears to not have been fully acknowledged until the introduction of the revised MRC framework (Medical Research Council, 2008), which stated: 'This document provides guidance on the development, evaluation and implementation of complex interventions to improve health.... and extending the coverage in the guidance of non-experimental methods and of complex interventions' (2008: 4). However, the actual innovation here seems not to be the combination of two different methods within the same study, but rather the research community's intense endeavour to structure and formalize this well-known but less formalized tradition under the umbrella term of 'mixed methods'.

Rationale for mixed-methods research

The increased attention on mixed methods can be partly explained by the recent academic focus on health and social care services as characterized by complex activities and interventions (Medical Research Council, 2008; Richards and Borglin, 2011; Thompson and Clark, 2012). Studies not embracing this complexity have been said to have 'little value in the complex world of practice' (Griffiths, 2012: 584). Additionally, senior researchers in the field (Chalmers and Glasziou, 2009; Mantzoukas, 2009; Rahm Hallberg, 2006, 2009; Richards et al., 2014) have highlighted the importance of moving the research field forward from descriptive and cross-sectional research, to research supporting an increased implementation of knowledge fit for the complex reality of health care.

Simultaneously, health services research, i.e. the study of how social factors, financing systems, organizational structures and processes, health technologies and personal behaviours affect access to health care, the quality and cost of health care, and health and well-being (Lohr and Steinwachs, 2002), has become increasingly interdisciplinary. This field has begun to recognize the necessity of using innovative methods such as mixed methods to help understand health services phenomena in a more in-depth manner (cf. Wisdom et al., 2012). During the same time frame the MRC framework was introduced (Medical Research Council, 2000, 2008), and its release has put mixed methods as a research design in the spotlight. Two authors of the MRC framework (Craig and Petticrew, 2013: 585) recently stated:

> We did not intend to break new ground, conceptually or theoretically, but to draw researchers' and research funders' attention to examples of good practice and to the value of some lesser-used designs. We sought to encourage a phased and where necessary, iterative approach to researching complex interventions.

If health care professionals' activities and interventions are considered as complex, it is natural that research questions within the field need to be investigated and answered with methods capable of dealing with this complex clinical reality. Since health services researchers focus on health care provision, their questions are therefore likely to address effectiveness and cost-effectiveness of both established and new interventions. Thus, designs that can capitalize on the strengths of both qualitative and quantitative methodologies by combining approaches in a single research study to increase the breadth and depth of understanding (Johnson *et al.*, 2007) are warranted. Taken together, all this has led to an intensified awareness and an increased knowledge about mixed methods as a design. Consequently, today more research questions than ever before are likely to need and gain from being addressed by mixed-methods designs neatly positioned within a framework such as the MRC's.

Creswell (2003) outlined the advantages of mixed-methods designs as: complementary, practical, strengthens credibility/trustworthiness and incremental (producing a stepwise increase of knowledge). *Complementary* is taken to mean that one method represents numerical data (quantitative) and the other textual data (qualitative). Thus, by integrating both types of data in the same study or programme of research, each of the method's limitations can be eliminated whilst their strengths remain. *Practical* reflects the fact that complex research questions demand that researchers use practical and methodological tools able to deal with complexity in the soundest way. Using both quantitative and qualitative data can support the hypothesis, the model or the researchers' interpretation. Therefore, if this is the case, the study's *credibility* and/or *trustworthiness* is supported. Finally, the advantage of *incremental* advances the idea that knowledge development within a subject occurs in a stepwise manner and is dependent on so-called 'feedback loops'. Within a mixed-methods design it is possible to build in a feedback loop as knowledge from one methodological strand can inform another. This means that both explanatory and exploratory research questions can be addressed and answered simultaneously. As the MRC framework (Medical Research Council, 2008) supports a process of 'development-testing-evaluation-implementation', the types of research situations (Box 3.1) said to be especially suitable for a mixed-methods design (Creswell and Plano Clark, 2011) will be part of the context when we develop and test different types of health care interventions.

BOX 3.1 EXAMPLE OF RESEARCH ISSUES SUITABLE FOR MIXED-METHODS DESIGN

- New and badly defined concepts or phenomenon.
- Findings from one method can strengthen findings from the other method; alternatively, one method's findings are difficult to interpret and the other method might help to explain the findings.
- Neither method alone will answer the study objective.

Theoretical point of departure

Nothing is quite as simple as many health service researchers might wish it to be, and mixed methods' youthfulness means that it is part of a challenging but creative field of tension, a field signified by evolving methodological development as well as animated paradigmatic discussions (cf. Johnson and Onwuegbuzie, 2004; Johnson *et al.*, 2007). This discourse becomes obvious when considering the different terms used: the 'silent revolution', the 'third research paradigm' and the 'third methodological movement'. By including the word 'third' the latter two include clear reference to the strict border between quantitative and qualitative methods that has been present for many decades. These theoretical discussions very much focus on different ways of viewing the world and include debates between those who state that paradigmatic departures are of no importance, and those stating that naturalistic and post-positivistic world-views are incompatible and cannot be present in the same study.

Whether individual health service researchers agree with the above or not, an understanding of the context in which mixed methods and hence the 'development-testing-evaluation-implementation' process suggested by the MRC (2008) exist seems to be important, not only because our ways of viewing the world as researchers tend to define what 'good research' is, but also because the polarization between quantitative and qualitative methods is still present within the health services research community, despite a number of position papers saying or calling for the opposite. Currently, if any ideological grounds are mentioned at all in writing about mixed methods, the philosophy of pragmatism is most commonly associated with mixed-methods research (Johnson and Onwuegbuzie, 2004; Johnson *et al.*, 2007). Mixed-methods designs originating in pragmatism are characterized by the importance given to the research objective, which governs the direction of the research. This means that here the objective of the study is more important than which methods are used to address it. Equally important is that the objective is approached from more than one, i.e. pluralistic, perspective. Consequently, researchers adopting this perspective generally reject the idea of needing to choose between a post-positivistic or naturalistic world-view. Pragmatism can also mean that research takes place in a social, historical, political or other context of importance. Induction is as important as deduction, with the consequence that theory can be both verified and generated. Pragmatism is (of course) also signified by being 'pragmatic', meaning that regardless of philosophy, the method or approach leading to the best evidence should be used (Johnson and Onwuegbuzie, 2004). Another core idea within pragmatism is that only those questions of importance for the greater good of the majority are worth investigating. Thus, the strategy, plan of action or design of research procedures for gathering, analysing and interpreting data, i.e. *methodology*, the nature of reality, what is real, i.e. *ontology*, and how we gain knowledge of what we know, i.e. *epistemology*, as well as the language of research, i.e. *rhetoric*, have their own stance (Table 3.1).

TABLE 3.1 Overview of the pragmatic world-view (adapted from Borglin, 2012)

Pragmatism	
Methodology	Mixed-methods design.
Ontology	Multiple ways of viewing, hearing and understanding the world.
Epistemology	Knowledge is *not* neutral as influenced by human interest. Hence knowledge is formed by both objective and subjective values.
Rhetoric	Meta-inference, inference quality and inference transferability.

It is important to note that there are several branches within pragmatism and others have different views than the one presented in this chapter. For example O'Cathain (2009; O'Cathain *et al.*, 2007) highlights that within health services research, mixed-methods approaches are often justified as being purely pragmatic rather than on ideological grounds. Hence, the connotation of pragmatic here simply means to help us as researchers to design and engage with the complexity of health and of the health care context in which the study takes place.

Research questions in mixed-methods research

Most people would agree that research originates from a problem or a question – a subject that has caused us to think and wonder about. Formulating or stating the research question or the research problem is one of the most important and intellectually demanding steps in the research process. In general, the research question reflects what the researcher wants to investigate. However, according to Onwuegbuzie and Leech (2006), the research question can also fulfil more functions. It can, amongst other things, form the frame within which the study is conducted and in this way can help to maintain focus during the study. Thus, the research question limits and defines the study's borders and, maybe most importantly, determines what types of data (quantitative, qualitative, mixed) are going to be collected.

In mixed methods, the research question can appear more challenging to develop than when a mono method is used. Unfortunately, the literature contains very little advice on how a mixed-methods research question can or should be developed. Onwuegbuzie and Leech (2006) are among the small number of authors discussing this issue, and they suggest that in contrast to a qualitative research question, a 'quantitative' research question is signified by being more specific and often falling within one of the following three categories: (1) descriptive; (2) comparative; (3) relational. Descriptive questions are used to quantify variation in one or more variables while comparative questions are used to compare two or more groups regarding some dependent variable. Correlational/relational questions focus on associations between one or more variables. In contrast, qualitative research questions tend to focus on discovery or illuminating processes or describe an experience and are often 'what and how'-type questions (Onwuegbuzie and Leech, 2006).

It is worth noting that in contrast to questions posed in mono-methods studies, the mixed-methods research question can be modified and/or changed during the study and additional questions can be added. Considering the iterative and pragmatic approach suggested by the MRC, one would think this should strike a favourable note with health services researchers when choosing designs. However, so far this has been rarely discussed in published research. According to Teddlie and Tashakkori (2009), question formulation within mixed-methods designs deals with unknown aspects of a phenomenon that can be answered by information presented both as textual data and numerical data. These authors suggest formulating an overarching mixed-methods question that includes sub-questions requiring a quantitative as well as a qualitative answer. Conversely, Creswell and Plano Clark (2011) suggest that researchers identify separate research questions for each strand and then develop a mixed-methods question that frames the integration of the results from both strands. A mixed-methods design, therefore, brings forth the possibility of answering specific questions related to the mixing of the two strands as well as answering the 'qualitative' and the 'quantitative' research question(s) independently These can include questions such as: 'To what extent do the different types of data explain each other?', and 'How can one type of data explain the other type of data?' and so on (Creswell and Plano Clark, 2011). A specific research example of this is the study by Mayoh *et al.* (2012) in which they mixed quantitative methods (questionnaires) with the aim of delivering a breadth of quantitative data to 'provide a level of quantitative depth' (2012: 24) in the discussion alongside in-depth interviews (qualitative methods) collected in phase two. This facilitated a more complete picture of the phenomena under investigation. They additionally used a mixed-methods question aiming to review and develop innovative mixed-methods research techniques. Mayoh *et al.* (2012) concluded that their findings indicated that something would have been lost or misunderstood regarding the phenomenon if only one method had been used in isolation.

Design principles and key decisions

The mixed-methods research process generally follows the same steps and principles as any other type of research design. The process is, however, not always linear, and as both the research question and design can change as the study proceeds, mixed methods are an especially suitable design for research developed using the MRC framework. Before going on to choose the specific mixed-methods design, researchers planning to conduct a mixed-methods study need to take a standpoint regarding some key decisions. These are: (1) the level of interaction between the strands; (2) the relative priority of the strands; (3) the timing of the strands; and (4) the procedures for mixing the strands (Creswell and Plano Clark, 2011).

The *level of interaction* can be independent or interactive. Independent implies that the two methods are mixed during the overall interpretation (i.e. when drawing conclusions), and that they are kept independent of each other in terms of the research question, data collection and data analysis. In the latter, there is direct inter-action in that the design and the methods are mixed before the final interpretation takes place. Interaction can, therefore, take place at different points and in different ways during the research process.

The *relative priority* of the strands refers to three possible weighting options, i.e. equal, quantitative or qualitative priority, and the choice will of course depend on the research questions, not least the priority given to the need to answer them.

Timing of methods can occur at several different stages in the research process. Where timing is concurrent, both methods are implemented during a single phase of the study. Sequential timing refers to implementing the methods in distinct phases where data collection and analysis of one method are finalized before data collection using the next method starts. Finally, in multi-phase timing, methods are implemented in several phases concurrently and/or sequentially. The latter type of timing is mainly used in studies conducted over more than two phases or research programmes combining concurrent and sequential elements.

The final decision deals with the *procedure for mixing* or the point of interface. Here the issue is at what point should the integration take place. Creswell and Plano Clark (2011) suggest the following possible points. The first is in study designs where the quantitative and qualitative strands are not mixed until after data collection and separate analysis of both data sets, i.e. *mixed during interpretation* (1). This involves drawing conclusions by reflecting on what was learnt from using both methods as well as comparing and synthesizing the result in a discussion. *Mixing during data col-lection* (2) means that the results of the first method used shape the design of the data collection in the second strand, for example by specifying the research questions, informing the sample and selecting participants, and informing the development of data collection protocols or instruments. *Mixing during data analysis* (3) occurs when researchers analyse each strand separately but then merge the two sets of results together in a combined analysis. This can be done in a matrix where data can be compared and interpreted. It can also be conducted by transforming one type of data into the other type (text to numbers, numbers to text).

Finally, there is the possibility of mixing at the design level or *mixing within a programme objective framework* (4). This should be of special interest for researchers designing their studies using the MRC framework, as mixing takes place in the development phase, i.e. when the researcher uses a theoretical framework to guide the overall design and within which the two methods are mixed. The programme objective guides the joining of multiple studies in a type of multi-phase project (Creswell and Plano Clark, 2011).

Mixed-methods designs

There are no standard classifications – typology or prototype – for different mixed-methods designs (Polit and Tatano Beck, 2012; Tashakkori and Creswell, 2007). Rather the different research communities, health sciences, sociology, education, etc. use varied classifications for different types of mixed-methods design, which when scrutinized appear to contain similar components. Creswell and Plano Clark (2011) have for example introduced six different prototypes for basic designs within mixed methods. These prototypes can generally be considered to differ according to: sequencing, i.e. in which order the qualitative and quantitative data collection occurs; in terms of priorities, i.e. what precedence the different methods of data collection and analysis will have; and finally in integration, i.e. where in the process the two types of data collected by the different methods will be combined and/or integrated – during analysis, interpretation or reporting.

In the following discussion, the four main designs – the convergent parallel design, the explanatory sequential design, the exploratory sequential design and the embedded design – will be briefly introduced and discussed. Additionally, the multi-phase design will be introduced as a promising design, especially for researchers who are planning to use the MRC guidance (2008) as a framework for their research.

Convergent parallel design

In the convergent parallel design the aim is to obtain different but complementary data about a central phenomenon. Textual and numerical data are collected simultaneously (concurrent) and with equal priority (equal status). However, the strands are usually kept separate during data analysis, and integrated first during the overarching interpretation of results. For example, in a study where the research question deals with understanding health care professionals' attitude towards research and its implementation in care, the researcher could choose to use a questionnaire together with a qualitative data collection method such as focus group interviews. This design strategy will help to gain an optimal understanding of the research problem and was initially referred to as a triangulation design. Within mixed methods the concept of triangulation, as opposed to triangulation in qualitative methods, is a process where the research question is investigated with both a qualitative and quantitative strand to achieve a more complete understanding of the research question (O'Cathain *et al.*, 2010). A health services research example of this design is that of Stirling and colleagues (2010). They used self-reported assessments on carer burden and stress as well as indications of service wants (quantitative data) followed by semi-structured interviews (qualitative data), to explore the relationship between different types of carer service need.

Explanatory sequential design

The explanatory sequential design is run in two distinctly separate phases, where the quantitative strand has priority and quantitative data are collected and analysed in the first phase. In the second phase the researcher uses the findings coming out from phase one to conduct the qualitative strand. This design is especially suitable when results from the first phase are hard to explain or to understand. Once again, if we use the example of the survey investigating health care professionals' attitude towards research, the results could show that among health care professionals, nurses with a degree-level education had a much more positive attitude towards research than nurses educated to a lower academic level. Taking these phase one findings into account, the qualitative strand in the second phase needs to be designed in such a way that we can arrive at in-depth knowledge and understanding to explain the quantitative findings. By conducting semi-structured interviews it would be possible to achieve a reasonable insight into why this was the case. A research example of an explanatory sequential design is that of Carr (2000) where in the first phase she assessed pain, anxiety and depression together with analgesic prescribing and consumption as well as pain documentation (quantitative data), while in the next phase semi-structured telephone interviews (qualitative data) were conducted to elucidate a greater understanding of the quantitative findings.

Exploratory sequential design

The exploratory sequential design aims to explore an under-researched phenomenon at depth in the first phase and then, in the second phase, to measure and/or classify the phenomenon under investigation. Here the qualitative strand is prioritized so that qualitative data are both collected and analysed in the first phase, as the findings are needed to inform us in phase two. For example, let us assume that no available measurement instrument exists to assess attitudes in relation to research and research implementation in clinical practice. By interviewing health care professionals in phase one we will gain knowledge about their experiences regarding contextual factors, facilitators, barriers towards research and possible consequences of research implementation. Thus, after phase one, we should be ready to develop a measurement instrument assessing attitudes towards implementation of research, which can be used in a larger population during phase two. A health services research example of an exploratory sequential design is that of Stoller *et al.* (2009) who, in the preliminary phase, focused on identifying decision-making factors influencing alcohol consumption in existing standardized instruments. In phase one, these researchers assessed the applicability of the decision-making factors (i.e. the 733 items addressing drinking decisions from the preliminary phase) by collecting and analysing data from semi-structured interviews, electronic illness narratives and Internet threaded discussions. The qualitative codes originating from the analysis were then compared to the decision factors. During phase two, they estimated the prevalence and association of post-diagnosis drinking using the new decision factors in telephone interviews.

Embedded design

In the embedded design the two strands are mixed at the outset in an a priori process to facilitate the maximum data to be collected. One type of data is used mainly in a supportive capacity (for example, only for the development of an intervention) while the other type will form the primary base for the study. Consequently, here the supplemental strand is added on to enhance the overall design. Let us look at the example of health care professionals and research once again. We now want to develop an intervention to help health care professionals create strategies for breaking down barriers and enhancing facilitators for implementation and use of research. We start by focus groups for example, to learn when and in what situation barriers are experienced. Using the results coming out of the focus group data we are now able to develop an intervention and test its effectiveness with an experimental design involving staff on different hospital wards. A research example of an embedded design is that of Wand *et al.* (2010) where in three distinct phases they used a framework to evaluate a new model of nursing practice as a means to obtain knowledge of how complex programmes work. In the first phase, they conducted a systematic literature review, focus group interviews and individual interviews. In the second phase an expert panel was used to refine the framework. In phase three the framework was implemented and evaluated (quantitatively) before the interpretation took place, based mainly on the qualitative results.

Multi-phase design

The multi-phase design, also sometimes known as the sandwich design, is, according to Creswell and Plano Clark (2011), a design that goes beyond the basic designs described above. This design is said to offer an overarching methodological framework in which concurrent and sequential components can be combined over a set period of time in a single mixed-methods project or programme to address an overall project objective. Thus, it is a step-by-step process of connected quantitative and qualitative studies sequentially aligned with each new approach building on what was learned previously. Consequently the multi-phase design is suitable for a set of incremental research questions. These design features make it particularly suitable for research guided by the MRC framework (2008), since the multi-phase design aims to support the development, adaption and evaluation of programmatic research. A health services research example of a multi-phase design is that of DeBar *et al.* (2011) who divided their programme into three complementary but distinct phases. First, they conducted a retrospective study using information from medical records to identify unique clusters of patients using allopathic and complementary and alternative therapies. Second, they collected interviews to explore allopathic providers' recommendations for acupuncture and patients' decisions to pursue and retain complementary and alternative therapy care. Third, they performed a prospective evaluation of health service costs and functional outcomes associated with the receipt of acupuncture.

The designs presented here aim to gain answers to different kinds of research question while offering us a framework for mixing, collecting and analysing data as well as for the interpretative research element. It is, however, important to remember that there are a number of different variants within each design, and to date the convergent parallel design is the most well-known design in mixed-methods research (Kettles *et al.*, 2011).

Sampling strategies in mixed-methods research

In any research project the sample is particularly important, as it is the sample that forms the basis for the data to be analysed, interpreted and reported. Hence, it is important to seriously and strategically consider who should participate, in what context will participants be recruited and how they are going to be chosen. In mixed-methods designs the possibilities to combine different samples and sampling strategies are both creative and almost infinite (Polit and Tatano Beck, 2012). Sampling techniques are as rigorous as in a mono-methods study. For example, power analysis to determine the size of the sample for the quantitative strand, the use of standardized instruments, plus other precautions such as saturation need to be taken into account here too.

In mixed methods it is not unusual for the same sample to participate in both strands, i.e. the qualitative and quantitative elements. Onwuegbuzie and Collins (2007) have put forward a categorization of mixed-methods samples determined by the relationship between the quantitative and qualitative components in a mixed-methods study: *identical*, *nested*, *parallel* and *multilevel* samples. The *identical sample* aims to include the same participants in both strands of the study, whereas a *nested* sample aims to include some participants, i.e. a subgroup from one strand. For example, some participants that scored high or low on a standardized assessment in the quantitative part of the study may be purposively sampled for the other strand too. In the *parallel* sample, participants are in either one or the other of the methods (quantitative/qualitative) but all participants are selected from a homogeneous population. Participants share the same characteristics and traits such as age, education, diagnosis, care situation, etc. In the *multilevel* sample, participants are not the same in the different parts of the study. Here, participants can be drawn from different populations and on different levels, i.e. a very heterogeneous sample in regards to characteristics and traits (Onwuegbuzie and Collins, 2007).

Collecting and analysing data in mixed-methods research

Data collection in mixed methods is no different from that in mono methods per se. Differences between quantitative, qualitative and mixed methods become particularly obvious during the data analysis phase. In mixed methods, data analysis should result in a meta-inference (Teddlie and Tashakkori, 2009). Thus, the integration of results coming from the two methods should result in a sum that is larger than the individual parts. The meta-inference needs to be motivated as well as explained, and the data analysis in a mixed-methods study can be *simultaneous*, *sequential* or *parallel* (Onwuegbuzie and Teddlie, 2003). *Simultaneous* data analysis means that the

TABLE 3.2 Seven-step analysis procedure (data taken from Onwuegbuzie and Teddlie, 2003)

Data	
1. Reduction	Numerical data are analysed with descriptive statistics and textual data are categorized in descriptive themes or categories.
2. Presentation	Data from both methods are organized and presented visually in matrixes and diagrams.
3. Transformation	Numerical data are transformed to textual codes that can be analysed by qualitative techniques; textual data are transformed to numerical codes that can be analysed by quantitative techniques.
4. Comparison I	The different types of data are explored for correlations.
5. Consolidation	The different types of data are integrated to one set of data.
6. Comparison II	Data originating from different sources are compared.
7. Integration	Numerical and textual data are integrated to one coherent whole and are analysed as one set of data or as two sets of data (numerical/textual) separately

data from each strand are integrated in the analysis phase to obtain a more complete picture of the results. *Sequential* data analysis is when data are analysed in order, with the aim to inform rather than to be integrated. One example of this is when the findings originating from numerical data (quantitative data) are used to guide the sample for an interview study (qualitative data collection) or where textual data are used to develop items for a questionnaire (quantitative data collection). *Parallel* data analysis implies that data analysis from both sets (numerical and textual data) occurs separately from each other and the findings from both data sets are only integrated during the interpretative phase (Onwuegbuzie and Teddlie, 2003). Currently, parallel data analysis is the most commonly used analysis method, closely followed by sequential data analysis (Östlund *et al.*, 2011). By integrating data collected in mixed-methods studies it is apparent that the practical procedures and finished product differ significantly between mono-method studies and mixed-methods studies. Different descriptions for the hands-on analysis of data exist and, for example, Onwuegbuzie and Teddlie (2003) have proposed a useful seven-step analysis procedure (Table 3.2).

One of the most significant elements of mixed methods is that integration is explicit and occurs at some, or more, points in the design. Strategies for how integration can take place are described by O'Cathain and colleagues (2010). Here the three most commonly used strategies for data integration of text and numerical data are: (1) triangulation protocol, (2) following a thread and (3) mixed-methods matrix. Methodological strategies for how to deal with those cases of integration where data are in conflict with each other are under development (cf. Moffat *et al.*, 2006).

Transferability of findings in mixed-methods research

The majority of established researchers within mixed methods seem to avoid concepts such as validity and trustworthiness. Teddlie and Tashakkori (2009) have put forward the concepts of inference quality and inference transferability. Inference quality should be viewed as an overarching criterion to evaluate the quality of the conclusions and interpretations from a mixed-methods study. It refers to the accuracy of the mixed-methods study's conclusion and semantically encompasses the quantitative concept of internal validity and the qualitative concept of credibility. Inference transferability is composed of the quantitative concept of external validity as well as the qualitative concept of transferability and deals with how reasonable the conclusions from the mixed-methods study are in a similar context, population or milieu.

Mixed methods – where are we now?

Different methods, standing alone, cannot lead health services researchers to the point where they have acquired a comprehensive understanding of health and social care or patient issues. Indeed, health service researchers cannot develop, test, evaluate and implement effective and feasible interventions without complex designs. Thus, methodologically sound mixed-methods research can improve our understanding of health services by providing a more comprehensive picture than single methods alone (Wisdom *et al.*, 2012). What can make mixed-methods designs specifically useful within the MRC framework, and what differentiates them from multiple methods is: (1) the possibility of developing the research question iteratively throughout the development-testing-evaluation-implementation phases of the framework. This is, however, not forgetting: (2) the advantages when answering complex research questions, of integrating one or all of the methods, analysis and findings. Together, these possibilities increase the likelihood that health services research in the future can deliver more detailed answers to important questions for developing health care for the greater good of patients and the public. Therefore, one might assume that the MRC framework (2008) should fit with mixed-methods designs like 'two peas in a pod'.

For example, the suggested place of mixed methods within the framework for complex interventions implies that the long-lasting conflict between qualitative and quantitative purists within health services research might be dwindling. Howes' (1988) incompatibility thesis, which states that qualitative and quantitative research paradigms including their associated methods cannot and should not be mixed, might finally be buried. As an example, and interestingly enough partially acknowledged by the MRC (2008), qualitative designs are now regarded as of increasing importance in order to recognize patient and public perspectives. Research structured by the framework has thus helped to clearly demonstrate the importance and the usefulness of qualitative study designs, in particular in exploring people's experiences of illness, health services and treatments, as well as in identifying need and evaluating the acceptability and feasibility of complex interventions. On the one hand, the introduction of mixed methods into the field has got us to the point that we may now have gained an in-depth understanding about certain issues. But on the other hand we have also gained insight into the fact that using qualitative studies alongside randomized controlled trials (RCTs) can reveal discrepancies between the two methods' results (O'Cathain, 2009). For example, Campbell and colleagues (2003) compared individual patient outcomes and found that people talking about improved health in the qualitative strand did not show a similar improvement on the scale used in the quantitative strand, and that the same was true in the other direction. In another study by Moffatt *et al.* (2006), a pilot study revealed a zero-effect size but in the concurrent qualitative component, participants described positive benefits of the intervention. Thus, it is important to understand that as a part of the methodological development, for every methodological step we go forward in complex designs, we are also likely to take some steps back.

One challenge is that few published studies to date, combining qualitative and quantitative methods developed from the perspective of the framework, describe using any of the established prototypes for mixed-methods designs, even though an analysis of their method clearly identifies the use of mixed-methods designs. A research example of this is Corry and colleagues (2013) who attempted to review and identify the approaches used by researchers to develop complex interventions in nursing research. They highlighted that the MRC framework (2000, 2008) appeared to be the most widely reported structure for developing complex interventions in this context. They further concluded that interventions developed within the MRC framework tended to provide a more comprehensive account of intervention development, and gave greater emphasis to theory and intervention modelling than research using other frameworks. If one conducts a more detailed scrutiny of the nine papers identified by Corry *et al.* (2013) as having used the framework, one can conclude that all of them described having used both quantitative and qualitative methods. Carefully analysing those few claiming to have used a mixed-methods design reveals further confusion. For example, authors may have reported their studies as following Creswell and Plano Clark's (2011) prototype A, but described prototype B in detail. Some authors reported their studies as prototype A, but offer insufficient information about prototype characteristics to critically assess the study's methodological rigour, or if it indeed actually was prototype A as reported in the title. This results in two important implications for the future. First is the impact of the further development of mixed-methods research within health services research and which designs are applicable. Second is the difficulty of gathering and synthesizing evidence coming out of mixed-methods research, given that conducting literature reviews is an important part of the recommended development phase within the MRC framework.

In regards to the first, reasonable questions to pose here have to be, do prototypes and/or typologies make or break us, and is our effort to create standard designs a facilitator or a barrier to solving important patient issues within health services research? One possible and pragmatic solution put forward has been to focus instead on the level of interaction between the strands, the relative priority of the strands, the timing of the strands and finally the procedures for mixing the strands, together with using reporting criteria such as 'Good Reporting of a Mixed-Methods Study' (GRAMMS) (cf. O'Cathain *et al.*, 2007) when designing and reporting mixed-methods studies. Adopting a transparent approach regarding these components is of vital importance, and is likely to solve some of the more urgent issues while simultaneously taking forward the development of mixed methods and the designs' usefulness.

In regards to the second, systematic reviews indicate that it is becoming more and more common to find published studies that have used a mixed-methods design within health services research. However, guidance on how to report and how to assess the quality (soundness) of published mixed-methods studies has so far received little consideration, even though attempts to develop quality criteria exist. One such example referred to earlier is GRAMMS, suggested by O'Cathain *et al.* (2007). The authors claim that good mixed-methods reporting should be signified by: clear justification for why a mixed-methods approach was used; transparency regarding design; suitable sampling, data collection and analysis; the justification at integration for data transformation; contradictory findings that are explained; convergent findings that are not related to bias between methods (O'Cathain *et al.*, 2007).

Published literature reviews imply that the present state of affairs is not encouraging. For example, Wisdom and colleagues (2012) reviewed five high-ranking health services research journals between the years 2003 and 2007, aiming to investigate the frequency of published mixed-methods articles. A further aim was to compare the reporting of methodological components to indicate a methodologically sound approach. Out of the 1,651 papers reviewed, only 47 papers were categorized as mixed methods (i.e. integrated or combined both quantitative and qualitative methods in a single study) but only five of those used the term 'mixed-methods' design or multi methods in the abstract or full text. Additionally, very few of the studies included the level of methodological detail one might expect to be required for a mono-method study to be accepted in a high-impact journal. Others have reported similar disconcerting findings (O'Cathain *et al.*, 2007; Östlund *et al.*, 2011).

Additionally, few authors seem to have taken on the challenge of offering detailed accounts of the analysis process or presenting visual examples of how data were and can be integrated. Controversially, it appears that within health services research, data integration is only stated to occur during the discussion part of the reporting. An explanation for this might be that the sequential parallel design seems to be the most commonly described. Integrating the two methods often appears to take place mainly in the discussion. The consequences of this are that very little guidance is available for researchers to follow, and we are not fully taking advantage of the integration feature throughout study designs. It might be that we are not at the point where we are able to fully grasp how to develop complex mixed-methods research questions. A reasonable question is how the clear lack of published methodological detail negatively affects the transfer of knowledge, as well as the development of mixed methods. Increasing the opportunity to publish, i.e. reporting study protocols, would clearly help to develop both the design and the methodological knowledge of the wider health services research community.

However, no research method is perfect and nor are researchers. Rather, research is about how you can think logically, systematically, and in a structured and analytical manner about the different methods, their weaknesses and how these can be eliminated or compensated for by another method. Mixed-methods designs demand time, money and human resources in the shape of researchers well acquainted with both quantitative and qualitative methods and methodology. These designs imply that a number of important decisions need to be made early while planning research programmes. These choices demand knowledge, methodological competence and teamwork by established and experienced researchers. Regardless of these challenges, the gain, when the questions are the right ones, is that both strands complement each other. Unlike in the past, different methods and methodologists are not competing with each other. Rather, the great advantage of mixed-methods research is that the strengths within one method can eliminate the weaknesses within another. Mixed-methods approaches, rigorously designed, logically executed and transparently reported fit particularly well within the MRC's (2008) process of 'development-testing-evaluation-implementation'. Taking on the methodological challenge of utilizing the design as a vital part of the complex interventions framework is likely to forward the quality and effectiveness of modern health care services as offered to patients and the public.

4

THE CRITICAL IMPORTANCE OF PATIENT AND PUBLIC INVOLVEMENT FOR RESEARCH INTO COMPLEX INTERVENTIONS

David A. Richards

Introduction

Although by no means a universal phenomenon, many societies are evolving away from patriarchal structures, not least the belief that what health care professionals 'prescribe' for patients is always right. 'Doctor knows best' is being challenged by the emergence of the information society (Webster and Robins, 1989), super-fast information technology and the growth of online social networking. People now expect to be consulted and involved when decisions about their health care are being made, and health care professionals know only too well that the outcome of any treatment is dependent on patient involvement and attitude. The MRC guidelines for developing and researching complex interventions (Medical Research Council, 2008) said almost nothing about the value of 'Patient and Public Involvement' (PPI) in research. This chapter will attempt to remedy that deficit by describing methods and models by which patients, informal carers and members of the public can and should be involved in all research, at all stages and in all elements of the process of developing, testing, evaluating and implementing complex interventions.

Learning objectives

- Recognize the importance of involving patients and the public in research.
- Understand how models of patient and public involvement have developed and evolved over time.
- Describe how patients and the public can contribute to the development, testing, evaluation and implementation of complex interventions.

Involving patients and members of the public in research: priority setting

Patient and public involvement, or the lack of it, is one reason cited by some authors (Chalmers and Glasziou, 2009) for research waste. The priorities of commercial research companies, academic researchers and clinical specialists are often dramatically different from the concerns of patients, members of the public and informal or formal carers of people struggling with distress, disability and disease. As noted by recent commentators (Macleod *et al.*, 2014: 103), researchers may prefer 'research that they find interesting rather than research that addresses issues of importance to the users of research'. Here, potential users of research are defined very broadly as 'policy makers, patients, professionals making practice or personal decisions, and researchers and research funders deciding which additional research should be done' (Chalmers *et al.*, 2014: 156). Data support this view. For example, when the research priorities of patients with osteoarthritis and clinicians providing care and treatment were compared to the type of studies actually being undertaken, it was found that whilst 91 per cent of patients favoured trials of non-drug treatments, in practice the reverse was true with 80 per cent of actual research being undertaken into the efficacy of drugs (Tallon *et al.*, 2000a), leading to a call for greater PPI in research agenda setting (Tallon *et al.*, 2000b).

One example of involving patients (and their carers and clinicians) in setting research priorities is the James Lind Alliance (http://www.lindalliance.org), named after one of the pioneers of clinical trials who discovered that vitamin C in the form of oranges and lemons was helpful in preventing scurvy in sailors. The James Lind Alliance brings patients, carers and clinicians together on an equal footing to work on specific health conditions (Partridge and Scadding, 2004). These condition-specific groups identify uncertainties in the treatment of these conditions and work to develop consensus on a priority list of around ten questions that they would like answering. These priorities are then made available for researchers to consult and for research funders to think about commissioning research.

A broader agenda for patient and public involvement

However, important as it is, involving patients and the public in research is more than merely inviting them to contribute to identifying the questions that need to be asked. Equally, PPI is also not at all the same as patients providing research data, even qualitative data from interviews or focus groups. This is not what is meant by PPI. Patient and public involvement in research should be considered in the context of a broader movement to include people in governmental policy-making. One of the earliest attempts to articulate involvement is Arnstein's well-known 'ladder of citizen participation' (Arnstein, 1969) in which she presented steps in participation from 'manipulation' to 'citizen control' as a continuum from a situation where professionals and policy-makers are completely dominant to one where lay people make the major decisions. Essentially, her ideas focus on the relative distribution of power between citizens and policy-makers in decision-making.

Several authors have presented extensions and critiques of Arnstein's work as applied to health care and health research. Tritter (2009) for example, locates involvement in a matrix of individual/collective, direct/indirect and proactive/reactive involvement. He also differentiates health services involvement depending on its aims – treatment decision-making, service evaluation, service development, education and training, and research – and raises concerns as to how the recasting of patients as consumers redefines PPI as the exercise of individual choice within the global marketization of health care. Whilst the ability to exercise choice has been limited by organizational factors in European systems of state-provided health care, it has been enshrined in US health care, albeit of course limited by ability to pay or to obtain sufficient insurance. Collective involvement, for example where people have equity of health services access, can be undermined when systems are set up that promote individual choice and can lead to some people getting quicker access to services than others. The fear is that people come to erroneously believe that the ability to exercise individual choice should define patient and public involvement (Gibson *et al.*, 2012). Once again, this is not what we should mean when considering PPI in research.

Early commentators have postulated that the value of PPI comes in terms of obtaining complementary insights to those of health professionals (Entwistle *et al.*, 1998). It is also suggested by these authors that lay involvement may improve the management of research, its interpretation, dissemination and implementation, as well as the setting of research agendas and priorities. The dilemmas voiced by Tritter and colleagues (Tritter, 2009; Tritter and Lutfey, 2009) cited earlier are also relevant when discussing the role of PPI in research, particularly the tensions between collective involvement (for example, of pressure groups) and individual patient involvement, and the extent to which either of these variants of PPI opinion can ever deliver a representative lay opinion (Entwistle *et al.*, 1998).

Importantly, a number of reviews have been published that have examined how people could be involved in research (Boote *et al.*, 2002; Oliver *et al.*, 2004). Oliver and colleagues (Oliver *et al.*, 2008) further analysed accounts of lay involvement in research and created a matrix where the degree of public engagement is set against the degree of engagement in the process of PPI by researchers themselves. In their model, they suggest that in a research agenda setting, researchers' actions around engagement can vary from minimal, through behaviour responsive to lay people's actions (such as responses to lobbying), to active invitations to lay people and/or lay groups to participate. However, lay people can also be more or less involved whatever researchers do; here Oliver *et al.* (2008) grade public engagement from minimal, through consultation, collaboration, to full lay control. For example, they report that consumer representation on a Cochrane review group was an example of effective collaboration, allowing lay members to bring broad perspectives to the process, whereas consultation could vary from effective participation in consensus-building exercises to mere response to written surveys, which was less effective at building real patient and public involvement.

Building on this work, some have advocated a more emancipatory approach so that 'true' participation is facilitated (Gibson *et al.*, 2012). In Gibson and colleagues' recent and highly sophisticated theory of PPI (Gibson *et al.*, 2012), involvement is conceptualized as more or less emancipatory in four distinct dimensions. In the first dimension – expressive/instrumental – PPI is influenced by the tension between the need for bureaucracies to involve patients and the public in strategic decision-making and lay people's own need to communicate their personal views and experiences. The second dimension refers to what is known as 'weak/strong publics', essentially the general ability of groups of people to influence decision-making. Thirdly, monism/pluralism refers to the value placed on different forms of social capital such as knowledge, for example the way in which medical knowledge may be given greater status than lay experiences of illness in decision-making. Finally, overseeing these three dimensions are the wishes of policy-makers to effect change or retain the status quo – referred to as the cross-cutting dimension of 'conservation/change'. Researchers can use these ideas when considering involving the public or patients in their research projects, essentially basing this activity on a good theory of involvement.

The impact of patient and public involvement

One important question raised has been whether PPI in its various forms does actually lead not only to more relevant research questions being asked but also to 'better' research, for example findings that are more relevant to patients and the public or research that is more 'successful' in terms of recruitment or other performance metrics. Of course, merely asking this question places us at the instrumental end of Gibson *et al.*'s first dimension (Gibson *et al.*, 2012), in that it neatly skips issues around the moral imperative to involve people in research into their health and addresses bureaucratic notions of benefit to the 'system'. Nonetheless, given Oliver *et al.*'s (2008) suggestion that greater participation requires effort on the part of researchers, it might not be unreasonable for researchers, policy-makers and research funders to ask the question.

In this respect, PPI can be seen as a complex intervention itself. In the case of PPI, because it has been introduced as a policy – for example, in the UK the National Institute for Health Research will not grant funds to researchers unless there is a programme of PPI built into the research programme – it is not open to a randomized experimental evaluation but is actually an example of a natural experiment (see Chapter 20). One study has been published using data from this experiment (Ennis and Wykes, 2013). Because study-monitoring data were available to the researchers during the time that PPI became more common, by charting the relationship to study success criteria and PPI they were able to analyse the extent of involvement as an independent predictor of study performance. In summary, this study showed that a greater level of PPI was associated with better recruitment into clinical studies.

The authors speculate that this may be because PPI has led to more participant-friendly information sheets, patient involvement has led to designs that are more 'patient-friendly', and participants are more willing to take part in research that has been endorsed by people with the same health condition as themselves.

Although these factors are speculative, the combination of moral and operational reasons for PPI should be sufficient to persuade researchers undertaking studies into complex interventions to actively engage patients and members of the public in their studies, not as study participants, but as partners in the research endeavour. By reflecting on the various models cited here, researchers can do much to avoid tokenism. Patients and the public can be involved at all levels from designing studies, writing participant information and consent materials and intervention design, to data collection, analysis and write-up. Patients can be equal partners on study committees and independent scrutiny panels and can work with researchers, funders and clinicians to help implement research findings. As researchers, we should think hard about whom to involve, either by responding to known patient advocates or actively soliciting new involvement from patients and the public. How to involve lay members and good practices for doing so – including fair payment to lay members of a research team – is the subject of some helpful guidance from INVOLVE (http://www.invo.org.uk), an organization specifically set up to provide support to researchers, patients and members of the public. Although it is UK-based, indeed funded by a major UK health research funder, its suggested principles for good practice are not UK-specific.

Conclusion

This chapter has provided a rationale for and a narrative on the development of patient and public involvement. The chapter has applied current emancipatory thinking to research involvement. From the perspective of the contributors to this book, we regard PPI as essential to high-quality research into complex interventions and we urge readers to incorporate PPI policies and actions into all parts of the research endeavour.

Further reading

INVOLVE. 2012. *Evidence Bibliography 4*. INVOLVE Coordinating Centre, Eastleigh. http://www.invo.org.uk/wp-content/uploads/2012/11/Bibliography4-complete.pdf.

SECTION 1
Developing complex interventions

Introduction to Section 1

Gabriele Meyer and Sascha Köpke

The development phase of a new intervention in health and social care is extremely important for its future success, irrespective of whether one is developing single-component or complex interventions. The MRC guidance uncompromisingly asks, 'Are you clear about what you are trying to do: what outcomes you are aiming for, and how you will bring about change?' (Medical Research Council, 2008: 4). It moves on with probing questions such as: 'Does your intervention have a coherent theoretical basis? Have you used this theory systematically to develop the intervention? Can you describe the intervention fully, so that it can be implemented properly for the purpose of your evaluation, and replicated by others? Does the existing evidence – ideally collated in a systematic review – suggest that it is likely to be effective or cost effective?' (Medical Research Council, 2008: 4).

The authors of the eight chapters in this section of our book highlight critical issues that determine the success of the important first step of developing a complex intervention, including as an early task the identification of the evidence base. One might assume that this is undertaken as a matter of course and a mandatory starting point for all clinical researchers during intervention development. Sadly, this is not always the case, as demonstrated by Clarke et al. (2010). The authors' consecutive enquiries in 1997, 2001, 2005 and 2009, analysing publications on randomized controlled trials in high-impact journals, revealed that the majority of publications of trials did not make an apparent systematic attempt to set the trials' results in the context of other trials. Rarely was the first trial addressing the question under investigation cited.

Decisions about health care require the full picture of evidence, not incomplete segments. *The Lancet* learned from this study and now asks authors of clinical trials to embed the reporting of their trial in a systematic review, ideally including meta-analysis. Although the bar for successful publishing is now set higher, the benefit to the users of evidence and scientific rigour is obvious.

Systematic reviews are the cornerstone of evidence-based health care, having the primary aim to overcome selective information-seeking and thus to help stakeholders in health care to make decisions based on solid foundations. Methods of systematically reviewing the evidence have become much more sophisticated during recent years. Reporting requirements have been upgraded, registration of systematic reviews has been introduced, scientific debates have been initiated about overlapping reviews, independent replication of systematic reviews has been introduced, as has consideration of a wider agenda in systematic reviews and meta-analyses in terms of breadth, timing and depth of the evidence. Different formats of systematic reviews have been developed, for example scoping reviews, snap-shot reviews, rapid reviews, integrative reviews, realist reviews, mixed-method reviews – to mention just a few. This section gives an overview of some of these new methods. Although it cannot cover all new methodological developments and every debate in detail, we aim to depict recent methodological discourse on this very important first step of developing a complex intervention. We do so by guiding readers through formats of systematic reviews which are useful for the identification of the evidence base within the development phase of complex interventions.

The section starts with a chapter exploring how systematic reviews identify, summarize and synthesize the relevant research evidence for the effects of any intervention – either simple or complex. Thus, we start smoothly, building on what many readers of our book possibly may have already come across. In their first chapter, Nicky Cullum and Jo Dumville make us particularly aware of the importance of systematic review protocols and their components. As generally in evidence-based health care, trustworthiness and reliability of evidence is paramount, so Cullum and Dumville focus the lens on how to minimize bias in the systematic review process.

The same authors then provide a second chapter on advanced approaches to evidence synthesis. Based on the premises of the first chapter, their focus now is on subgroup analyses and meta-regression of primary studies, which may be used to explore heterogeneity as a starting point when designing new complex interventions. They further discuss the potential of individual patient data meta-analyses rather than aggregate study meta-analyses and describe how overviews of reviews – known as umbrella reviews – as well as mixed-treatment comparison meta-analyses can be used to determine the relative effectiveness of interventions that have not been compared in head-to-head comparisons.

In the next chapter, Sascha Köpke, Jane Noyes, Jackie Chandler and Gabriele Meyer address a number of challenges encountered when preparing systematic reviews of complex interventions. So far, there is no gold standard and the authors could not instruct readers to rely on the *Cochrane Handbook*, since it still does not include firm guidance on how to deal with complex intervention synthesis. However, the authors refer to recent methodological contributions concerning the definition of key questions and the building of appropriate search strategies, together with methods to optimally describe intervention components including control interventions, as well as dealing with interdependencies between different outcome measures.

The next contribution comes from Jo Rycroft-Malone and Christopher R. Burton who provide an introduction to the synthesis of qualitative research within the context of research and development of complex interventions. Researchers engaged in complex interventions consistently agree that qualitative and quantitative research methods should go hand in hand in both development and evaluation phases. However, not much has been written about this topic and the authors' advice, illustrated by examples in this chapter, is a significant contribution to the body of knowledge.

Karin Hannes (Chapter 9) moves beyond separate quantitative and qualitative reviews towards mixed-method synthesis. Hannes discusses when this review format should be considered, reflects on the appropriate methodological synthesis approach and defines appropriate questions for different phases in mixed-methods reviews. She finally presents a clearly structured example on how to design and conduct a mixed-methods review.

After this rich information about the art of evidence synthesis and its different formats, the section moves on to outcome and process modelling. Susanne Buhse and Ingrid Mühlhauser discuss the selection of appropriate outcome measures which is without doubt critical for proper assessment of the effects of an intervention. The authors discuss the difference between patient-relevant outcomes and surrogate marker outcomes and the fallacies of the latter, and highlight the value of patient-reported outcomes and the assessment of intervention-related negative consequences. Furthermore, Buhse and Mühlhauser briefly address composite outcomes, multicomponent as well as interdependent outcomes and conclude with a discussion about the clinical relevance of outcomes.

The chapter by Charles Abraham and colleagues outlines an evidence-based approach to designing interventions aiming to change individual health-related behaviour patterns. Such interventions are most often complex. Abraham and colleagues introduce the Intervention Mapping framework (which we will revisit in Section 4) and focus on the understanding of change processes. The authors present a valuable example of theory-driven complex intervention development with helpful key recommendations for developers of behaviour change interventions.

The section is completed by Walter Sermeus, who focuses on modelling the processes in complex interventions. The overarching aim is to unravel the complex intervention's 'black box' and here Sermeus gives us insights using examples and model-based instruction. He explains how consensus on the components of the complex intervention might be achieved, how clinical activities can be clustered into key interventions, how the process could be organized and how process and outcome indicators can be derived. Finally he discusses approaches that try to take into account the degree of acceptance and willingness for change, critical when designing an intervention that will be fit for implementation.

Any framework for developing complex interventions must be iterative and reflexive, going back and forward between steps. Nonetheless, after spending time reviewing, theorizing and modelling, intervention developers will need to move to a testing phase. This first section prepares the ground for what is to follow, as intervention developers move to the generation of new evidence covered in Sections 2 and 3 of our book.

5

SYSTEMATIC REVIEWS OF THE EFFECTS OF INTERVENTIONS

Nicky Cullum and Jo Dumville

Introduction

In order to make informed decisions about implementing health care interventions or embarking on new research, including intervention development, we need high-quality summaries of all relevant, existing research. This chapter explores how systematic reviews identify, summarize and synthesize the relevant research evidence of the effects of any intervention – whether simple or complex.

Questions about whether interventions are effective and how effective they are relative to alternatives are fundamentally questions of causality, i.e. is this effect caused by this manoeuvre? The best research design for addressing this type of question is the randomized controlled trial (RCT) which allows comparison of the effects of alternative approaches in people with a particular health problem. Randomization is a powerful tool because it prevents selection bias (in this context that is the bias that arises when comparison groups have not been assembled at random and have different prognostic profiles at baseline). When participants in RCTs have been properly randomized the results cannot be confounded, although there may be chance prognostic factor imbalances that can be corrected using appropriate analyses. However, whilst single RCTs are important, decisions about which interventions or new research to implement should be informed by *all* the available RCTs that have tackled the same or similar questions. Systematic reviews are the solution as they identify, collate, synthesize and analyse all relevant studies using the scientific method.

Learning objectives

By the end of this chapter and associated reading you should be able to:

- Discuss why systematic reviews are an important aid to decision-making about the implementation of either interventions or new research.
- Analyse why a protocol is an important step in a systematic review and what the components of a protocol should be.
- Discuss steps to minimize bias in the systematic review process.

Conducting a systematic review

Below we provide a synopsis of the systematic review process (see Figure 5.1) and recommend further detailed reading before beginning your own review. Two particularly useful (and freely available, online) resources are *The Cochrane Handbook for Systematic Reviews of Interventions*, which is regularly updated (Higgins and Green, 2011), and guidance from the Centre for Reviews and Dissemination (Centre for Reviews and Dissemination, 2009) as well as the PRISMA statement (Liberati *et al.*, 2009). Whilst PRISMA is concerned with how to *report* systematic reviews it is well worth reading before you start to do one. These tools cover the basic principles of why and how to conduct any type of systematic review.

Developing a focused, answerable question

The defining characteristic of a systematic review is that it uses a scientific method to answer a *focused* and *answerable* question; this is true of any systematic review whether the interventions of interest are considered complex or not (Petticrew *et al.*, 2013a). The most tried and tested method of focusing a question for primary research or review is the PICO method (Fineout-Overholt and Johnston, 2005) which helps frame uncertainty and requires us to name our parameters of interest in advance. In PICO, P represents the *patient population* of interest, I refers to the *intervention of interest*, C, the *comparator* and O is the *outcome of interest*. This focused question will then drive all other aspects of the review methodology including the search strategy, the nature of the eligible studies and the analytical approach. Quite how the PICO approach is used in the context of complex interventions reviews will partly depend on the purpose of the review. PICO will still be useful if your objective is to synthesize the evidence and determine the average intervention effect (or range of effects) and RCTs will be the optimal study design to include (Petticrew *et al.*, 2013a). Where the objective of the review is to explore and understand complexity, authors whilst still requiring explicit research questions, may explore how and why interventions or their components work and PICO may be a less useful approach. The driving questions may be more concerned with *when*, *how* and *why* interventions work rather than *if*, and exploration of contextual factors may be particularly important. Such research questions require evidence from a broader range of study designs and approaches to be synthesized including qualitative research and process evaluation (Petticrew *et al.*, 2013b). Further guidance on

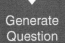

Generate
Question

- Develop focused, answerable question using PICO

Write Protocol

- Provide rationale for area of interest
- State PICO question and relevant primary and secondary outcomes
- Present inclusion and exclusion criteria particularly on the types of study, participants and careful definition of interventions you are including
- Design search strategy
- Plan study selection process and data extraction, including what will be extracted and where you will extract data to
- Plan data synthesis and analyses
- Publish protocol and register review

Conduct
Review

- Initiate study database searches to obtain a list of titles and abstracts (where possible) of potentially eligible studies
- Screen identified studies (and relevant reference lists) against eligibility criteria – ensure this is undertaken by two reviewers. Record reason for exclusion especially when basing decisions on full-text articles
- Complement database searches with searches for unpublished material, e.g. by contacting experts and searching trial registration databases. Also consider searching the reference lists of relevant studies – such as those of included studies and previous systematic reviews. Again another reviewer should be involved in inclusion/exclusion decisions
- Extract data following the methodology outlined in the protocol and only for pre-specified outcomes. Contact study authors to request missing details where possible. Ensure interventions are fully described
- Following your protocol and interrogating your data, decide on the narrative synthesis structure and whether meta-analyses are appropriate and if so whether a fixed or random-effects model will be considered in each case
- Present clear and proportionate interpretation of results

FIGURE 5.1 Overview of systematic review process

developing research questions for complex interventions is provided by Squires and colleagues (Squires *et al.*, 2013b).

Given that the scope of this chapter is specifically systematic reviews of effectiveness, this chapter will focus on research questions in the PICO format best answered by an RCT study design. The methodological features of a systematic review presented are of universal relevance; however, the analytical approaches described here are most relevant for quantitative data analysis.

Drafting a protocol for the review and having it peer reviewed and published

Systematic reviews, like primary research, should be driven by pre-specified protocols, with the protocol containing as much detailed methodological information as possible prior to seeing the data. Review protocols help to reduce bias and ensure transparency and rigour and are the detailed advanced plans in which you must:

1   Provide a rationale for your topic of interest.
2   Clearly state your question or objective in a clear format, e.g. PICO. All elements of the PICO are specified in the question including the primary outcome for the review. The primary outcome should be important and meaningful to those most affected by your review question (e.g. patients with the particular condition) rather than the outcome that is most likely to be have been measured or reported in the existing research.
3   A good protocol states clear, well-defined and unambiguous eligibility criteria for the kinds of studies that will be included in the review. For many reviews these will typically also follow the PICO format with the addition of study design, language and publication status. When reviewing complex intervention studies it is vital to think carefully about the operational definition of the eligible intervention(s) and their components. This and related issues are interrogated in an extremely important paper by Glasziou and colleagues (Glasziou *et al.*, 2010). Systematic reviews, like trials, should be registered in advance in the PROSPERO database (http://www.crd.york.ac.uk/PROSPERO/). Registration avoids unplanned review duplication and facilitates comparison of review conduct with what was planned in the protocol (Abaid *et al.*, 2007).
4   Construct a search strategy. Undertaking a search for a systematic review is a specialized activity for which reviewers are advised to work with information scientists who are expert in designing and running maximally sensitive search strategies in appropriate databases. Readers are referred elsewhere for detailed guidance (Centre for Reviews and Dissemination, 2009; Lefebvre *et al.*, 2011). It is particularly important for complex intervention reviews that you anticipate the many varied ways the intervention may be described or named in the primary studies for your search. Failure to give this sufficient consideration will result in studies being unintentionally excluded from your review.
5   Plan how study selection will proceed and be documented. Ideally two people undertake this selection process using an agreed approach (possibly using an algorithm), usually involving (i) screening titles and abstracts from the searches'

outputs to identify potentially eligible studies and (ii) obtaining full text copies of potentially eligible studies to screen in detail against the eligibility criteria.

6   Pre-define a data extraction strategy (include variables) and a procedure including how you will assess risk of bias. The term 'risk of bias' is preferred to 'study quality' when referring to the strength of the individual studies because it refers specifically to internal validity (and the risk that this has been compromised due to study design or conduct). Two reviewers, ideally working independently, are essential to minimize bias and mistakes. If two independent reviewers are not available then as a minimum there should be a second reviewer checking the data extraction and risk of bias judgement. You will need to predetermine which variables relating to risk of bias you will extract and how you will define them (Higgins *et al.*, 2011a, 2011b).

7   Plan how you will undertake data analysis including your key measure of treatment effect. Binary outcomes (e.g. dead or alive) are usually represented as relative risks (otherwise known as risk ratios) or odds ratios (Deeks *et al.*, 2011). Where outcomes are continuous (e.g. body weight or blood pressure), your effect measure is likely to be a difference in group means. Planning your data analysis at the protocol stage is a crucial means of minimizing bias. Your data analysis plan will be driven by methodological considerations and your review questions rather than the data. Thought will need to be given to how you will assess between study heterogeneity and how you will deal with it in analysis; what kinds of interventions you may consider grouping together and whether you will use risk of bias assessment in deciding which studies to meta-analyse (you may decide, for example, to exclude all studies from meta-analyses that do not have blinded outcome assessment) (Hróbjartsson et al., 2012).

Conduct the review

Follow the steps outlined in your protocol and carefully document your decisions and findings, including your search results. If studies are highlighted that require deviation from the original protocol (for example if you identify a group of studies which address a comparison that was not anticipated in the protocol), before deviating from pre-specified plans you should assess the extent to which you might introduce any bias into the review process. If there seems to be no strong risk of bias associated with protocol deviation you can go ahead provided you document your decision and are explicit in the review that a particular strategy was determined *post hoc*.

The process of study selection, decisions taken and rationales should all be documented. The reasons for excluding every study which at first glance would seem eligible must be clearly recorded and will appear in the published review (or be otherwise available). This would usually involve justifying exclusion of those studies which needed to be seen in full text before the exclusion decision could be made.

When you have identified your eligible studies you can begin to extract data (as they relate to all elements of PICO in the included studies). Only extract data for the outcomes you pre-specified in the review protocol (and for the time points you pre-specified were important) to avoid reporting bias (Kirkham *et al.*, 2010). How you use your extracted data depends on the nature of your review and the software you are using. Cochrane reviews are conducted using RevMan software from protocol stage to publication and updates (see http://ims.cochrane.org/revman, accessed 22 July, 2013). However, if you are writing your review in word processing software and conducting statistical analysis in statistical software you will need to enter your data into the statistical package. Whichever method you use it is important to have your extracted data available in a format that can be interpreted by others; it may not be published in full but an editor or reader of your review may want to see the detail.

Once you have extracted the required data from your eligible studies you are able to make decisions about your analysis and the type of synthesis that you will undertake. You will follow the approach that you specified in your protocol. It may be inappropriate to undertake any meta-analysis, for example if the studies you have identified have evaluated interventions that are too different or have very different lengths of follow-up. Whether meta-analysing your data or not, it is extremely important that you report the results in clear, unbiased language whilst ensuring you are faithful to your original protocol in terms of the outcomes presented. A common mistake (whether or not a review includes meta-analysis) is for reviewers to simply present the plethora of results reported by the original researchers, forgetting that they only pre-specified one or two of the reported outcomes in their review protocol.

The key feature to start with for a narrative synthesis of quantitative research is the structure of the results section. Again this is largely driven by your original PICO question and is usually structured by nature of the comparisons and then the results for the pre-specified outcomes reported under each comparison heading. The narrative of the results section will lay out study results, the precision of effect estimates (using 95 per cent confidence intervals), indicate sample sizes, study results and the risk of bias of individual studies and overall the risk of bias associated with your main outcomes. This information, using a combination of words and numbers, should be clearly and concisely reported so that the reader gains a coherent picture of the available evidence relevant to the review question. The reviewer should explore any patterns emerging from the data and bear in mind that the quality of a body of evidence is influenced by factors such as risk of bias in the original studies, unexplained heterogeneity in results, imprecision of the results, any indirectness of the evidence (such as existing trials only having recruited a very narrowly defined sample of participants) and any publication bias that might be influencing the identification of studies. These features are all part of GRADE (Guyatt *et al.*, 2011) and are key factors that should influence the interpretation of a body of evidence.

Meta-analysis

Pooling data from similar studies in meta-analysis increases statistical power and precision, thus reducing the risk of Type II errors. Whether or not meta-analysis is appropriate in any given situation depends on whether more than one study compares the same or sufficiently similar interventions in a similar context. If you have at least two studies that are sufficiently similar (in a clinical and experimental sense), then meta-analysis may be possible.

If meta-analysis seems appropriate, start with your primary outcome in order to derive a pooled effect estimate. The process of undertaking meta-analysis involves two stages: calculation of a study-level treatment effect for each study and then calculation of a weighted overall treatment effect across the studies. There are several software programs that do meta-analysis, including RevMan which is the freely available Cochrane Collaboration software (Cochrane Collaboration 2012) and Comprehensive Meta Analysis (http://www.meta-analysis.com, accessed February 14, 2014).

The output of your meta-analysis will tell you whether any difference in outcomes between the treatments is greater than that expected by chance, along with the precision around your estimate of effect. The other important information this pooling provides is a statistical estimate of heterogeneity. Heterogeneity refers to the nature and amount of variation in the results of the included studies. Heterogeneity can be due to obvious differences in study participants (clinical heterogeneity); differences in study design and methods (methodological heterogeneity); or may be detected as statistical heterogeneity but not easily explained.

Two common pieces of information about heterogeneity produced from a meta-analysis are the results of a Chi^2 test for heterogeneity and the I^2 statistic. The I^2 statistic is reported as a proportion of variation in study results that is due to heterogeneity rather than chance (Higgins *et al.*, 2003). Since the importance of any heterogeneity needs to be assessed by the author, I^2 values should be assessed on a case-by-case basis. Generally an I^2 over 40 per cent may represent moderate heterogeneity, over 50 per cent substantial heterogeneity and over 75 per cent considerable heterogeneity (Higgins *et al.*, 2003). There is much debate about whether it is advisable to pool studies at all in the face of high levels of heterogeneity, and there is no consensus (Ioannidis *et al.*, 2008).

Another important decision influenced by heterogeneity is whether to pool using a fixed-effect or random-effects model (Riley *et al.*, 2011). In the presence of obvious heterogeneity it makes sense to apply a random-effects model, which allows for the true effect to vary between studies – viewing the studies included in the meta-analysis as a random sample from studies displaying a distribution of results. It is also important to bear in mind the implications of fixed or random-effects meta-analysis when interpreting review results (Riley *et al.*, 2011). Another way to investigate heterogeneity is by subgroup analysis and meta-regression (see the following chapter). Authors of systematic reviews should help readers interpret the results, especially of meta-analyses. Numerical results can be seductive but they must be considered in the light of the risk of bias at study and out-come level *and* other features of the quality of evidence such as precision and indirectness (Guyatt *et al.*, 2011; Higgins *et al.*, 2011a, 2011b). Again you are referred to the reporting expectations detailed in PRISMA (Liberati *et al.*, 2009). Increasingly reviewers are urged to use the GRADE approach to summarizing the quality of the evidence for a particular question and Cochrane reviewers are now expected to publish these as Summary of Findings Tables (Guyatt *et al.*, 2011; Langendam *et al.*, 2013).

Summary

A systematic review of research evidence is a scientific approach to summarizing the results of similar studies that focus on a shared question about the effectiveness of alternative interventions for a common health problem. This approach is driven by a need to guard against bias at all stages of the review process.

A key initial step in producing a systematic review is the production and peer review of a protocol. A review protocol anticipates all the main methodological decisions involved in conducting a review and either makes the decisions in advance or creates decision rules where there is uncertainty (e.g. what to do where reviewers do not agree on study inclusion). When the systematic review concerns complex interventions it is crucially important to pre-specify the characteristics and particularly the components of complex interventions that will determine the study inclusion criteria.

Sometimes deviation from your review protocol is necessary; however, this should be done only when you are content that the protocol change will not intro-duce bias into the review; such decisions should be clearly reported and explained in the review.

Search results and study selection decisions with explanations should be care-fully recorded and published or made available for reasons of transparency.

Thorough data extraction is essential for complex intervention reviews where it is particularly important to fully specify the components of the interventions in the primary studies and the contexts in which they were delivered (Glasziou *et al.*, 2010). The outcomes data extracted, analysed and reported should follow your pre-specified protocol and not go beyond this (for example by adding multiple time points or outcomes).

Meta-analysis should only proceed after careful consideration of all forms of heterogeneity and risk of bias.

It is important that authors of reviews give careful consideration to interpret-ation of results, particularly in the light of the volume and quality of the research. GRADE represents the internationally accepted, gold-standard approach to inter-pretation of the evidence in this context (Guyatt *et al.*, 2011; Langendam *et al.*, 2013).

Further reading

Agency for Healthcare Research and Quality. 2014. *Methods Guide for Effectiveness and Comparative Effectiveness Reviews.* January. http://effectivehealthcare.ahrq.gov/ehc/products/60/318/CER-Methods-Guide-140109.pdf.

Anderson, L. M., Petticrew, M., Chandler, J., Grimshaw, J., Tugwell, P., O'Neill, J., Welch, V., Squires, J., Churchill, R. and Shemilt, I. 2013. Introducing a series of methodological articles on considering complexity in systematic reviews of interventions. *Journal of Clinical Epidemiology*, 66: 1205–8.

Bastian, H., Glasziou, P. and Chalmers, I. 2010. Seventy-five trials and eleven systematic reviews a day: how will we ever keep up? *PLoS Medicine*, 7: e1000326.

Chalmers, I. and Glasziou, P. 2009. Avoidable waste in the production and reporting of research evidence. *The Lancet*, 374: 86–9.

The Campbell Collaboration Resource Centre. http://www.campbellcollaboration.org/resources/training/The_Introductory_Methods.php.

6

ADVANCED APPROACHES TO EVIDENCE SYNTHESIS AND ITS APPLICATION TO INTERVENTION DESIGN

Nicky Cullum and Jo Dumville

Introduction

We saw in the previous chapter how a pre-planned, methodical and scientific approach to reviewing primary research evidence is essential in order to avoid bias and mistakes. We will now build on that chapter to explore new innovations in evidence synthesis.

Typically, systematic reviews that investigate whether interventions are effective analyze pair-wise, head-to-head comparisons of treatment alternatives and do so using the aggregate (i.e. study-level) data. These kinds of analyses work well if there are several studies with low between-study heterogeneity and (collectively) sufficient statistical power to minimize risk of a Type II error. This set of circumstances is probably relatively rare with complex interventions, nonetheless there are good examples where we are able to see a signal above the noise. One example is a Cochrane review of interventions to reduce falls in older people living in community settings (Gillespie *et al.*, 2012). This review is large and complex and includes 159 studies, most of which are evaluations of complex interventions. The analysis found evidence that several complex interventions reduce falls and fall-related injuries (Gillespie *et al.*, 2012). Home safety assessment and modification reduced risk of falling (pooled relative risk of falling 0.88, 95 percent confidence interval 0.80 to 0.96) and exercise interventions significantly reduced fall-related fractures (pooled relative risk 0.34, 95 percent confidence interval 0.18 to 0.63) (Gillespie *et al.*, 2012). However, there are frequently circumstances in evidence synthesis where standard approaches to meta-analysis (as outlined in the previous chapter) are inadequate. These circumstances include where analyzing aggregate, study-level data is too restrictive and meta-analysis of participant level data from multiple studies (individual patient data, or IPD meta-analysis) can offer important advantages. Alternatively a traditional meta-analysis of complex intervention studies may yield promising findings but leave us feeling that if we were to harness the most powerful elements of a range of complex interventions in a new intervention (which could be evaluated) we might be able to yield greater patient benefit. Methods such as subgroup analysis and meta-regression may help us in these situations. Alternatively the research landscape in your area of interest may be exceedingly messy with few replications of head-to-head comparisons and it may be impossible to identify the likely *most effective* intervention from existing evidence – in this case network meta-analysis may help. Finally there may already be several systematic reviews of interventions for a particular condition and an overview of reviews or umbrella review may be needed. This chapter will introduce each of these more advanced methods.

Learning objectives

By the end of this chapter and associated reading you should be able to:

- Understand how subgroup analysis and meta-regression of primary studies (randomized controlled trials, or RCTs) may be used to understand heterogeneity and design new complex interventions.
- Understand the differences between study-level meta-analysis and IPD meta-analysis and identify where IPD meta-analysis may be beneficial.
- Understand how network meta-analysis can be used to determine the relative effectiveness of interventions that have not been compared in head-to-head comparisons.
- Describe the difference between a traditional systematic review and an umbrella review or overview.

Subgroup analysis and meta-regression

Subgroup analysis and meta-regression are techniques that can be deployed to investigate the reasons for between-study differences in the estimates of treatment effects, otherwise known as heterogeneity. Given that the precise nature of complex interventions for a given purpose is likely to vary across studies, as are other characteristics such as the patient population and context, it is probably most surprising when heterogeneity is *not* detected. When synthesizing the evidence we often want to know whether the intervention is more or less effective in certain kinds of participants and/or whether complex interventions with particular components or characteristics are more or less effective. Those variables which influence the intervention effect are typically known as 'effect modifiers'.

Subgroup analysis

Subgroup analysis in the context of systematic reviews (as opposed to within trials) usually involves stratifying the included studies and classifying them by the characteristic of interest. Such analyses should be pre-specified in a review protocol and be based on a rational prior hypothesis. For example one might want to examine whether a complex educational intervention for promoting a healthy diet in people with diabetes has a differential effect in people who are newly diagnosed compared with those with long-standing diabetes. However, the extent to which you can undertake subgroup analysis with study-level data is usually limited, depending as it does on there being clear differences between studies for the variable of interest (in this case, time since diagnosis). Importantly, great care must be taken in interpreting the results of subgroup analyses; one cannot just compare the effect estimate between the subgroups and conclude that any difference between them is due to a differential effect of the intervention (see Deeks *et al.*, 2011). There is much more scope for subgroup analysis within IPD (as opposed to study-level) meta-analysis. There are excellent texts on subgroup analysis available and it is important to remember the increased risk of Type I errors if several are undertaken (see Deeks *et al.*, 2011; Fu *et al.*, 2008).

Meta-regression

Meta-regression can be of particular value in the context of complex intervention reviews since it facilitates the identification of particular study characteristics (e.g. intervention components) that are influencing the outcome (Thompson and Higgins, 2002). The value of this technique can be illustrated in the context of complex interventions by examining a review undertaken of collaborative care in depression which set out to identify the effective components of the intervention (Bower *et al.*, 2006). The review was driven by recognition that the management of depression could be improved and that a collaborative approach to care seemed to be effective. There were many manifestations of collaborative care for depression and it was unclear which aspects and approaches were important. The team developed and tested a taxonomy of intervention content and used it to classify the collaborative care intervention in each study included in their meta-analysis (Bower *et al.*, 2006). They then applied random effects meta-regression to the study data using the eight intervention variables (the explanatory variables in the regression) for the outcome variables of anti-depressant use (28 studies) and reduction in depressive symptoms (34 studies). Although it was not possible to identify an intervention component that predicted anti-depressant use, the team was able to identify intervention variables that predicted reduction of depressive symptoms and these included the professional background of the staff involved in care (Bower *et al.*, 2006). There are important caveats that must be borne in mind when employing meta-regression. In this context, random effects, rather than fixed-effect, meta-regression should be employed because there is an implicit acknowledgement of between-trial heterogeneity in the approach (Thompson and Higgins, 2002). Furthermore, the exploration of effect modifiers using meta-regression is observational and there is always the possibility of confounding (Deeks *et al.*, 2011). Notwithstanding these points, meta-regression (which requires a minimum of ten studies) clearly offers a rational approach to the selection of potentially more effective intervention components which can then be incorporated into a new complex intervention that can be evaluated. Indeed, the meta-regression conducted by Bower and colleagues (2006) and summarized above informed the development of a new collaborative care treatment for depression. This complex intervention was evaluated in initial pilot (Richards et al., 2008) and fully powered (Richards et al., 2013) RCTs and shown to result in significantly lower depression scores at 12 months follow-up compared with usual care.

Individual patient data meta-analysis

When trying to summarize everything that is known about the effectiveness of an intervention at a particular point in time, there are sometimes situations in which the available, published data from RCTs feel somewhat inadequate. You may find similar trials that have not reported the same outcome or not at the same time point, you may not like the published statistical analysis for a given trial, or participants may have been excluded from analysis that you feel should have been included (e.g. if the original trialists did not undertake an intention-to-treat analysis). IPD meta-analysis involves (usually) entering into a new collaboration with the original trialists and developing a new protocol together with a view to presenting a re-analysis of all the participant data from the original trials in one meta-analysis (Riley et al., 2010). For example, an IPD meta-analysis project involving one of us explored the relative effects of four-layer compression bandaging and short-stretch bandaging for people with venous leg ulcers. This approach enabled us to reinstate previously excluded participants, harmonize the outcome measures analyzed, deploy a more appropriate statistical technique than several of the studies had previously used, and identify a treatment effect that was previously masked by the lack of all the above (O'Meara et al., 2009). IPD meta-analysis is likely to be particularly beneficial in complex intervention reviews as it will enable more sophisticated analysis such as meta-regression to identify effect modifiers (factors that influence how an intervention works) and the intervention components that seem influential. An example of this approach in complex interventions is a review of very early mobilization (VEM) after stroke (Craig et al., 2010). At the time of the review only two trials of VEM had been undertaken, with a combined sample size of only 103 participants. These two trials had different primary outcomes: death at three months (Bernhardt et al., 2008) and Rankin score at three months (Langhorne et al., 2010). The IPD meta-analysis of the two trials adopted the primary outcome of independence at three months as measured by a modified Rankin score ≤ 2 and Barthel Index ≥ 18 (Craig et al., 2010). Because the research group had access to the patient-level data they were able to undertake multivariate analysis and adjust for any imbalance in prognostic factors at baseline (this would be impossible with study-level data). They were also able to identify a beneficial effect of VEM on independence at three months (using the modified Rankin scale) compared with standard care (adjusted odds ratio 3.11, 95 percent confidence interval 1.03 to 9.33). Other examples of

IPD meta-analysis in the context of complex interventions include a review of community occupational therapy after stroke (Walker *et al.*, 2004), acupuncture for chronic pain (which involved data from 17,922 participants) (Vickers *et al.*, 2012) and outcomes for depression treated by brief psychological therapies (Bower *et al.*, 2013). Detailed guidance for the conduct of IPD meta-analysis is beyond the scope of this text and can be found elsewhere (Stewart *et al.*, 2011; see also http://ipdmamg.cochrane.org/resources, accessed 9 May 2014).

Umbrella reviews (overviews of reviews)

Systematic reviews address questions that are focused in terms of population, interventions and outcomes. This means that for any specific condition there are a number of potential systematic reviews, each focusing on different interventions. For example if a decision-maker turns to the research evidence to answer the broad, but valid, question: *Which wound dressing is the most effective for healing foot ulcers in people with diabetes?* they will find several reviews, each focusing on the effects of different dressing types, e.g. hydrocolloids, alginates and foams (Dumville *et al.*, 2013a, 2013b, 2013c, 2013d). Where there are 'collections' of systematic reviews centred on a common, core theme, one way of helping decision-makers draw 'overall' conclusions about the best intervention (in this case, the best dressing) is to conduct an overview of reviews. These 'umbrella' reviews or overviews have a different methodology to a standard systematic review in that it is not individual studies that are identified for inclusion but all relevant systematic reviews. These overviews are relatively new and there are variations in how they have been conducted; good examples of protocols and completed reviews can be found in the Cochrane Library, e.g. Flodgren *et al.* (2011) and Ryan *et al.* (2011). Ryan and colleagues (2011) undertook an umbrella review investigating interventions to improve safe and effective medicines use by consumers. The authors note that some interventions were at the simpler end of the continuum (such as changing medicine formulation) and some interventions were complex (being variously composed of education, self-monitoring, counselling and self-management programs, etc). In order to identify relevant reviews for the overview the authors developed a taxonomy of different interventions components. This taxonomy was used to make both inclusion and exclusion decisions as well as to map further synthesis. Using this taxonomy the overview authors were able to identify common components across a range of intervention types and comment on the effectiveness of specific strategies across the 75 included systematic reviews (Ryan *et al.*, 2011).

Network meta-analysis and networks of evidence

Umbrella reviews seldom conduct any further detailed data analysis. Rather, like the systematic reviews they include, they present pair-wise meta-analysis in which data are synthesized from multiple trials evaluating the same two interventions.

Whilst this process provides important pooled-effect estimates for these head-to-head comparisons, it does not necessarily answer the decision-maker's broader question which is ultimately: of all the available interventions for this condition, *which is the best*?

An analytical approach that synthesizes all the available evidence from RCTs is called network meta-analysis (sometimes also known as a mixed-treatment comparison or mixed-treatment meta-analysis). This is an extension of standard meta-analysis and allows estimation of relative treatment effects for both direct (pair-wise) and indirect comparisons whilst at the same time preserving the randomization. Such network meta-analyses can be complex to structure and run (Barth *et al.*, 2013; Elliott and Meyer, 2007; Salanti, 2012); however, they are increasingly common – not least because when run in a Bayesian framework the final output can be a summary of treatments ranked by the probability of each being the 'best' treatment in terms of the outcome being evaluated (Salanti *et al.*, 2011). Examples of this approach include a network meta-analysis of treatments for sciatica (Lewis *et al.*, 2013) and one of alternative wound dressings for diabetic foot ulceration (Dumville *et al.*, 2012). The potential for network meta-analysis to evaluate complex interventions is a growing area of interest, especially as it extends the scope for meta-regression. Welton and colleagues (2009) used network meta-analysis (which as they note is a form of meta-regression) to quantitatively explore the relative effects of various intervention components that formed psychological interventions (for coronary heart disease) (Welton *et al.*, 2009). Again the particular value of a network approach over a standard meta-regression was that it allowed relative estimates to be calculated where components were linked indirectly as well as directly. The work started with a systematic review to identify relevant studies which were then grouped based on a taxonomy of six different interventional components. The studies were then linked and compared in a network. From the analysis the authors found that interventions with a behavioural component had the strongest effect on all-cause mortality (mean log odds ratio −0.58; 95 percent credible interval −1.13 to −0.05) (Welton *et al.*, 2009).

Summary

Use of subgroup analyses and/or meta-regression, where valid, can help explain outcome heterogeneity based on study characteristics, including intervention components, and/or population characteristics. Identification of such effect modification is important when considering the design and delivery of treatments. Within a review, subgroup analysis involves stratifying and classifying the studies by the characteristics of interest and then comparing outcomes for each group. In this way the approach is observational so caution is required when considering observed associations as evidence of causality. Subgroup analyses should be kept to a minimum to reduce the chance of Type I errors and they should be specified a priori and based on current wisdom and existing evidence.

An extension of subgroup analyses at the study level is meta-regression, which again uses study-level covariates and outcomes. Here, as in a standard regression, the outcome of interest can be regressed simultaneously onto multiple covariates of interest and the number and magnitude of associations observed. Whilst a useful technique, meta-regression does not maintain randomization, i.e. the data are observational and findings are at risk of confounding.

Meta-analysis and subsequent meta-regression can be enhanced by the use of IPD data which enhance the usability of data for any meta-analysis, e.g. by standardizing outcomes and minimizing missing data. Undertaking IPD analysis is not necessarily straightforward as data custodians for all included studies need to agree to collaborate and share their data.

'Umbrella' reviews or overviews have a different methodology to a standard systematic review in that it is not individual studies that are identified for inclusion but all relevant systematic reviews. By identifying and summarizing all relevant reviews around a specific research question overviews are able to provide the reader with a more complete overview of the current evidence.

Most meta-analyses are limited to pair-wise comparisons. However, from a decision-making perspective the more relevant question is often 'of all the available interventions for this condition, *which is the best*?' Network meta-analysis is a powerful analytic tool that allows estimation of relative treatment effects for both direct (pair-wise) and indirect comparisons whilst at the same time preserving the randomization.

These advanced analytical approaches allow more detailed exploration of the data collected in systematic reviews in terms of summarizing data, exploring heterogeneity and incorporating indirect data into relative effect estimates. All the approaches detailed in this chapter may also be of particular value in helping to identify the 'active ingredients' of complex interventions.

Further reading

Dickens, C., Katon, W., Blakemore, A., Khara, A., Tomenson, B., Woodcock, A., Fryer, A. and Guthrie, E. 2014. Complex interventions that reduce urgent care use in COPD: a systematic review with meta-regression. *Respiratory Medicine*, 108: 426–37.

Grant, E. S. and Calderbank-Batista, T. 2013. Network meta-analysis for complex social interventions: problems and potential. *Journal for the Society for Social Work and Research*, 4: 406–20.

Riley, R. D., Lambert, P. C. and Abo-Zaid, G. 2010. Meta-analysis of individual participant data: rationale, conduct, and reporting. *British Medical Journal*, 340: c221.

Shepperd, S., Lewin, S., Straus, S., Clarke, M., Eccles, M. P., Fitzpatrick, R., Wong, G. and Sheikh, A. 2009. Can we systematically review studies that evaluate complex interventions? *PLoS Medicine,* 6: e1000086.

7

EXPLORING COMPLEXITY IN SYSTEMATIC REVIEWS OF COMPLEX INTERVENTIONS

Sascha Köpke, Jane Noyes, Jackie Chandler and Gabriele Meyer

Introduction

The development of a complex intervention inevitably requires the preparation of a systematic review of the existing evidence in order to inform all steps of the development and evaluation processes. Beyond the general methodological challenges of systematic reviews and meta-analyses, systematic reviews of complex interventions pose specific challenges. In particular, the reporting of primary studies of complex interventions is often not sufficient to produce meaningful summaries of the research evidence (Guise *et al.*, 2014). As a consequence, systematic reviews of complex interventions regularly provide insufficient information. Frequently, randomized controlled trials of complex interventions that have been developed and evaluated carefully through different development phases are combined with trials of insufficiently developed interventions. Studies evaluating the efficacy of an intervention for the first time are often combined with studies that transfer a programme to another context. In view of these difficulties, this chapter addresses a number of challenges encountered when preparing systematic reviews of complex interventions.

We also introduce the methodological work undertaken by members of Cochrane as part of the Methodological Investigation of Cochrane reviews of Complex Interventions (MICCI) project, including development of the 'iCAT-SR' tool for assessing and describing intervention complexity in included trials, the 'CERQual' tool for assessing the confidence of synthesized findings to explain intervention complexity and heterogeneity, and methodological work to determine the relative benefits of using qualitative evidence that is either related or unrelated to trials included in systematic reviews.

Learning objectives

- To understand important challenges encountered when preparing systematic reviews of complex interventions.
- To recognize the importance of carefully defining study inclusion criteria and review questions in systematic reviews of complex interventions.
- To be aware of some of the challenges posed by combining different study types and data in syntheses of complex interventions.

Background

Recently, a number of methodological publications have dealt with the challenges of systematic reviews of complex interventions, although this discussion is not new. In 2007, Lenz *et al.* used examples of their own complex educational programmes to show that 'Meta-analysis does not allow appraisal of complex interventions in diabetes and hypertension self-management' (Lenz *et al.*, 2007: 1375). The authors assessed 14 systematic reviews and meta-analyses and showed that although reviewed interventions were classified as complex or multidimensional, systematic reviews did not adequately consider complexity, leading to different conclusions from the same evidence base. For example, different approaches to literature searching led to different publications being included when ostensibly reviewing the same intervention. Classification of interventions differed between and within reviews. Furthermore, in meta-analyses the influence of single intervention components was derived without considering differences in underlying theoretical concepts. Finally, outcome measures were not reviewed in terms of the aims of the interventions.

In another example, we have shown that by not considering challenges related to complex interventions, the Cochrane review on hip protectors for preventing fractures in older people (Parker *et al.*, 2006; Santesso *et al.*, 2014) provides inadequate results that are not suitable to inform clinical practice (Meyer and Mühlhauser, 2006). The same has been shown for the two Cochrane reviews on accidental fall prevention (Mühlhauser *et al.*, 2011). Although there are now more than 150 randomized controlled trials included in these reviews (Cameron *et al.*, 2012; Gillespie *et al.*, 2012), results remain vague and the authors suggest that more research is needed. It is clear that standard review and meta-analytic methods are insufficient to arrive at a clear-cut synthesis of evidence and subsequent clinical guidance.

Further to the realization that standard systematic review methods struggle to synthesize evidence from trials of complex interventions, in 2009 Shepperd *et al.* called for the development and evaluation of 'methods to improve the descriptions of complex interventions [...] with the expectation that they will complement existing systematic review methodology' (Shepperd *et al.*, 2009: 4). In the US, the Agency for Healthcare Research and Quality (Guise *et al.*, 2014) has recently published a research White Paper aiming to identify the challenges of conducting systematic reviews of complex multicomponent health care interventions.

As a consequence of these issues being raised, Cochrane funded the MICCI project to explore some of the challenges of and develop the methods for mixed-method evidence synthesis. The methodological work will inform a chapter on complex interventions for the *Cochrane Handbook* (http://methods.cochrane. org/projects-developments/methodological-investigation-cochrane-reviews-complex-interventions-micci). Aspects to be considered in this context will include a better understanding of heterogeneity and the use of qualitative data to understand intervention complexity. As a basis for the chapter, a series of articles have recently been published in the *Journal of Clinical Epidemiology* (66(11), 2013) (see Anderson *et al.*, 2013 for an overview).

Key challenges to systematic reviews of complex interventions

Developing key questions

The essential first step of a review of complex interventions is to clarify the key review question(s) and the complexity of the review, mapping these to various aspects of intervention complexity and sources of evidence. Reviews of complex interventions may be more or less complex, depending on the question to be answered (Petticrew *et al.*, 2013a). Key questions should clarify 'the clinical logic, potential linkages, and what information is being sought' (Guise *et al.*, 2014: 6). Although interventions such as fall prevention may have the same intention, differences could be present in the class of intervention (e.g. group vs. individual training), the components included (e.g. endurance vs. resistance training) and aspects of components (e.g. intensity and duration of components). The *Cochrane Handbook* (Chapter 5.3) asks authors to consider these factors as key components of a well-formulated question in complex interventions and to decide whether it may be feasible to restrict questions to specific aspects (Higgins and Green, 2009).

The standard PICO question framework (population, intervention, comparator, outcome) described in Cullum and Dumville's first chapter in this section can be extended to include time and setting and other phenomena of interest to explore complexity and heterogeneity and help to decide on the level of complexity of the question being asked. PICO has also been adapted by Booth (2011) for developing questions on phenomena of interest to explore complexity and heterogeneity using qualitative evidence. This reflects the fact that questions about the overall effectiveness of interventions have to be broadened when asking more complex questions about reasons for interventions' success or failure, which may need a theory-driven approach. More elaborate description of these aspects can be found in Guise *et al.* (2014: table 2), Petticrew *et al.* (2013a: table 2) and Squires *et al.* (2013b: table 1).

Building appropriate search strategies

Depending on the key questions to be answered, there may be different challenges concerning appropriate strategies to identify adequate sources of evidence. The review by Lenz *et al.* (2007) has shown that systematic reviews frequently do not apply adequate search strategies to retrieve all available evidence for an intervention and that relevant publications may not be found using standard search methods. Information on the implementation of complex interventions is difficult to assess, as many may be implemented as part of quality improvement measures across different health care organizations (Guise *et al.*, 2014).

Booth (2011) has developed guidance on searching for qualitative evidence to help explain implementation factors and explore heterogeneity. One aspect of the MICCI project was to explore the relative benefits of identifying trial sibling studies (i.e. studies within or alongside the trial) versus unrelated qualitative studies, as searches that include qualitative studies unrelated to the original trial may have the potential to identify research that could help explain the impacts of complexity on implementation and outcomes.

Clearly, there is not one appropriate method to derive as much relevant information as possible, but snowballing techniques including contacting experts in the fields should be used as described by Greenhalgh and Peacock (2005). In addition, structured approaches like the empirically derived search strategies described by Hauser *et al.* (2012) can be used.

Describing the complex intervention

A systematic review of complex interventions should focus on the sources of complexity, and review authors must be aware of interventions' various relationships and interdependences. They should aim to identify these sources in order to understand how an intervention works within its context (for example, geographical, cultural, social environment, organizational and political systems). Chapter 1 in this book by Richards outlines different approaches to describing complexity, including complexity of the intervention itself, implementation, context and participant response (Anderson *et al.*, 2013).

These areas of complexity have to be acknowledged by systematic reviewers who must aim to prospectively identify potential sources of heterogeneity and detect these in included studies in order to systematically analyse the influences of heterogeneity. Pigott and Shepperd (2013) have visualized important features of complex interventions that potentially lead to heterogeneity (Figure 7.1).

As a result, reviewers should aim to describe the key components of the intervention as clearly as possible. This may include conducting primary research to derive this information, such as interviews and surveys among trialists, practitioners and patients. For example, Langhorne and Pollock (2002) used questionnaires and case studies among trialists to describe common elements of the complex intervention 'stroke unit care'. The use of 'logic models' may also be useful, in order to describe in detail how the intervention may work (Pigott and Sheppard, 2013). Anderson *et al.* (2011) have provided a concise summary of logic models to capture complexity in systematic reviews.

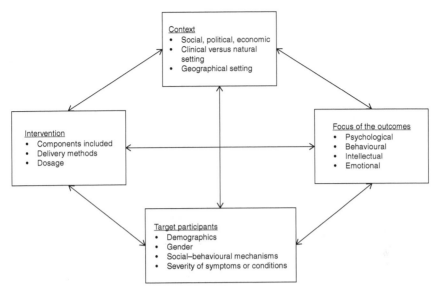

FIGURE 7.1 Features of a complex intervention that can lead to heterogeneity (Pigott and Shepperd, 2013). Reprinted from *Journal of Clinical Epidemiology*, 66(11). Copyright (2013), with permission from Elsevier

Systematic reviews of complex interventions must consider studies from all phases of the development and evaluation of the complex intervention, which requires inclusion of different study types including qualitative studies and process evaluations that describe and untangle distinctive features of the complex intervention (Craig *et al.*, 2008). Moore and colleagues (this volume, chapter 23) summarize new guidance on process evaluations that will hopefully lead to improvements in both conduct and reporting in this area.

Recently, reporting guidelines have been published aiming to advise authors about the reporting of important information on complex interventions and to help readers (including systematic reviewers) to identify gaps in reporting. These include the template for intervention description and replication (TIDieR) guideline (Hoffmann *et al.*, 2014) that aims for a clear description of interventions to allow their replication, and the CReDECI guideline (Möhler *et al.*, 2012) covering the whole process of complex intervention development and evaluation.

When incorporating qualitative evidence to explore patient experiences, implementation factors and explain heterogeneity, it is important to specify phenomena of interest that can be addressed with qualitative evidence. The Cochrane 'CERQual' tool has recently been developed for assessing the confidence in synthesized qualitative findings exploring phenomena of interest and was used for the first time in a mixed-methods integrated Cochrane review using a logic model (Glenton *et al.*, 2013).

Finally, the combination of quantitative and qualitative data in systematic reviews certainly requires an expanded set of skills (Guise *et al.*, 2014). The overall description of data synthesis methods is beyond the scope of this chapter; however, these issues are tackled by others in this section of the book. Although there is little consensus on the type or scope of qualitative evidence to include in a synthesis, the chapters in this volume by Rycroft-Malone and Burton (Chapter 8) and Hannes (Chapter 9) articulate how to undertake reviews of qualitative and mixed-methods studies, respectively. These methods are also discussed by Noyes *et al.* in chapter 20 of the *Cochrane Handbook* (Higgins and Green, 2009) and by the Centre for Reviews and Dissemination (2009). Finally, the Cochrane Qualitative and Implementation group provide detailed supplemental guidance on the integration of qualitative and quantitative evidence (Noyes and Lewin, 2011).

Importantly, reviewers will often come to the decision that meta-analytic methods are not suitable and descriptive methods may be more appropriate. Petticrew *et al.* (2013b) summarize various approaches to synthesize complex interventions including commonly used methods like meta-regression, multivariate meta-analysis and network meta-analysis, as well as broader approaches like hierarchical models and causal diagram-based analyses. Importantly, all these approaches initially require the reviewer to identify key components of the intervention and understand possible interactions, for example by using 'logic models' (see e.g. Turley *et al.*, 2013a).

Describing the control intervention

When assessing the effects of a complex intervention, the effects of the control intervention, which might be a placebo intervention or (optimized) standard care, need to be considered. It is certainly important to acknowledge the quality of care provided regularly. This might result in different effects for the same programme in different health care settings. For example, a fall prevention intervention that had shown strong effects in England failed to be effective in the Netherlands, a result that might be explained by the different levels of standard care in both systems (Bleijlevens *et al.*, 2008).

Identifying appropriate outcome measures

The importance of addressing adequate and patient-relevant outcome measures has been the subject of many discussions, leading for example to the GRADE framework (http://www.gradeworkinggroup.org), where outcome measures are classified according to their importance. Confidence in the effects of the interventions is assessed for each outcome across studies. This way of reporting is now mandatory in Cochrane reviews, presented in summary of findings tables (http://www.editorial-unit.cochrane.org/mecir). Unfortunately, this approach does not usually account for the specific challenges of complex interventions. For example, Lenz *et al.* (2007) have shown that the interpretation of regularly used primary outcome measures such as the HbA1c measured in diabetes education studies, needs to be considered in terms of other outcomes (for example, the incidence of hypoglycaemia and use of co-medication). Therefore, pooling of results for the same outcome measures across different complex interventions is often inadequate. Alternatively, interdependencies between different outcome measures, processes and study aims should be analysed and reported transparently.

Summary

There has been a lot of discussion about the most adequate approaches to performing systematic reviews and meta-analyses of complex interventions. Some authors generally question the feasibility of squeezing complex interventions into a tight analytical framework that might not be suitable and ultimately lead to uninformative results or even detrimental recommendations. We have outlined here that there are distinctive challenges that require reviewers to broaden their view and to have a detailed look at all available evidence for the whole process of developing and evaluating complex interventions. Decisions about approaches should acknowledge intervention aims. Importantly, decisions about the scope and methods of the systematic review depend on the available information, which should be assessed in view of clinicians' and patients' needs. Important decisions to be made include the type of evidence to be searched and the choice of methods to describe or synthesize it. This will usually require a combination of different study types including quantitative and qualitative data. Transparent reporting is certainly a key issue to allow readers to apply the findings to specific contexts.

Further reading

Centre for Reviews and Dissemination. 2009. Systematic reviews: CRD's guidance for undertaking reviews in health care. University of York, Centre for Reviews and Dissemination. http://www.york.ac.uk/inst/crd/pdf/Systematic_Reviews.pdf.

Grant, A., Treweek, S., Dreischulte, T., Foy, R. and Guthrie, B. 2013. Process evaluations for cluster-randomised trials of complex interventions: a proposed framework for design and reporting. *Trials*, 14: 15.

Noyes, J., Popay, J., Pearson, A., Hannes, K. and Booth, A. 2008. 20: Qualitative research and Cochrane reviews. In: J. P. T. Higgins and S. Green (eds), *Cochrane Handbook for Systematic Reviews of Interventions Version 5.0.1* (updated September 2008), chapter 20. http://www.cochrane-handbook.org.

Wells, M., Williams, B., Treweek, S., Coyle, J. and Taylor, J. 2012. Intervention description is not enough: evidence from an in-depth multiple case study on the untold role and impact of context in randomised controlled trials of seven complex interventions. Trials, 13: 95.

8

THE SYNTHESIS OF QUALITATIVE DATA

Jo Rycroft-Malone and Christopher R. Burton

Introduction

This chapter introduces readers to the synthesis of qualitative research within the context of research and development of complex interventions. By drawing on examples from the literature, this chapter will outline how qualitative evidence synthesis should and could be part of the process of complex intervention design.

Learning objectives

- Understand the contribution of qualitative evidence syntheses to complex intervention development.
- Discuss some common approaches to conducting qualitative evidence syntheses, and their strengths and limitations.

Background

Complex interventions are prone to adaptation through dynamic implementation processes, and effectiveness may be contingent on contextual conditions and the responses of practitioners and patients. Qualitative evidence syntheses have a potentially important function in developing insights into 'which' aspects of complex interventions work, and 'how' these interventions work in the real world, and therefore how they might best be developed. Evidence synthesis may occur in the early stages of complex intervention research programmes, informing intervention design and implementation, where, for example, barriers and enablers to implementation may be hypothesized and accounted for. In this way, they have the potential to construct a complex intervention's 'theory of change' which can explain the impacts observed through, for example, experimental evaluation.

Specifically, qualitative evidence synthesis can inform the development of complex interventions by:

- Identifying potential intervention components.
- Developing additional insights into the underpinning evidence base, for example in establishing the differences and similarities in reported interventions and in their theoretical perspectives.
- Identifying barriers and enablers to the implementation of interventions.
- Identifying the theory/ies underpinning interventions in order to make more informed decisions about selection and evaluation of outcomes.
- Understanding the organizational, clinical and policy contexts in which complex interventions are implemented.

Conducting qualitative evidence syntheses

Scope and scale

Qualitative evidence reviews, whilst sharing some common principles, vary in terms of their aims and scope, breadth and depth. Typically, however, reviews of complex interventions are likely to be more involved than reviews of interventions that are less complicated. For example, the need to explore the action and impact of different intervention components will probably necessitate the need to explore multiple sources and types of evidence, and from within these sources, build explanations about how interventions operate in different contexts.

Reviews should follow a predetermined and written protocol, which ideally should be made publicly accessible. Readers are signposted to the available standards for the reporting of different types of qualitative evidence reviews, which also provide useful checklists for conducting reviews.

- Enhancing transparency in reporting the synthesis of qualitative evidence: ENTREQ (Tong *et al.*, 2012) http://www.biomedcentral.com/1471–2288/12/181.
- RAMESES publication standards: meta-narrative reviews (Wong *et al.*, 2013a) http://www.biomedcentral.com/1741–7015/11/20.
- RAMESES publication standards: realist synthesis (Wong *et al.*, 2013b) http://www.biomedcentral.com/1741–7015/11/21.

Description, characteristics and contribution of different qualitative evidence review approaches

Table 8.1 summarizes the features of some common approaches to conducting qualitative evidence syntheses, and provides examples for further information. As shown, each approach has more or less potential to unpack issues of complexity,

TABLE 8.1 An overview of selected approaches to synthesizing qualitative evidence about complex interventions

	Thematic synthesis	Meta-narrative reviews	Realist review/synthesis	Meta-ethnography
Question/ aim/ scope	– Provides a description of what works and potentially how – Question often framed in terms of whether and how different interventions might work	– Provides an explanation (i.e. narrative) about the way in which different interventions have been studied and what effect this might have – Particularly suited to topics where there is a difference of opinion about the nature of what is being studied and what the best empirical approach to studying it might be – Asks questions such as: 'which research traditions have considered this topic area?', 'how has each tradition conceptualized the topic?', 'what theoretical approach did they use?', 'what insights can be drawn by combining and comparing findings from different traditions (Wong et al., 2013a, 2013b)	– Provides an explanation about why an intervention works or not, and how in what circumstances – Pays particular attention to the conditions in which interventions work – Theory-driven and interpretative – Often includes the question: 'what works, for whom, how and in what circumstances?' – Starts with the construction of a programme theory – including context (c), mechanism (m) and outcome (o)	– Provides insights and an interpretative explanation about how different contexts (including behaviours and actions of people) affect how interventions might work – Attempts to preserve the interpretative properties of the primary data/study – Question often framed around the need to better understand the topic of interest – e.g. to determine barriers and facilitators, to understand the meaning of …

Search strategy/ approach	– Systematic and comprehensive searching of all relevant databases – Snowballing for grey/ unpublished literature	– Exploratory scoping review undertaken – Purposive – to find evidence that will make a contribution to understanding the review question – Looking in different literatures – Iterative – backwards and forwards citation tracking, and snowballing	– Exploratory scoping review undertaken – Purposive and theoretical – i.e. the strategy is based on the programme theory being tested through the review process – Iterative and ongoing throughout the review	– Purposive, based on the review question – Can be broad or more focused depending on approach to sampling until saturation
Data extraction and relevance	– Data extraction based on pre-defined criteria/ concepts – Quality and relevance judged through the application of appraisal tools, and each study given a strength of evidence 'weighting' – Studies not reaching a threshold, excluded	– Unable to be prescriptive – decisions made about data extraction and inclusion based on the usefulness in producing an account – Might include, for example, how research questions framed, preferred methodologies, key actors in unfolding the tradition, significant findings that shaped subsequent work	– A bespoke data extraction [template] is developed based on the information needed to test and refine the programme theory/ies – Contribution of data based on two criteria: *Relevance* – whether it contributes to theory testing and/or building *Rigour* – whether the method used is credible and trustworthy	– Extraction based on answering the review question – Inclusion of evidence determined by tests of relevance and rigour and trustworthiness – Judgements often made on quality appraisal (e.g. CASP)

(cont.)

TABLE 8.1 (cont.)

	Thematic synthesis	Meta-narrative reviews	Realist review/synthesis	Meta-ethnography
Analysis and synthesis	– Coding of text in primary studies – Codes organized into descriptive themes – Further interpretation to develop analytical themes	– Development of a storyline that includes mapping specific meta-narratives and interpretative analysis – Comparing and contrasting the meta-narratives – Deliberative and iterative process	– Looking for common patterns of contexts and outcomes – and then seeking to explain these through the mechanisms by which they occurred – Deliberative and iterative process	– Layered synthesis conducted through the identification of key metaphors and a series of translations – Reciprocal translation – translation of concepts from individual studies – Refutational synthesis – exploring and explaining the differences/contradictions between studies – Lines of argument – based on cross-study patterns and threads
Output	– New interpretations that go beyond those from the original, individual studies	– Summary of key meta-narratives – Highlighting points of key contestation and commonality	– Refined theory – about why and how an intervention may or may not work in particular circumstances	– New insights about the topic under review – Can result in new frameworks/models or hypotheses
Examples	Lipworth *et al.*, 2010	Greenhalgh *et al.*, 2004	McCormack *et al.*, 2013; Wong *et al.*, 2011, 2013b	Pound *et al.*, 2005

TABLE 8.2 The contribution of qualitative evidence synthesis to complex intervention research

Approach	Contribution
Thematic synthesis	– Summaries across descriptions of interventions – Barriers and enablers of implementation – Testing of theory (e.g. through framework approach)
Narrative and meta-narrative	– Interpretative summaries across descriptions of interventions – Scoping and interpretation of intervention impacts, stakeholder perspectives and implementation – Intervention theory development
Meta-ethnography	– Explanation of how different interventions might have an impact – particularly in relation to the context of their implementation – Intervention theory development – Descriptions of implementation context – e.g. barriers and facilitators
Realist review	– Intervention theories of change and contingencies – Understanding complexity of implementation and impacts

how context might influence intervention implementation and for theory testing and development. Of course review teams might naturally align themselves with a particular approach because of their epistemological stance and associated understanding about the construction of knowledge.

Lipworth *et al.*'s synthesis provides a *thematic synthesis* of a pool of qualitative studies which explore lay people's understanding of cancer risk (Lipworth *et al.*, 2010). This can be contrasted with Greenhalgh *et al.*'s *meta-narrative review* of innovation of health care organizations that emphasizes the integration of theory and evidence in extending theoretical understanding, rather than a summary of emerging issues (Greenhalgh *et al.*, 2004). Wong *et al.*'s (2011) *realist synthesis* focuses on the complex problem of using legislation to ban smoking in cars carrying children (Wong *et al.*, 2011). In this case, the purpose of the synthesis was to 'road-test' legislation as a policy intervention prior to its implementation drawing on evidence in this, and related public health and safety issues. Together with McCormack *et al.*'s synthesis on change agency as an implementation strategy, this highlights the contingent nature of theory in realist synthesis (McCormack *et al.*, 2013). In both cases, the syntheses are structured around questions in the form of 'what works for whom'. These syntheses typically draw on broad literatures guided by the underpinning theory, rather than a tightly defined pool of studies defined by a clinical topic. Pound *et al.*'s *meta-ethnography* also demonstrates how synthesis across studies provides a framework to reflect on the nature of research within a given area, including the linkages across studies (Pound *et al.*, 2005).

The potential contributions of each approach to synthesizing evidence about complex interventions are summarized in Table 8.2. Broadly, approaches to evidence synthesis can be descriptive, aggregative or interpretative, where new insights can be gained through ongoing analysis throughout the review process (Gough et al., 2012).

The examples of syntheses indicated earlier provide rich information on the structure of complex interventions, and how they may work in different contexts, which will be valuable in both intervention development and implementation, as summarized in Table 8.2.

Realist review: illustrating the method

This section outlines the process undertaken to complete a realist review to determine how a complex implementation intervention (change agency) operates and impacts. The review methods and findings are fully described elsewhere (Rycroft-Malone et al., 2012; McCormack et al., 2013).

Aim/scope: the broad purpose of this review was to determine what interventions and strategies are effective in enabling evidence-informed health care. The specific aim of the review was refined through a process of stakeholder engagement with a knowledgeable community of practice, which resulted in review questions: what change agency characteristics work, for whom do they work, in what circumstances, and why?

Initial programme theory development: through a process of 'digging into' the literature, workshops and discussions, a number of theory areas were developed through a process of concept mining and mapping. A number of review questions were developed by the team through a deliberative process based on the content of these theory areas – these provided the focus for the review.

Searching: the search of the literature was purposive in order to scrutinize the initial programme theories. Search terms were compiled in conjunction with relevant indexing terms and multiple databases were searched. For pragmatic reasons, grey literature was not searched for in this review. Screening was intentionally inclusive to include all potential papers relevant to testing the programme theory/ies.

Inclusion/exclusion: the test for inclusion in this review was: is this evidence 'good and relevant enough' to facilitate testing/scrutinizing the theories about the characteristics, context and impact of change agency?

Data extraction: the programme theories were made visible through the data extraction forms in that they were populated with evidence in 'fields' directly relevant to the theory/ies being tested. For example, there was a field in the data extraction pro-forma that enabled the reviewers to capture information on the characteristics of change agents, including how these might impact on their ability and success in promoting evidence informed health care. Typically, each piece of evidence that is reviewed has information that is relevant to a number of different areas in the pro-forma; equally, there were areas that did not get populated.

Synthesis: in this review, the approach to synthesis was based on the principles of realist evaluation and was both inductive and deductive, including:

• organizing extracted data into relevant evidence tables;
• looking across the evidence tables to look for patterns;
• creating chains of inference within these patterns;
• formulating hypotheses based on these patterns of inferences.

Development of the narrative: the findings from this review were formulated to be consistent with the theory areas guiding data extraction and analysis. Findings, for example, included a change agent's potential in creating the conditions for evidence-informed health care, including in leadership and creating supportive cultures. Positive attitude, respect, positivity and credibility seem more likely to be able to build up a critical mass of leadership influence, solicit the required resources from leadership and facilitate the necessary supportive culture. There was evidence to suggest that 'fit' between a change agent's characteristics and context (setting) may lead to their greater potential impact.

The findings from this review begin to uncover some of the key features of change agency interventions, including the characteristics of change agents that may have more impact than others, how the role is enacted and how different contexts may impact on both role enactment and effect. Therefore findings from a realist review such as this have the potential to unpack the mechanisms of action of this complex intervention, and inform the development of change agency interventions.

Summary

The development of complex interventions poses some challenges to researchers, specifically in understanding how they work through their components parts in different contexts, and issues of implementation, fidelity and impact. There are a range of available approaches for the synthesis of rich qualitative evidence which reflect the different approaches to qualitative research, and the methodological starting points of reviewers. Each of these approaches may contribute different explanatory perspectives which may aid the design and evaluation of complex interventions in health care. Being clear about the purpose or intended contribution of a synthesis of qualitative evidence should indicate which approach will have maximum utility.

9

BUILDING A CASE FOR MIXED-METHODS REVIEWS

Karin Hannes

Introduction

In previous chapters, approaches to synthesizing quantitative and qualitative evidence have been discussed and presented. Attempts to combine these two strands of review evidence present unique challenges for authors of systematic reviews. Not only do they require a good theoretical and practical understanding of how an intervention might work or may cause change, they will also need an understanding of what potential facilitators or moderators need to be considered for a successful roll-out and what issues may impact on the overall outcomes defined. The dissemination of mixed-methods reviews via international non-profit organizations such as the Cochrane and Campbell Collaboration is fairly recent. The Cochrane Library, one of the largest databases of systematic reviews, currently contains over 5,000 effectiveness reviews. Examples of qualitative evidence syntheses in the library are still scarce. Recent examples include the review from Glenton and colleagues (2013) on barriers and facilitators to the implementation of lay health worker programmes to improve access to maternal and child health, presented as a supplement to an effectiveness review, and that from Turley and colleagues (2013b) on slum upgrading strategies, integrating textual and numerical data. These examples have sparked an interest in review authors to start submitting review protocols that position themselves within the mixed-methods review discourse (Hurley *et al.*, 2013). A recent example of a Campbell review combining insights from numerical outcome measures and contextual data is that from Berg and Denison (2013) addressing female genital mutilation and cutting in African countries. We expect that the number of mixed-methods type of reviews will increase significantly in the coming years.

The need for a more comprehensive type of review, taking into account different layers of research evidence, has grown stronger in the context of trying to evaluate the effects of complex interventions and the recognition that there is no such thing as a simple intervention or a simple review question, particularly in health care. Most interventions are indeed complicated. They challenge review authors to address multiple components, multiple agencies and multiple simultaneous or alternative strands of evidence. Over time, review authors have developed strategies to respond to this challenge: the use of programme theory to build up a logic model underpinning reviews of effectiveness or the development of scoping reviews to identify qualitative research evidence that may inform question formulation, inclusion criteria or the development of logic models (Harris *et al.*, 2011).

It becomes even more interesting when review authors are challenged to choose a path to the success of an intervention that is cyclical in nature, where outcome measures or moderators that impact on the effect of an intervention cannot fully be anticipated in advance and specific targets of the review, as well as the means to achieve them, tend to emerge during the review process (Rogers, 2008). In this case, relevant strands of evidence may interact with and mutually affect each other, thereby potentially reshaping the review question, the expected outcome measures and the findings of the synthesis as a whole. In other words, review teams may no longer fully control the direction of their review and may need to consider a more iterative approach to synthesis, in which they allow different strands of evidence to directly influence each other. It follows that decisions on the direction of the review process should be guided by the questions that emerge during the process.

Learning objectives

- Briefly outline what a mixed-methods synthesis is.
- Explain why we need to consider this.
- Evaluate when we need to consider it.
- Choose an appropriate methodological approach to synthesis.
- Define appropriate questions for different phases in a mixed-methods review.

The what, why, when and how of a mixed-methods review approach

What is a mixed-methods synthesis?

Harden and Thomas (2005) were among the first to launch the term 'mixed-methods review' in an article exploring methodological issues in combining diverse study types in systematic reviews. The term refers to a meta-methodology that advances the idea of systematically integrating, or mixing, quantitative and qualitative findings from original research reports or articles. Mixed-methods types of review generally promote the inclusiveness of contextual and experiential aspects of health care interventions and the delivery of health care. The basic premise of a mixed-methods review approach is that an integration of insights generated via studies addressing different types of questions contributes to a more synergistic, holistic utilization of research evidence.

Why do we conduct them?

For some review authors, the reason for conducting mixed-methods reviews originates from the desire to compare, validate and triangulate review results. It allows them to build on the strengths of one particular method to compensate for the weaknesses of another. For example, qualitative evidence may be used to provide illustrations of context for effect measures reported in the review. Research accounts on lived experiences can be presented in conjunction with outcome measures or to follow up on some of the unexpected results that require a more in-depth exploration. Heterogeneity in an effectiveness review may prompt the search for explanations in qualitative studies, or vice versa; potential relations between concepts outlined in theoretical frameworks developed in a qualitative evidence synthesis could further be explored in a quantitative type of review. A strong argument for the mixed-methods type of reviews is that the combination of quantitative and qualitative evidence enables review authors to view problems from multiple perspectives, in other words to address fundamentally different questions while looking at the same phenomenon. In this case, merging insights from quantitative and qualitative research evidence enhances and enriches the meaning of a singular perspective and allows review authors to develop a more complete understanding of a problem.

When do we need to consider them?

Not all types of systematic review project are in need of a mixed-methods review approach. For example, questions related to understanding the meaning of a particular phenomenon, such as how people make sense of a particular chronic disease or why they behave or feel the way they do, may be explored in a stand-alone qualitative evidence synthesis. In line with the arguments presented above, mixed-methods review approaches are most suitable for phenomena and problems in which (a) one particular synthesis approach, by itself, is inadequate to develop a complete understanding, (b) qualitative insights can help to explain or elaborate on quantitative findings and (c) quantitative review evidence can further generalize, test or confirm qualitative findings. Mixed-methods approaches dealing with the latter two issues most likely present themselves as a *sequential* type of review, either exploratory (b-qualitative evidence is synthesized first) or explanatory (c-quantitative evidence is synthesized first). Review authors who aim to achieve a complete understanding of their research phenomenon might opt for a *concurrent* type of review, looking at the different strands of evidence simultaneously and, where appropriate, working with textual and numerical data insights in different phases of the review process. This is often referred to as a multi-phase type of review.

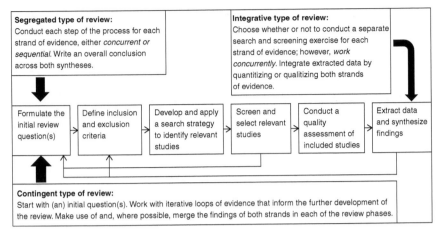

FIGURE 9.1   A stepwise approach to conducting mixed-methods reviews

How do we conduct them?

Attempts to mix quantitative and qualitative meta-methodology have raised the methodological stakes. Several authors have pleaded for the careful planning of mixed-methods reviews, particularly in relation to choosing an appropriate mixed-methods synthesis design (Sandelowski *et al.*, 2006; Heyvaert, Maes and Onghena, 2013). Procedural guidance on how to efficiently combine insights from quantitative and qualitative research studies in a review is scarce. However, most mixed-methods review approaches follow the linear approach outlined in Figure 9.1.

Depending on the type of design, the review process will differ slightly. In their most basic form, mixed-methods reviews present themselves to the reader as two separate reviews, quantitative and a qualitative, published alongside each other (Heyvaert *et al.*, 2014a, 2014b) or as a *segregated* review design, merging some of the insights of both evidence strands in the end phase of the review process (Sandelowski *et al.*, 2006). The approach builds on the idea that qualitative and quantitative studies are different entities and therefore ought to be treated separately.

A second mixed-methods review option presented by Sandelowski *et al.* (2006) is the *integrative* type of mixed-methods review, grouping primary research studies by findings rather than by designs. The analytic emphasis of such reviews is on transforming or translating findings to enable review authors to combine them. Quantitative data are 'qualitized' or qualitative findings are 'quantitized'. This is an approach that has been used, for example, in Bayesian approaches to mixing methods (Roberts *et al.*, 2002; Voils *et al.*, 2009). The approach subscribes to the theory that qualitative and quantitative studies can address the same research questions and purposes and do not warrant separate syntheses.

A third approach to mixed-methods reviews promotes a *contingent* review design that presents a cycle of research synthesis studies conducted to answer specific review questions. This review type works well for complex interventions reviews, because it allows design-related decisions to grow organically, based on the type of questions that emerge (Sandelowski *et al.*, 2006). In what follows, we will introduce a worked example of a contingent type of mixed-methods review.

A theoretical example of a contingent mixed-methods review design

A research inquiry into the most beneficial promotion programme to stimulate breast feeding will be used as an example to illustrate how different types of question may reveal themselves to an author team in the context of a review on complex interventions. Saini and Schlonsky's (2012) outline of the various stages in a review process is used to structure the worked example (Figure 9.2).

Phase 1

In the beginning phase of a mixed-methods review, authors are mainly concerned with defining the core review questions and identifying the contextual factors that assist them in developing a review question that matches the expectations of the target group. Very often, qualitative questions related to the meaningfulness and appropriateness of an intervention are used to inform the development of a logic model. Appropriateness in our particular case refers to the extent to which the breastfeeding programme fits with or has the potential to fit with what is considered the state of the art, from the perspective of both the reviewer and the mothers involved, or how it matches these mothers' expectations. Meaningfulness relates to the personal opinions, values, thoughts, beliefs, positive or negative experiences and interpretations from the mothers (Pearson *et al.*, 2005). Logic models outline the theory of change that underpins the mixed-methods review as well as the moderator variables that are known to impact on the breastfeeding intervention evaluated. Authors may want to take into account successful and less successful components of the programme that are known up front, such as a supporting environment or the adequacy of the information provided. In addition, the scoping exercise will inform the development of relevant questions or the type of subgroups (e.g. first-time mothers versus others) that need to be considered in the effectiveness review. Subgroup analyses may reveal important variations in the benefits (or harms) achieved.

Phase 2

In the middle phase, the focus shifts from the conceptual level via scoping to an exploratory level via a more systematic approach to studying the literature. Evidence from qualitative studies may provide additional important information on the type of moderators and facilitators that actually impact on the intervention. Inquiries

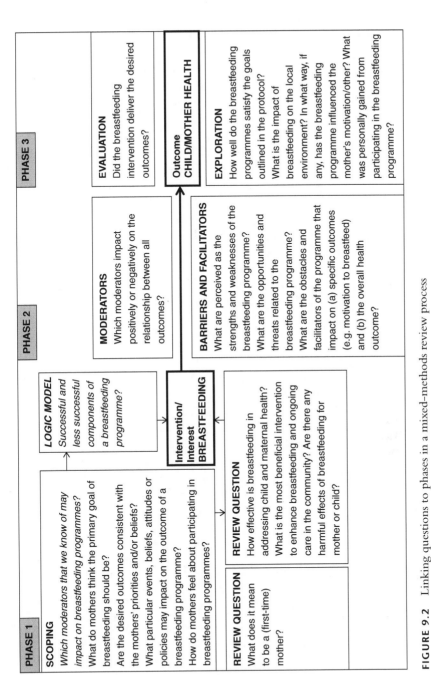

FIGURE 9.2 Linking questions to phases in a mixed-methods review process

into conditions and circumstances that may impact on the outcome of a review are crucially important. They may reveal conflicting or contradictory evidence for which a strategy on how to deal with these conflicts needs to be developed. These types of inquiry relate to the feasibility of the intervention. Feasibility is the extent to which the breastfeeding intervention is practical and applicable (Pearson *et al.*, 2005). It focuses on aspects of process and implementation and emphasizes particular obstacles in applying the intervention, issues that positively (or negatively) impact on a successful roll-out of a programme or the strengths and weaknesses of the programme itself. Examples of process-related factors that may impact on the outcome measures include the impact of characteristics of the health care provider or the mothers themselves, or the broader ecological context at play, such as how supportive the government is of breastfeeding in general. These elements may provide insight into why a particular intervention did not (fully) meet the expectations of the reviewers in terms of effectiveness or which elements might have been overlooked in compiling the logic model that underpins the breastfeeding intervention (see phase 1). In most cases, review authors engage with this type of information once the set of effectiveness studies considered for inclusion in the review has been defined. They may search for information on these aspects in the included articles or actively screen the literature for any sibling studies that have been published alongside the trials.

Phase 3

In the end phase, review authors will most likely present pooled estimates of effectiveness or, in the absence of a statistical meta-analysis, a narrative summary of the results of individual studies. Review authors may be interested in pulling in qualitative research evidence that allows them to explore reasons for potentially unexpected results (such as a programme that did not deliver the desired outcome) or heterogeneity in results (programmes that lead to different results in different subgroups, settings or situations). In addition, issues of relevance and applicability expressed by mothers caring for an infant may help to clarify what was personally gained from a programme, how they benefit or which elements have been helpful, advantageous or good for them. A richer discussion of the evidence retrieved on the impact of breastfeeding programmes can be obtained from studying potential contextual issues that may need to be addressed in order to promote a large-scale roll-out of a breastfeeding programme and/or to support claims for the potential transferability of the results to other settings and populations, for instance to a non-Western population of young mothers.

Summary

We support the claim that mixed-methods synthesis approaches are useful in the context of complex interventions. With an emphasis on phases that occur in a mixed-methods review process, we deliberately move away from the instrumental focus on 'mixing' evidence synthesis approaches that leaves potential review authors with the impression that differences between quantitative and qualitative approaches to synthesizing research evidence are merely technical and can be overcome by choosing the appropriate mixed-methods review design. Instead, we encourage review authors to consider which configurations of methods, techniques and approaches make sense to answer not only the predefined research questions but also those that emerge during the review process. The clear distinction between 'meaning' studied from a qualitative perspective and 'effectiveness' measured in quantitative parts of the example review reconciles a phenomenon such as breast-feeding to an exclusive quantitative or qualitative research paradigm. It is in addressing issues of feasibility and appropriateness of the intervention that we create an opportunity for both strands to meet and for the development of a shared vocabulary between reviewers representing different research traditions. It is recommended that teams working towards a publication of their review clearly report their rationale for conducting a mixed-methods review, reconstruct their iterative loops for the reader (or at least provide an indication of their mixed-methods design), outline the general review approach and describe the strategies by which the quantitative and qualitative strands of evidence will be merged, connected or integrated.

Further reading

Bennett, S., O'Connor, D., Hannes, K. and Doyle, S. 2013. Appraising and understanding systematic reviews of quantitative and qualitative evidence. In: T. Hoffmann, S. Bennett and C. Dell Mar (eds), *Evidence-Based Practice across the Health Professions*, 2nd edn. Chatswood, NSW: Churchill Livingstone, chapter 12.

Heyvaert, M., Hannes, K., Maes, B. and Onghena, P. 2013. Critical appraisal of mixed methods studies. *Journal of Mixed Methods Research,* 7: 302–27.

Pluye, P. and Hong, Q. N. 2014. Combining the power of stories and numbers: mixed methods research and mixed studies reviews. *Annual Review in Public Health*, 35: 29–45.

Pluye, P., Hong, Q. N. and Vedel, I. 2013. Toolkit for mixed studies reviews. http://toolkit-4mixedstudiesreviews.pbworks.com.

10

DEVELOPMENT OF COMPLEX INTERVENTIONS

Outcome modeling

Susanne Buhse and Ingrid Mühlhauser

Introduction

As described previously in Chapter 1 by Richards, complex interventions consist of a number of components that may act interdependently, and whose development, testing, evaluation and implementation encompass multiple methodological phases. One of the most important aspects of this research process is the selection of appropriate outcome measures with which to assess the effectiveness of the intervention. Researchers have to define which indicators are most relevant for the group receiving the intervention and how these indicators can be assessed using valid and reliable measures of outcome. To do so, researchers must identify not only the desired primary outcome of the intervention but also model the intermediate processes and pathways by which they postulate that the intervention will achieve its desired effect. This chapter outlines key considerations in choosing indicators and measures of outcome.

Learning objectives

- To understand the difference between patient-relevant outcomes and surrogate markers.
- To appreciate the value of patient-reported outcomes.
- To consider the importance of measures to assess intervention harms.
- To reflect on the use of composite, multicomponent and interdependent outcomes.

Outcome modeling

Modeling the outcomes of a complex intervention and deciding on which measures to use to assess them are part and parcel of the overall process of modeling

TABLE 10.1 Explanation of terms and illustrative examples

Outcome measure	Explanation	Example
Patient-relevant	Reflects how a patient feels, functions or survives.	Mortality, activities of daily living.
Patient-reported	A report on patient's health condition that comes directly from the patient.	Health-related quality of life.
Surrogate	A substitute to patient-relevant outcomes (intermediate outcome).	HbA1c, blood pressure, cholesterol levels, bone mineral density.
Composite	Includes two or more relevant outcomes that can be objectively defined.	Combination of fatal and non-fatal cardiovascular disease events.
Multidimensional	Comprises two or more separate parameters that are combined to a single construct.	Informed choice (composed of knowledge, attitude, decision).
Interdependent	Interdependent parameters, which should be considered when interpreting results.	HbA1c in relation to treatment goals as well as modes and intensity of treatment.

the intervention. It is also intimately connected with the decision we need to make about which design to use in researching the effect of a specific intervention. Sermeus (Chapter 12) describes the process of modeling the intervention. This process can help us to identify what the expected outcomes should be, together with confounding factors that need to be controlled for. Modeling the outcome, therefore, is not something to be done in isolation from modeling the intervention. They are closely linked to each other. However, what follows in this chapter is a more detailed account of the process of outcome modeling. Table 10.1 provides an overview of various types of outcome measure we might consider in our outcome modeling process.

Patient-relevant outcomes

A patient-relevant outcome is defined as a 'characteristic or variable that reflects how a patient feels, functions, or survives' (Biomarkers Definitions Working Group, 2001). The American Food and Drug Administration (FDA) and the European Medicines Agency (EMA) provide disease-specific guidance that supports research-ers in defining and justifying patient-relevant outcome measures. Morbidity and mortality are typical patient-relevant outcome measures (FDA, 2007; EMA, 2008). However, an isolated interpretation of these endpoints can be misleading. An intervention that leads to a decreased disease-specific mortality could be accompanied by an increase in all-cause mortality, outweighing the positive effects of the intervention for the specific condition. For example, a decrease in cardiovascular mortality could be outweighed by an increase in cancer-related mortality. Further, improving survival rates at the cost of poor neurological health may not be considered beneficial overall from a patient's perspective.

One example illustrates the use of patient-relevant outcomes for the evaluation of complex interventions. A recent Cochrane review summarized evidence that patients treated in stroke units are more likely to survive and have a higher degree of independence (Stroke Unit Trialists' Collaboration, 2013). A stroke unit consists of multiple interdependent components such as a specific multidisciplinary care team, stroke-specific monitoring devices, acute care standards and processes of early management and rehabilitation (Langhorne and Pollock, 2002). They should not be evaluated only on neurologic status and death. Outcomes such as health-related quality of life (HRQL) and dependency on and requirement for institutional care are also important outcome measures.

Identifying patient-relevant outcomes

In order to identify patient-relevant outcomes, literature searches can be used to retrieve research on equivalent or similar topics and identify outcome measures around relevant concepts such as patients' needs, perceptions and attitudes. In addition, focus groups or face-to-face interviews may help to identify relevant outcomes. Patients and members of the public can also be involved in the development of outcome measures, for example by participating in the design and validation of knowledge tests. As noted by Richards (Chapter 4), patients are experts when it comes to the evaluation of the applicability, feasibility and usability of complex interventions.

Patient-reported outcomes

A patient-reported outcome (PRO) is defined as 'any report of the status of a patient's health condition that comes directly from the patient, without interpretation of the patient's response by a clinician or anyone else' (FDA, 2009). PROs encompass heterogeneous constructs, such as health perception, functioning, perceived symptoms, satisfaction and HRQL. Using PROs, researchers can obtain valuable information from the patients' perspective.

The definition, modeling and interpretation of PROs can be challenging in that PROs can appear to contradict a clinical outcome. For example, people may feel satisfied with treatment whilst clinical outcomes are poor, or the converse might be observed. One possible reason might be that patients have unrealistic expectations of treatment outcome, an issue that could be addressed by giving evidence-based patient information that includes reliable information on the expected outcome. Equally, satisfaction might be related to the quality of care delivery not the outcomes of that care, and PROs can provide valuable information on *how* treatment is being delivered as well as *what* treatment is provided.

PROs can be used additionally or complementary to other relevant outcome measures, strengthening the interpretation of findings. However, in conditions where there is an absence of reliable clinical biomarkers, for example depression and many other mental health disorders, patient-reported outcomes are actually the principal way in which the effectiveness of interventions can be assessed and they are often used as primary outcomes in clinical trials.

Surrogate markers and their potential fallacies

Surrogate outcome parameters are typically used in clinical trials to obtain evidence for efficacy earlier and more easily. Surrogates can be metabolic parameters, for example LDL-cholesterol or blood glucose, blood pressure, X-ray images or bone density. Surrogates may also represent an intermediate step leading to the relevant outcome. They can be regarded as intermediate endpoints (Mangiapane and Velasco Garrido, 2009), and are often used to predict patient-relevant long-term outcomes. For example, blood pressure and LDL-cholesterol are used as surrogate endpoints for stroke and myocardial infarction, respectively.

Nevertheless, the role surrogates play in the appraisal of the overall clinical outcome is questionable. There are examples of misinterpretation with serious consequences. For example, hormone replacement therapy has a positive effect on serum cholesterol and blood glucose levels in postmenopausal women, but actually raises the risk of myocardial infarction and stroke (Rossouw *et al.*, 2002). Equally, treatment with beta-carotene restores normal serum vitamin A levels in smokers but long-term administration increases lung cancer mortality (Cortés-Jofré *et al.*, 2012).

Conversely, surrogate parameters may be essential for the development and evaluation of complex interventions. Parameters such as knowledge or attitudes are typically used to evaluate intermediate effects of educational interventions. Nonetheless, surrogates should be interpreted with caution when used as an outcome measure in clinical trials. The assessment of endpoints, such as knowledge and attitudes, is based on the hypothesis that good knowledge or decisions congruent with individual attitudes improve patients' involvement in health decisions. However, this hypothesis remains theoretical until patient involvement is measured as an independent outcome and knowledge and attitudes are shown to mediate levels of actual patient involvement. Clearly, the overall effects of complex interventions should be evaluated by using relevant outcome parameters, and only validated surrogate endpoints should be used. For example, patient-reported knowledge is not a substitute for a knowledge score achieved by using a validated test. Table 10.2 provides an example of modeling the outcome measure 'patient understanding'.

TABLE 10.2 Example: modeling of 'patient understanding' as an intermediate outcome

Background	Educational intervention XYZ aims at enhancing patients' participation in decision-making. Patient information is a prerequisite for decision-making. It should be decision-relevant, evidence-based and understandable.
Objective	Patients achieve in-depth understanding of information.
Development of a knowledge test	The assessment of 'understanding' should be valid and reliable:
	• Definition of core issues based on the education material and evidence-based patient information.
	• Operationalization of items of a questionnaire.
	• Piloting: assessment of face-validity (content relevance, content coverage) and understandability by using concurrent think-aloud interviews, revision if necessary.
	• Specification of answering format, scaling and weighing.
	• Pretests within the target group focusing on item-difficulty (exploration of floor and ceiling effects), revision if necessary.

Assessing harms

Every intervention may have adverse effects and it is by no means assured that all heath care actions will be benign. However, harms are rarely reported in trials on complex non-pharmacological interventions (Ethgen *et al.*, 2005). Interventions in complex systems may induce unintended effects that may be difficult to identify. Therefore, accompanying changes in care or settings should be meticulously documented alongside implementation of a study. For example, in a study of telephone triage for same-day appointments in primary care, although the intervention decreased doctor workload more patients attended the emergency department following triage than in the usual care group, an unintended negative consequence of the complex triage intervention (Richards *et al.*, 2002).

Composite, multidimensional and interdependent outcomes

A composite endpoint includes two or more relevant outcomes that can be objectively defined. Composite endpoints are often used to reduce the sample size required in studies of conditions with low event rates. In trials of cardiovascular disease prevention, a combination of fatal and non-fatal events forms a typical composite endpoint. However, combining 'hard' and 'soft' endpoints can be inappropriate and misleading (EMA, 2008). Let us assume that in a trial of a complex intervention, results for a composite endpoint 'disease-specific mortality and admission to hospital' reach statistical significance, indicating that the intervention has an overall benefit. However, the results may be mainly due to a decrease in hospital admissions, just one element of the composite outcome. If there were an associated increase in pre-hospital mortality, because more patients die before they reach the hospital, we would actually assess the intervention as harmful rather than beneficial.

Unlike composite endpoints, multidimensional endpoints comprise two or more separate components combined in to a single construct. A good example is Marteau et al.'s (2001) measure of 'informed choice' which includes three components: knowledge (poor, good), attitude (positive, negative) and choice (uptake, non-uptake of the intervention). These are assessed separately and then combined. An 'informed choice' is achieved if an individual demonstrates good knowledge and makes a decision congruent with the decision-relevant attitude.

Study outcomes may also be measured by interdependent parameters in which case their interdependency has to be kept in mind when interpreting study results. As an example, in diabetes care blood glucose or HbA1c values can only really be interpreted alongside information on individual treatment goals, dietary restrictions, quality of life, intensity of medication, therapeutic strategies, body weight and hypoglycemia. In this example, biological parameters and parameters of care have an interdependency. Improvement of blood glucose values may be associated with more or less intensive drug therapy, which in turn depends on the degree of patient adherence to non-drug therapy or prescribed medication (Lenz et al., 2007).

The clinical relevance of outcomes

Reliability and validity are essential quality features of all assessment instruments as is responsiveness, an important aspect of validity that describes the ability of an instrument to record changes in clinical endpoints. However, the interpretation of changes may be difficult, especially when using patient-reported or intermediate outcome measures. We need to be aware that a study result with statistical significance is not necessarily clinically relevant. For example, a difference in HbA1c level of 0.2 percent due to lifestyle or drug interventions may be statistically significant, but does not affect micro- and macrovascular outcomes.

The concept of minimal clinically important difference (MCID) or minimal important difference (MID) should be used to facilitate interpretation of the data. It is defined as 'patient derived scores that reflect changes in a clinical intervention that are meaningful for the patient' (Jaeschke et al., 1989: 407) or 'the smallest difference between two measurement results that a patient considers relevant' (Brettschneider et al., 2011). Defining a MCID or MID can be a challenge, since it varies across different interventions, study populations and other contextual factors. In terms of PROs, the FDA established the term 'responder' in order to focus on meaningful changes at the individual level (FDA, 2009). There are multiple statistical approaches to estimate important clinical differences and responder thresholds, for example anchor-based estimates (using external clinical or patient-based indicators that reflect changes) and distribution-based methods (distribution of observed scores) (FDA, 2009).

In addition, the relevance of an outcome for an individual person depends on factors such as severity and attitudes, since risks and outcomes are perceived differently by different people. For example, a small increase in the risk of a harmful side effect might be perceived as more relevant than a small risk reduction in the primary outcome measure. Equally a 50 percent relative mortality risk reduction says nothing about the relevance of the absolute risk reduction in the adverse event or condition. Concepts such as absolute risk reduction, number needed to treat and the risk of adverse effects are required so that clinicians and patients can deliberate on the pros and cons of an intervention and make an informed and meaningful decision about acceptance and adherence.

Summary

The evaluation of complex interventions requires that we define indicators to reflect both intervention processes and their outcomes. These indicators can be operationalized into various outcome measures. Relevant and objective outcome measures are essential for patients but sometimes difficult to assess, and outcome measures that focus on intermediate effects play an essential role in the evaluation of complex interventions. Intermediate outcomes can explain the mode of functioning for the active components of a complex intervention and allow interpretation of processes, intervention mediators and context-related interdependencies. The assessment and interpretation of intervention effects requires appropriate and validated instruments as well as considerations of clinical and patient relevance.

Further reading

The Patient-Centered Outcomes Research Institute (PCORI). http://www.pcori.org.

Williamson, P. and Clarke, M. 2012. The COMET (Core Outcome Measures in Effectiveness Trials) initiative: its role in improving Cochrane reviews [editorial]. *Cochrane Database of Systematic Reviews*, ED000041. http://www.thecochranelibrary.com/details/editorial/1797057/The-COMET-Core-Outcome-Measures-in-Effectiveness-Trials-Initiative-its-role-in-i.html.

11

DESIGNING INTERVENTIONS TO CHANGE HEALTH-RELATED BEHAVIOUR

Charles Abraham, Sarah Denford, Jane R. Smith, Sarah Dean, Colin Greaves, Jenny Lloyd, Mark Tarrant, Mathew P. White and Katrina Wyatt

Introduction

Individual behaviour patterns affect health, mortality and the cost of health service delivery. For example, rising levels of obesity are associated with increasing prevalence of cardiovascular disease, type 2 diabetes and cancers. In the UK, population prevalence of being overweight and obese is predicted to cost an additional £50 billion in health care costs by 2050 (Foresight, 2007). In this chapter we outline an evidence-based approach to designing interventions to change individual health-related behaviour patterns that can potentially improve public health.

Learning objectives

- Understand the principles of designing individual-level behaviour change interventions using the Intervention Mapping framework.
- Illustrate how change techniques included in interventions should be selected on the basis of a logic model of underlying modifiable mechanisms that regulate individual behaviour.
- Describe how implementation issues shape the intervention design process to ensure adoption and accurate implementation of interventions in routine practice.
- Explain the difference between outcome and process evaluations and the relationship between (i) logic models describing mechanisms underpinning behaviour change (see learning objective two) and (ii) process evaluations.
- Illustrate how the Information, Motivation Behavioural Skills model can be used in mapping modifiable mechanisms and selection of change techniques.

Designing behaviour change interventions

Developing, implementing and evaluating behaviour change interventions can be complex and a number of frameworks offer guidance on how to manage this process. 'Intervention Mapping' (IM; Bartholomew *et al.*, 2011; http://www.interventionmapping.com) provides a helpful guide to systematic evidence-based design of behaviour change interventions (see also Van Achterberg, Chapter 29 for examples of Intervention Mapping in implementation science). IM involves six planning stages briefly summarized in Table 11.1.

Needs assessment involves identification of the health, or well-being, problem, the behaviour patterns exacerbating that problem and the context in which behaviour change needs to occur to generate health/well-being gains. Often needs assessment should begin by examining best current practice and identifying why it is failing to promote desired health-prompting behaviour patterns (de Bruin *et al.*, 2010). This process facilitates stage two of the IM process, that is, definition of behavioural objectives specifying which behaviours need to be changed by whom and in which contexts. These objectives, in turn, clarify what needs to be measured to discover whether the intervention had the desired effects. In stage three, modifiable determinants or mechanisms underpinning the target behaviours are mapped. These may include changes in knowledge, beliefs, skills or access to resources including social support. These underpinning mechanisms (or regulatory processes) constitute the logic (or programme) model of the intervention. This may also be called the 'change theory' underpinning the intervention. At this stage designers specify *how* they think an intervention will work. This, in turn, determines the nature of the 'process evaluation' (see below).

Once modifiable mechanisms are specified in a logic model these can be mapped onto change techniques which have been found to successfully alter these mechanisms in previous studies (Abraham and Michie, 2008). Thus the logic model specifying targeted mechanism changes determines the content of the intervention. Hence, a good knowledge of the theoretical and applied behaviour change literature is needed for optimal behaviour change intervention design. This may warrant external consultation.

Delivery formats (e.g. written documents, websites and multi-media technology, or face-to-face interaction on an individual or group basis) are critical to intervention implementation. Replication and implementation fidelity necessitate production and publication of accurate, detailed manuals describing the intervention and its delivery in detail. To promote adoption and faithful delivery of interventions over time, it is crucial that stakeholders are involved in intervention development, including the planning of delivery methods in stage 4. If the motivations and resources of those who will deliver the intervention are not considered then an intervention found to be effective in a methodologically rigorous evaluation may not be implemented and so have no real-world impact on health or well-being.

Once developed, interventions should be piloted to ensure that the intervention is acceptable to the target population and sustainable in context. If resources

TABLE 11.1 Six stages of Intervention Mapping

Planning stage	Planning tasks
1. Needs assessment	Decide what (if anything) needs to be changed. For example, what is the health problem?
2. Objective setting	Specify primary and secondary outcome objectives. These are the criteria by which the efficacy or success of the intervention will be judged. A primary objective might be a health outcome. Change in a behaviour pattern could be a primary or secondary objective.
3. Identification of change mechanisms and techniques	Designers should identify which processes or mechanisms are responsible for current unwanted behaviour patterns and/or which processes would need be changed to instigate and maintain new desirable behaviour patterns. Techniques that have been found to change these processes can then be selected as the active ingredients of the intervention.
4. Delivery methods	Having identified mechanisms and techniques, designers must decide how best to deliver the intervention content, e.g. using leaflets, texts, posters or face-to-face interaction. This critically depends on the implementation context and audience.
5. Implementation	How will the intervention be delivered in practice? Who in the relevant context will deliver it and how? Are the necessary resources and skills in place and can the intervention be maintained over time?
6. Evaluation	The questions that the evaluation must answer should be clarified early in the design process. For example, the outcome evaluation must clarify whether the intervention changed the specified behaviour patterns in context (see stage 2). The process evaluation must clarify whether the intervention changed the targeted mechanism of change (see stage 3).

necessary for delivery of the intervention are not available or sustainable then the intervention may have to be redesigned to enable faithful implementation in everyday practice. Thus planning implementation of the intervention in stage 5 is critical to intervention impact on routine practice and health. Pilot or feasibility studies can also be used to clarify whether the planned evaluation is practical. For example, can sufficient intervention and control participants be recruited? Can outcome and process measures be taken as planned?

Even if an intervention is found to be efficacious when evaluated (e.g. in a trial), it will have no impact on health if it is not adopted, and implemented accurately in practice. RE-AIM is an evaluation framework focusing on the external validity of interventions (Glasgow *et al.*, 1999), that is on whether or not they have real-world impact. The framework defines five factors that relate to the successful integration of an intervention into real-world settings, namely: Reach, Effectiveness, Adoption, Implementation and Maintenance.

Evaluation is placed at stage 6 but, in practice, must be anticipated early in the design process. An outcome evaluation tests whether the intervention succeeded in changing its specified outcomes (stage 2). Such evaluation typically involves comparison of outcomes among those who received the intervention and those who did not. This may involve a non-intervention control group or another intervention group (as is the case when an intervention is compared to routine care) – or both. Typically, post-intervention levels of outcome measures are compared, controlling for pre-intervention levels.

Whether an intervention suceeds in changing primary objectives, it is important to know whether it was delivered, implemented and received as intended (e.g. classes took place and were taught as described in the manual, and participants engaged with the intervention). If we are to understand why an intervention does or does not work and whether it would work if implemented elsewhere, it is also critical that evaluations clarify whether observed effects were generated by the mechanisms specified (in stage 3 of the planning process). These questions are addressed in process evaluations. So the logic or mechanism model underpinning the selection of change techniques also determines which measures of mechanism should be included in the process evaluation. For example, if an intervention to reduce alcohol use was based on changing normative beliefs about others' drinking and approval of drinking then the process evaluation would assess change in both these beliefs (often referred to as descriptive and subjective norms, respectively). It is possible for an intervention to meet its objectives (e.g. reduced alcohol intake) but not by the mechanisms it sought to target (e.g. normative beliefs did not change). It is also possible for an intervention to successfully change underlying mechanisms but not change the primary outcomes. In both cases, findings from process evaluations suggest that the initial mapping of underlying mechanisms may have been incomplete or mistaken. Understanding this can help improve future intervention design. An example illustrating application of Intervention Mapping is described in Box 11.1.

BOX 11.1 THE HEALTH LIFESTYLES PROGRAMME (HeLP)

HeLP is a school-based intervention designed to prevent weight gain among 9- and 10-year-olds. The intervention was designed and implemented in accordance with an Intervention Mapping approach.

A needs assessment (IM stage 1) revealed that an acceptable, engaging school-based intervention that could prevent weight gain in 9- and 10-year-olds was needed (Wyatt *et al.*, 2011).

In accordance with IM steps 2 and 3, the primary objective was specified as being weight maintenance while secondary objectives were reducing fizzy drink intake, reducing screen time (e.g. television and gaming systems) and increasing the proportion of healthy to unhealthy snacks consumed. The focus for all three of these objectives was on replacing unhealthy behaviours with more healthy alternatives.

HeLP sought to change a variety of determinants and regulatory processes underpinning these target behaviours, including normative beliefs and self-efficacy.

As HeLP was designed to impact the whole school environment, it was believed that engaging the senior management team and teachers as well as the children and their families was crucial in achieving behaviour change. Behavioural objectives and modifiable regulatory processes were mapped for each target group (Lloyd et al., 2011).

Discussions with children, teachers and parents led to the selection of a combination of intervention approaches including drama workshops, classroom lessons and parent assemblies. In the drama workshops children co-created scenes with the actors, who played characters with whom the children identified such as 'Active Amy' and 'Snacky Sam'. School children discussed the challenges that these characters faced and offered the characters support and advice relevant to diet and physical activity. These intervention components deliver a range of change techniques that are mapped out in the HeLP manual (Lloyd et al., 2011). Information is provided to teach children about healthy eating, skill-building sessions to help children select healthy alternatives, and communication skills training to help children communicate effectively with others. The use of characters, with whom the children identify, and role play are effective means of building communication and developing problem-solving skills in an engaging and supportive environment. Providing children with the opportunity to 'act out' scenes enables them to demonstrate healthier behaviours and see the possible consequences of making changes.

Following the development of HeLP, an exploratory trial was used to test the acceptability of the materials and delivery methods as well as the feasibility of a larger evaluation (Lloyd et al., 2012). Interviews and focus groups with children and teachers allowed reflection on, and refinement of, acceptability of change techniques, delivery formats and measurement methods. A published protocol describing intervention and trail design is available (Wyatt et al., 2013).

Understanding change mechanisms and selecting mechanism-targeted change techniques

There are a multitude of theories of behaviour change, many of which specify overlapping regulatory processes (e.g. Abraham et al., 1998). Many – or few – regulatory processes may underpin behaviour patterns that need to be changed. So any one theory or model may not specify all – or any – of the regulatory processes that need to be targeted in an intervention.

The Information, Motivation, Behavioral skills (IMB) model (Fisher and Fisher, 1992) proposes that behaviour change occurs when individuals are well informed, highly motivated and have the skills necessary to perform the behaviour. Assessing whether the target group has the information needed to change their behaviour, is motivated (or not) and has (or has not) the relevant skills is a useful way to begin to identify the change mechanisms that need to be targeted in intervention design.

If a behaviour is easy to perform (i.e. the individual has the skills) and highly motivating, then information alone may be enough. For example, advertising free influenza vaccinations will prompt many (but not all) of those who are eligible to obtain the vaccination. Easily understood and accessible information is a key element of behaviour change practice but may not be enough to prompt change.

If knowledge has not been translated into a stable motivation to take action to change, then interventions must focus on motivating people, and there are many theories available that specify the modifiable beliefs that underpin motivation. For example, in a workshop aiming to 'identify a finite set of variables to be considered in any behavioral analysis', Fishbein *et al.* (2001: 3) identified five key processes (or mechanisms) underpinning motivation to perform any particular behaviour or set of behaviours. They concluded that a strong intention is likely to develop when an individual (i) judges that the advantages (or benefits) of performing the behaviour outweigh the perceived disadvantages (or costs); (ii) perceives the social (normative) pressure to perform the behaviour to be greater than that not to perform the behaviour; (iii) believes that the behaviour is consistent with his or her self-image; (iv) anticipates the emotional reaction to performing the behaviour to be more positive than negative; and (v) has high levels of self-efficacy, that is, believes that they could competently perform the behaviour. Any or all of these mechanism could be selected as crucial at stage 2 of the Intervention Mapping process and then measured in the process evaluation (in stage 6)

Sometimes well-informed, motivated individuals fail to take appropriate action because they lack the skills to undertake an action, or the skills needed to change impulsive regulation of an unwanted behaviour pattern. Hence health care staff may need hand-washing instructions to ensure they prevent infection spread and smokers may need training in self-regulation in order to successfully change their behaviour. There are a wide variety of skills relevant to health-related behaviour change, including motor skills (e.g. learning how to use an asthma inhaler), social skills (e.g. learning how to negotiate condom use with a seual partner) and self-regulatory skills (e.g. learning how to monitor one's own behaviour and relate that monitoring to success or failure defined by previously agreed goals).

This mapping of modifiable processes that underpin behaviour patterns provides the foundation for selection of change techniques to be included in intervention design. So, for example, if a person is well informed but does not perceive the social (normative) pressure to perform the behaviour to be greater than that not to perform the behaviour, then a technique that will change normative beliefs should be selected. The intervention might, for example, include provision of normative feedback informing participants of how others like them are behaving or how others they value approve or disapprove of a behaviour pattern. Providing students with information about (i) other students' alcohol consumption and (ii) other students' views on alcohol consumption could change intervention recipients' normative beliefs – so putting in place one key foundation of motivation to reduce alcohol intake. The process evaluation would then measure changes in normative beliefs while the outcome evaluation measured changes in drinking behaviour (the primary outcome).

Alternatively, if the target group is already informed and motivated, change is unlikely to occur as a result of using techniques that enhance knowledge or motivation. For example, women attending weight-control classes are already motivated to lose weight so it may be that they lack certain skills to translate motivation into action. Luszczynska *et al.* (2007) found that training people to improve planning, via formulation of if–then plans, could enhance weight loss among motivated women. If–then plans identify a situation in which the person wants to change their usual behaviour (the 'if') and pair this with a commitment to make a new response within the person's capability (the 'then') (Gollwitzer and Sheeran, 2006). For example, 'If cake is served at lunchtime, then I will decline and remind myself how much better I will feel later in the afternoon.' Of course, which techniques are needed in an intervention depends on the initial mapping of mechanisms underpinning the behaviours the intervention seeks to change (Abraham and Michie 2008).

Conclusions and recommendations

We conclude that it is possible to design, implement and evaluate individual-level behaviour change interventions. However, to do so successfully requires careful, systematic planning as advocated by the Intervention Mapping framework. Box 11.2 provides a set of summary recommendations for intervention designers.

BOX 11.2 KEY RECOMMENDATIONS FOR BEHAVIOUR CHANGE INTERVENTION DESIGNERS

- Ensure that an intervention is necessary before spending time and resources on its development.
- Identify and clearly specify the target recipients/users of the intervention and the particular behaviours that are to be changed.

- Use relevant research to identify mechanisms of behaviour regulation that need to be altered. The IMB model can provide a useful framework for this work.
- Select and describe change techniques based on analyses of the regulatory mechanisms or determinants that need to be changed.
- Select a mode of delivery – or delivery format – for the selected change techniques that will facilitate accessibility and usability for the target recipients.
- Ensure correspondence between mode of delivery, change techniques and targeted behavioural mechanisms.
- Carefully consider the context and environment in which the intervention is to be implemented, including available personal, interpersonal and physical resources.
- Co-create intervention materials with intended users and implementers to optimize ownership, adoption and sustainability.
- Pilot intervention materials before use.
- Make sure those delivering the intervention have appropriate training to ensure fidelity of delivery.
- Evaluate interventions in terms of outcomes (including behavioural outcomes) and underpinning mechanisms.

Futher reading

Abraham, C., Conner, M., Jones, F. and O'Conner, D. 2015. *Health Psychology*, 2nd edn. Hove: Routledge and Psychology Press.

Bartholomew, L. K., Parcel, G. S., Kok, G., Gottlieb, N. H. and Fernandez, M. E. 2011. *Planning Health Promotion Programs: An Intervention Mapping Approach*. San Francisco, CA: Jossey-Bass.

12

MODELLING PROCESS AND OUTCOMES IN COMPLEX INTERVENTIONS

Walter Sermeus

Introduction

In this chapter, we focus on probably the least studied and understood element of developing a complex intervention: modelling the complex intervention by putting together all 'active components' that are known to have an effect based on empirical evidence or theory. A first problem is that a complex intervention is often defined as a 'black box'. The problem with the black box type of intervention is that, when it works, we don't know why it works, which makes it more difficult to replicate. And when it doesn't work, we don't know how to fix it. A second problem is that the complex intervention might indeed generate some overall significant effect and you can find this good enough. But is this the best intervention possible? And can it be optimized? A third problem is that we see a high variability of success in the implementation of a complex intervention because of different contexts and constraints. It requires that right from the start of developing the complex intervention, the later implementation should be modelled as well.

Learning objectives

- Understand how to model multiple active components into a complex intervention.
- Understand how to optimize a complex intervention.
- Understand how to integrate later implementation into the model.

The aim of modelling a complex intervention

Box 12.1 (based on Campbell *et al.*, 2000) shows the aim of modelling a complex intervention and what a model should describe. There exists a wide range of different modelling tools that are often linked to specific disciplines such as economical models, mathematical statistical models or scale models in architecture. The types of models we are looking at here are conceptual or theoretical models that are used to develop, understand and simulate complex interventions. Models may be fully descriptive or may use a graphical representation. Examples are flowcharts, activity diagrams, entity-relationship (ER) diagrams, process maps, mind maps and network diagrams. Preferably they make use of an unified modelling language to provide a standard way to visualize the design of a system (Booch *et al.*, 2005). Models can be static, making use of widely available software tools to visualize conceptual models in flowcharts such as Visio and Smartdraw. They can also be dynamic. Examples include mathematical modelling techniques, such as System Dynamics (SD), covered in depth by Pitt, Monks and Allen (Chapter 32), that are specifically developed to help managers improve understanding of their processes. They allow us to incorporate all kind of estimates and feedback loops into the model that enhances the understanding of an intervention and allows simulation of the different scenarios (e.g. for optimization).

BOX 12.1 MODELLING A COMPLEX INTERVENTION

The aim of modelling a complex intervention is to unravel the black box. More specific aims are to:

- provide the conceptual foundation for the intervention;
- identify gaps in prior scientific literature;
- inform the choice of intervention components and show clearly what role each component is to play in the intervention process;
- guide the specification of a priori hypotheses;
- guide optimization of the intervention;
- identify barriers that should be solved;
- provide a framework for interpretation of unexpected results.

A model should describe:

- the active components in the complex intervention, how they work, why they might be active components and in what effect they result;
- the right outcome measures that are used to evaluate the effect of the complex intervention;
- how active components relate to each other;
- all important mediators and moderators;
- theories underpinning the relations and effects;
- theories and empirical evidence related to the implementation of the complex intervention.

Modelling multiple active components into a complex intervention

One of the most critical decisions is to compose a complex intervention out of the existing evidence. How many activities should we select? How do we transform these 'more general' research findings (type 'A has an effect on B') into an implementable multicomponent intervention? Modelling scenarios have been developed by Berry *et al.* (2009), Lodewijckx *et al.* (2012), Vanhaecht *et al.* (2012) and Nabitz *et al.* (2006). Berry *et al.* (2009) describe a method of modelling highly reliable care for use within one hospital, the Geisinger Health System in Pennsylvania, USA, called ProvenCare. The first application was described for coronary bypass surgery (CABG). They identified three phases: (1) review and validation of best practice evidence; (2) redesign of the process; and (3) implementation. Lodewijckx *et al.* (2012) describe an eight-step method to build the clinical content of an evidence-based care pathway, which they apply for COPD exacerbation, for use in a multi-center, multi-country context. They identify eight different steps: (1) specification of the care population and composition of an expert panel; (2) literature review and identification of clinical activities and outcomes; (3) getting consensus through an international Delphi study; (4) final selection of clinical activities; (5) process flow-chart and describing grouping into key interventions; (6) detailed description; (7) translation into a set of process and outcome indicators; and (8) piloting. Vanhaecht *et al.* (2012) describe a seven-phase method to design, implement and evaluate care pathways: (1) screening phase; (2) project management phase; (3) diagnostic and objectivation phase; (4) development phase; (5) implementation phase; (6) evaluation phase; and (7) follow-up phase. Phases (1) to (4) are interesting for the development of complex interventions. Nabitz *et al.* (2006) use the EFQM (European Foundation of Quality Management) excellence model to redesign treatment processes based on nine building blocks: (1) leadership; (2) policy and strategy; (3) people management; (4) partnerships and resources; (5) processes; (6) customer results; (7) people results; (8) society results; and (9) key performance results.

The different models help us to understand a general approach to build a complex intervention. A critical element in all these models is that the approach is more circular than linear. It means that development, piloting, implementation and evaluation might in theory be sequential steps, but in practice the development is more incremental. A draft version might be piloted and lead to changes in the design of the intervention. The Deming cycle or Plan-Do-Check-Act (PDCA) cycle is an iterative four-step management method used for the continuous development of a complex intervention. Although the development phase is highly focused on the plan phase of the cycle where goals and processes are defined, it is permanently linked to the other phases of the cycle. Therefore, a six-step modelling scenario for modelling complex interventions is proposed.

1. Installing a project team and formulating the key objectives of the complex intervention

All models start with installing a project team. This team is limited in number, ideally five to seven people, and consists of a representative of all actors involved in the intervention. It is recommended that a facilitator with experience in process (re) design joins the group. Also, a representative of the management of organizations where the intervention would take place should be invited. The team is in charge. This core team is supported by a larger working group involving more stakeholders, preferably also patient and public representatives. The main reason for creating this larger group is to get ownership and broad support. A critical task is in formulating key objectives. Is the aim to improve quality or to reduce costs? What are the main target groups? Inclusion and exclusion criteria should be defined. What is the scope of the intervention? Is it focused on all activities or just a selection? What are the main outcomes?

2. Getting consensus on the components of the complex intervention

The ideal input for modelling a complex intervention is a list of clinical activities from literature review-based guidelines, with gradings of evidence. The difficulties with these lists are that they are often too lengthy, that conflicting evidence may be in place, that there is no consensus among clinicians as to what to do and what not to do, and that some of these activities may be difficult to implement in practice or are rather costly. Other information may come from focus groups with patients or professionals. The main purpose of this phase is to get consensus on which activities should be taken into account as part of the intervention and evaluation. This choice can be made by the project team or the larger working group. An interesting suggestion is made by Lodewijckx *et al.* (2012) to work with an international interdisciplinary panel of experts not involved in the study. The advantage of the local team is ownership and time. The disadvantage is that local conflicts and power play can disturb team working. The advantage of a larger international panel is that it creates a large supportive platform for action. Lodewijckx *et al.* (2012) involved 35 experts from 15 countries. They were contacted because of their role in international organizations or first authors in leading publications in this domain. In the COPD exacerbation study, the panel was composed of 19 medical doctors (mainly pneumologists/respiratory physicians), eight nurses (mainly nurse specialists) and eight physiotherapists.

It is also recommended to involve patients or patient groups and the public in any consultation (see Richards, Chapter 4). A good example is given by Dancet *et al.* (2013) for fertility care patients.

To get consensus, Lodewijckx *et al.* (2012) used a two-round Delphi study with ratings of the relevance of including components in the intervention. A score from 1 to 6 was used, varying from 'low impact on outcomes and thus not relevant' (1) to 'high impact on outcomes and thus highly relevant' (6). For the outcome indicators, experts were asked to rate how sensitive to change they believe the listed outcome indicators would be when implementing the intervention. It was again scored on a six-point scale going from 1, 'low sensitive to change and thus not relevant', to 6, 'high sensitive to change and so highly relevant'. Consensus for inclusion was defined as 75 per cent of the panel members evaluating that activity or outcome as relevant (score 5 or 6) for inclusion. For the COPD exacerbation pathway 26 of the 72 activities (36 per cent) and 10 of the 21 outcomes (48 per cent) were selected for inclusion. Based on all existing information (grading of the evidence for each of the activities, the results of the Delphi study overall and per discipline) the core team can then discuss the final selection in a face-to-face consensus meeting.

3. Clustering of clinical activities into key interventions and building a process flow

This is a crucial step as it makes the intervention work. Clinical activities are grouped based on their clinical coherence (e.g. measurement of basal metabolic index, advice on malnutrition and supplementary nutrition are clustered into a nutrition key intervention), the performance by a specific team member (e.g. breathing exercises and positioning by the physiotherapist) and time constraints (e.g. all activities regarding discharge management). In the COPD study, the 77 initial clinical activities were grouped into 38 key interventions, categorized into three core processes (diagnostic, pharmacological and non-pharmacological management). All these interventions were mapped into a process flow diagram. An example of a process flow for CABG (Berry et al., 2009) is given in Figure 12.1. The design of the 'ideal' process flow is carried in brainstorming sessions within the core team and the wider working group. Current process flows can be observed where it might be helpful to discuss and understand variations. What is seen is that each discipline has a reasonable understanding of the processes in their area, but not how the entire process is interlocked. A process flow diagram helps to understand the interdependency of all actors involved.

4. Get the process organized and allocate resources

Based on the ideal process flow, the necessary resources should be allocated, and the tasks and roles of all actors might be reviewed. This is the reason why a manager should be part of the core team, to evaluate the organizational impact of the intervention.

5. Detailed description of the key interventions

A detailed protocol of the intervention is written as a whole. It means that individual components (often based on guidelines) need to be reconsidered. Berry et al.

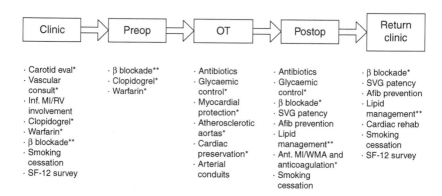

FIGURE 12.1 Example of a process map for elective coronary artery bypass graft ProvenCare high-level process flow. *Practice variation; **Non-existent previous practice. Afib, atrial fibrillation; Ant, anterior; Eval, evaluation; Inf, inferior; MI, myocardial infarction; OT, operating theatre; RV, right ventricle; SF, Short Form; SVG, saphenous vein graft; WMA, wall motion abnormality (Berry *et al.*, 2009)

(2009) give a good example. The reduction of length-of-stay for CABG to 3–4 days cannot be combined with the aggressive control of perioperative hyperglycaemia by insulin infusion until the third post-operative day to reduce the risk for deep sternal wound infection. It means that length-of-stay should be longer or insulin treatment should be shorter.

6. Translation into a set of process and outcome indicators

A set of process and outcome indicators should be developed to verify compliance to key interventions and to follow up the impact on outcomes. In the COPD study, 24 process and 15 outcome indicators were developed. This includes description of the indicator, relation to the intervention, type of indicator (baseline, process, outcome), nominator and denominator, data collection method, data elements and data reporting. Berry *et al.* (2009) argue for an 'all-or-none' measurement strategy where several data elements are measured. If, for example, a patient receives three out of four required interventions, the criterion is not met. No partial credits are given (Nolan and Berwick, 2006).

Modelling and optimization of complex interventions

Although you may carefully select all components to build a balanced intervention, you will never be sure that the composition is the right one or whether your selection has too few or too many components. Many intervention packages are evaluated as a whole and might indeed lead in the best case to a statistically significant effect but there is no guarantee that they are optimized. It is possible that you could have a better effect or use fewer resources if they were optimized.

Collins *et al.* (2007) propose an alternative way of building, optimizing and evaluating health interventions before undertaking the final RCT with all components included, called the multi-phase optimization strategy (MOST). They define three phases: a screening phase, a refining phase and a confirming phase.

The screening phase is based on the existing research literature or experience of involved professionals as described in the previous paragraph. The main objective is to explore which intervention components are active and contributing to positive outcomes and should therefore be included in the intervention. The main difference with other approaches is that in MOST trials, decisions are taken based on results (estimated effect size, costs) of randomized experiments and not on the basis of subjective decisions. To do so, they use a factorial design in which many interventions are randomly allocated simultaneously. If only a few components are evaluated simultaneously, then a full factorial design can be used. If many components need to be evaluated (e.g. six, which would lead to 2^6 or 64 different combinations), a fractional factorial design might be more appropriate. Collins *et al.* (2005) show how a full six-factor factorial design with 64 combinations can be redesigned in a fractional factorial design with 16 conditions, with the capability to provide main effects estimates for each of the six independent variables and to provide estimates for the selected interactions. The screening phase results in a draft version of the intervention with a selection of the most effective components.

The next phase, the refining phase, evaluates the optimal dose of any of the intervention components. Again a factorial design strategy is used. At the end of this phase, the investigator has identified the optimized final draft interventions with a set of active components at their best dose. In the final, confirming phase, the optimized intervention is evaluated in a standard RCT to evaluate whether the intervention, as a package, is effective and whether the effect is large enough to justify implementation.

Alternative approaches include adaptive or stepped care interventions and time-varying adaptive interventions. In adaptive interventions the dose of the intervention components may vary in response to the characteristics of the individual client/patient or environment/organization. These varying characteristics are called tailoring variables (Collins *et al.*, 2007). A time-varying adaptive intervention looks at the sequencing of intervention components. Sequential Multiple Assignment Randomized Trials (SMART) are used to develop and evaluate time-varying adaptive interventions in which each individual is randomly assigned to conditions several times.

Integrating implementation into the modelling of complex interventions

So far we have focused mainly on the rational side of the health intervention: what is working and what is not? What are the active components? How are these components interrelated? But the degree of acceptance and willingness for change might be important factors to take into account as early as possible in designing a multicomponent intervention. Maier's Law postulates that the effectiveness of an intervention is the result of the quality of the intervention multiplied by the acceptance of the intervention ($E = Q \times A$). So, even when the quality of the intervention is theoretically high, the effect might be zero if acceptance is zero. A suboptimal intervention might be preferred as this would lead to greater acceptance. The strategy should be to influence the acceptance level of an intervention by choosing complementary interventions targeted at increasing willingness to change.

The first approach is to evaluate the impact of an intervention to individuals (patients or health professionals) and organizations. A useful model is the Normalization Process Model (NPM) (May *et al.*, 2009). May *et al.* define normalization as the willingness to integrate the new innovation into daily practice. It is the opposite of rejection, in which people refuse to implement the new innovation. It is different from adoption, in which people pretend to use the new innovation but in fact do not. It is clear that when the impact of the new intervention on the daily lives of people is very high, the resistance to change might be high too, which would require much more effort to implement the change. See May (Chapter 30) for further details.

A second approach that is used in PRIME studies (Process Modelling in Implementation Research) (Walker *et al.*, 2003) is that every component is unravelled using psychological theories that are helpful to describe, understand and influence the behavioural change of the individual health professional or patient: motivational theories, action theories and stage of change theories.

A third approach is to evaluate the reach and adoption of an intervention (Box 12.2). The RE-AIM framework developed by Glasgow *et al.* (1999) has five useful domains (Reach, Effectiveness, Adoption, Implementation and Maintenance) and evaluates the way the intervention is really practised, has a measurable effect, is well adopted by organizations and providers, has good compliance, and is well integrated into the health system. If the intervention is widely spread or not well used in practice, a root cause analysis could be useful to evaluate the bottlenecks for implementation and to revise the intervention to get better acceptability.

BOX 12.2 CASE STUDY: A LEAN CARE PATHWAY FOR CATARACT SURGERY

Van Vliet *et al.* (2010) describe the introduction of a lean care pathway for cataract surgery in the Rotterdam Eye Hospital. The main goal was to improve quality of care while reducing costs. The intervention consisted of four major components based on the existing evidence and lean management: (1) a one-stop pre-assessment; (2) the formulation of a surgical plan based on the patient record instead of seeing the patient; (3) a next-day telephone review by a nurse; and (4) a final review four weeks after surgery by an optometrist. Follow-up by an ophthalmologist is the exception and only for those cases where there is a strong indication. Therefore decision rules were developed to refer patients to eye surgeons when required. The implementation of the new pathway was successful: 58 per cent of the patients were seen in a one-stop pre-assessment (compared with 32 per cent before). For 68 per cent of the patients, the surgical plan was formulated on the patient record compared with only 12 per cent before. Sixty per cent had a telephone review by nurses, compared with earlier when 100 per cent of the patients were seen by the cataract surgeons themselves. Forty-two per cent had their final review by an optometrist. Although the results are impressive, they are less so than expected. Based on the decision rules, 90 per cent of the patients' surgical plans could have been based on the patient record only; 82 per cent of the patients could have had their review by telephone; and 84 per cent of the patients could have had their final review by optometrists.

A root cause analysis revealed the reason for this. Although they appreciated that they could do more surgery (performance increased by 18 per cent) and waiting times decreased, eye surgeons missed the contact they previously had with their patients. They missed seeing the results of their work. They missed the patients' gratitude. So acceptance was not high and they took any opportunity to deviate from the preset decision rules. They insisted that they wanted to see patients personally, mainly to confirm the refractive aim of the surgery. They ordered self-reviews (reviews by patients themselves), mainly during Friday surgery sessions, because on Saturdays no nurses were available to conduct telephone reviews. As optometrists were a shared resource in the hospitals, administrative staff booked optometrist reviews when they were available. If not they booked a review by the ophthalmologist.

Based on the root cause analysis, the documentation of the refractive aim was shifted to ophthalmic screening in the pre-assessment phase. Optometrist capacity was increased. Telephone review by nurses was also organized on Saturdays. And most importantly, eye surgeons received a copy of the booking appointment when patients were seeing the optometrist for final review so that they could also come along to say hello. This was highly appreciated by surgeons as well as patients, and increased the acceptability and delivery of the intervention.

Conclusion

There is growing understanding that the design of a complex intervention should get much more attention. If the new intervention is not well enough designed, then the overall effect will be weak. If it is not understood clearly how the intervention works, it will be difficult to replicate it and find consistent results. If the degree of acceptance is low, the effect will also be rather low. If the process flow is not well designed with a lot of flexibility and freedom in how the intervention is applied, the effect will be highly variable and strongly dependent on the context. The modelling scenario, described here, gives guidance on how to build a complex intervention by evaluating the existing evidence, installing a project team, getting consensus among stakeholders on crucial components, modelling them in a process flow to provide the necessary resources and describing them in concrete detail.

Many complex interventions have too many components. The result is that the intervention is more complex, less understood and therefore much harder to realize. The MOST approach is therefore very useful. It makes us realize that adding components increases complexity exponentially. Evaluating the acceptability of the intervention and taking away potential barriers will leverage the overall effect. Also, these 'facilitating' components should be part of the intervention. The more these elements are built into the intervention from the start, the less dependent the intervention will be on the context and the more it will reduce the variability of the effect.

Investigating feasibility and undertaking pilot testing of complex interventions

Introduction to Section 2

David A. Richards

As we turn the page to the beginning of this next section we have come to the point in describing any programme of research where we can no longer avoid addressing the need to collect primary data. In the last section we addressed how one might go about identifying the building blocks to develop a complex intervention. We discussed theory selection or postulation, various methods of evidence synthesis, outcome measure selection and the modelling of both the intervention and research implementation processes. One might imagine that this should be sufficient effort to go ahead and evaluate our proposed intervention using the best possible design adapted to the particular intervention and its contextual circumstances.

Unfortunately, we would be wrong. One of the major drivers behind the development of guidance for researching complex interventions (Medical Research Council, 2008) was the recognition in the clinical trials community that too many trials were failing to deliver clear results. Too little preparatory empirical work on intervention design, methodological choices and research procedures can lead to failed studies – not failed in the sense of producing a negative result; negative results are important findings in their own right – but failed because they did not deliver clear results. Poor design choices, low levels of recruitment, significant attrition, lack of intervention fidelity, and interventions unacceptable to those delivering or receiving interventions can all lead ultimately to research projects that deliver inconclusive results. In this regard they are both wasteful (Chalmers and Glasziou, 2009) and unethical.

Consuming resources (often although not exclusively publicly funded), seeking the involvement of patients or members of the public in experimental interventions, subjecting them to the burden of increased assessment, and asking busy clinicians to engage in different and unfamiliar complex behaviours, only to have to report, 'more research is needed' is a disaster for research funders, investigators, participants and the health and social care community. Many of these problems and their invidious effects can be eliminated or at the very least minimized by prior feasibility and pilot testing of complex interventions.

The MRC guidance pays much attention to recommending how to prevent the potential problem of failed trials. In this section of this book we expand on this guidance and offer a series of short chapters addressing solutions to the major pitfalls facing any complex interventions researcher.

We start with a chapter written by Lora Giangregorio and Lehana Thabane, who give an overview of the role and function of feasibility and pilot trials. They consider definitional differences, if indeed they exist, between studies that test the feasibility of an intervention and those that pilot a full trial. They make the hugely salient point that by undertaking pilot or feasibility studies, investigators can improve the chances of a large, expensive study successfully achieving its objectives. They also point out that feasibility and pilot studies start from carefully constituted questions, have explicit criteria for success, and should be reported with all the thoroughness of any other piece of clinical research.

The next few chapters address some of the issues raised by Giangregorio and Thabane in more detail. First, Rod Taylor and colleagues consider methodological uncertainties. What sort of design should one use in a feasibility or pilot trial and how can this help us determine the best design for a full-scale trial? They take us through the common methodological uncertainties (recruitment, randomization, retention/drop out, blinding and data collection/outcome assessment) and provide examples of methods we can use to monitor each of these methodological issues. They address one of the main contentious issues in this stage of the complex interventions research process – to randomize or not – and show how different uncertainties can be addressed using different processes. They also expand on Giangregorio and Thabane's point about the need for explicit success criteria and give us clear examples of these as applied to the pilot or feasibility stage of the research programme.

Obioha Ukoumunne and colleagues then take us into a more technical world in which they show us how to estimate the parameters that may be used to calculate sample sizes for large-scale trials. They describe how the use of recruitment and retention rates in pilot trials can provide much-needed information for the design of full evaluations. They also provide us with a method to use pilot outcome data – binary or continuous – and the relationship between pre- and post-intervention data to estimate the sample size required in a future evaluation. One of the oft-heard questions in pilot trial design is, 'how many participants do I need?' These chapter authors help us to understand how one might answer this question. By gathering sufficient pilot data we are able to estimate the parameters on which trial evaluations can be powered with reasonable certainty, depending of course on factors such as the uncertainty around these estimates and issues such as likely clustering.

We then move on to the chapter by Shaun Treweek whose work on understanding barriers to and facilitators of recruitment into clinical studies provides important lessons for anyone considering undertaking an evaluation of a complex intervention (Treweek *et al.*, 2010). Here we have moved from methodological ambiguity to procedural uncertainty. He describes how either failing to recruit sufficient participants or problems with participant retention, can produce inconclusive results. As a consequence, the possibility of demonstrating important benefits to patients can either be overlooked or at the very least there can be delays in demonstrating the benefits of an intervention while we await further trials. In his chapter he describes what we know about barriers to recruitment and retention, and outlines strategies that investigators can apply to ensure participant recruitment is 'to time and on target'. He shows how feasibility and pilot studies can be used to predict and avoid recruitment and retention problems in any subsequent fully powered clinical trial of a complex intervention.

Our next contribution comes from Nancy Feeley and Sylvie Cossette who move us away from issues of research design and back to those pertaining to the intervention itself – clinical uncertainties. Given that feasibility and pilot studies generally address uncertainties of design, clinical content and research procedures, their focus on clinical uncertainties reminds us that no amount of theoretical modelling in the development phase can necessarily assure us that patients and health care providers will find the proposed intervention either acceptable or indeed feasible. They distinguish between research efforts to determine whether the intervention can actually be delivered as planned (feasibility) and work to test whether intervention recipients and providers view the intervention as appropriate or relevant (acceptability). These authors really get to the heart of complex interventions development and testing by showing how to pull apart the proposed intervention and subject it to rigorous investigation – not at this stage to test its effectiveness but specifically to determine its tractability and suitability for evaluation. To do this they emphasize the importance of gathering and analysing mixed-methods data.

All this information on methodological, procedural and clinical uncertainty can feel overwhelming. Therefore, we finish this section by including a chapter describing how one research team were able to use a modest amount of research funding to prepare the ground for a full-scale evaluation. To do so, they had to address multiple uncertainties around procedure, method and intervention design. This chapter is used to show how it is possible to undertake a pilot feasibility trial that addresses methodological uncertainty around future trial design, the sample size required to power a full trial, recruitment procedures and the acceptability of the intervention for recipients and providers. We have included it here so that readers can appreciate that, no matter how daunting, careful work at the feasibility and piloting stage can really reap rewards. As the chapter outlines, this work enabled the research team to undertake a full-scale clinical trial of their complex intervention successfully in an area where many other trials have failed to deliver.

All the chapters in this section, but especially the last one, lead us neatly to one place. Feasibility and piloting is not an end in itself. It is part of a story – the development, testing, evaluation and implementation of complex interventions. There are now three possible options: (1) the results of feasibility and piloting show that the intervention is unacceptable or impossible to evaluate and researchers may choose to withdraw from further work on it; (2) the intervention requires further development, in which case the proper reaction is to return to the previous development stage perhaps to re-examine the theoretical or pathway model, or to conduct further advanced syntheses to search for knowledge on intervention components and their effects; (3) if all has gone well, move to full-scale evaluation. Ultimately, option three is the prize. Only by the proper and fair testing of new complex interventions can they be prepared for implementation into routine practice for the benefit of those whose well-being will be improved by receiving or applying the interventions to their health problems. We have already covered the development of complex interventions in Section 1 of this book. At the end of Section 2, therefore, we move to the next stage – evaluation.

13

PILOT STUDIES AND FEASIBILITY STUDIES FOR COMPLEX INTERVENTIONS

An introduction

Lora M. Giangregorio and Lehana Thabane

Never fly the 'A' model of anything.
— Second World War pilot officer Edward Thompson
of 433 (RCAF) Squadron

Introduction

The consequences of flying an 'A' model plane may appear obvious, but what is the harm in letting your brilliant research idea 'fly'? Researchers can fall victim to the planning fallacy, where they underestimate the time, cost and potential pitfalls or risks of executing a research study, and fail to test the 'model A' of the study (or elements of the study that are new or untested in the researchers' hands) before full-scale execution.

Landing a plane smoothly requires a good pilot. The same could be said for launching a clinical trial of a complex intervention. Conducting a pilot or feasibility study is often an essential step in the planning and implementation of a clinical trial. We would like to introduce the concepts 'pilot study' and 'feasibility study' in the context of clinical trials, and provide examples relevant to researchers planning complex interventions.

Learning objectives

- Be able to define pilot and feasibility studies.
- Appreciate the role of feasibility and pilot studies in complex interventions research.
- Understand some of the key considerations for the design of pilot or feasibility studies.

Definitions and objectives of pilot or feasibility studies

One definition of the word 'pilot' in the online Oxford Dictionary (http://www.oxforddictionaries.com/definition/english/pilot?q=pilot) is: 'test (a scheme, project, etc.) before introducing it more widely'. A pilot study has also been defined in epidemiology and statistics dictionaries as a small-scale 'test of the methods and procedures to be used on a larger scale if the pilot study demonstrates that the methods and procedures can work' (Last, 2001); or 'investigation designed to test the feasibility of methods and procedures for later use on a large scale or to search for possible effects and associations that may be worth following up in a subsequent larger study' (Everitt, 2006).

The concept of a feasibility study is not unique to clinical research. In fact, feasibility studies are often part of project planning and management in business and engineering ventures, where the goals include developing your ideas into a practice, product or service, identifying the strengths and weaknesses of the venture, as well as informing the plan for business operation and growth, which may include an evaluation of process or revenue needed to meet operating expenses (Georgakellos and Macris, 2009). It can also be used to provide convincing evidence of the viability of the business plan to investors, which in research is analogous to convincing grant reviewers that your team is capable of conducting the research as proposed. In essence, before launching a clinical trial, one needs to think carefully about the potential obstacles that would prevent the trial from being a success (e.g. low recruitment, poor retention), or the pieces of information needed to finalize the study design (e.g. variability in outcome measures). Pilot or feasibility studies are designed to address these potential roadblocks or information needs.

Pilot study versus feasibility study – are they the same thing?

Feasibility studies and pilot studies are often used as synonyms, but have also been defined as distinct entities (Arain *et al.*, 2010). Although several of the characteristics of each, or the rationales for doing them, are similar, the following descriptions outline our interpretation of the distinctions between pilot and feasibility studies that have been suggested previously (Arain *et al.*, 2010).

A *pilot study* is often defined as a small-scale study or smaller replica of a study to test the proposed study design or methodology. A pilot study will employ the same protocol as the main trial being planned and will have an assessment of the primary outcome similar to the main trial. A pilot study tests how well the main study processes will *work together* when the trial protocol is launched, and often evaluates outcomes related to those processes, e.g. recruitment rates, timelines for assessment, successful intervention delivery or follow-up.

A *feasibility study* is 'pre-study' research that is done to gather pieces of information needed to formulate the plan for the main study. The research questions asked in a feasibility study are usually centred around discrete aspects of the study processes or design, e.g. the number of potentially eligible participants and the number who agree to participate, ability to retain participants throughout the follow-up period, the estimated variability in an outcome measure in the population of interest, estimated timelines for study visits or assessments, or adherence of team members to the protocol (Haynes *et al.*, 2006). However, a feasibility study may not necessarily be a randomized trial, or resemble the protocol for the main trial, or assess the same outcomes.

Whether or not pilot and feasibility studies are synonymous, they have a similar aim: *to inform the development and conduct of a planned research project.* Regardless of your position on the need for a distinction between the terms, the emphasis should be placed on carefully defining the research question(s) you are addressing. The research question(s) will dictate the design of the pilot or feasibility study. Some questions about study process or methodology are best tested in the context of a smaller-scale version of the full protocol. However, for some research questions, it may be possible, or more appropriate, to answer them without testing the entire protocol. For example, a more realistic estimate of a screening to recruitment ratio for a trial with seven clinic visits may be obtained if you are testing whether people will agree to participate in a pilot with seven clinic visits, rather than if you simply test to see whether it is feasible to get them to agree to one clinic visit. However, obtaining an estimate of the number of potentially eligible participants for a trial may simply require a feasibility study that monitors a population for a discrete period of time and records how many participants are eligible. In other words, the importance of testing 'feasibility' aspects in a small replica of the full trial, or pilot, depends on what you are testing.

BOX 13.1 COMPLEX INTERVENTION DESIGN EXAMPLE

You are designing a clinical trial of a complex intervention with three components – each participant will have a session of motivational interviewing delivered by a physical therapist, will attend a group-based education session and will be asked to complete a written action plan for exercise. The intervention will be delivered on one occasion, and you are evaluating its effect on quality of life and activity levels six months later. You would like to test the feasibility of intervention delivery, with process outcomes of time taken to deliver each component (and variability around that estimate) and percentage of components completed. You could recruit a convenient sample of individuals comparable to your target population to receive the intervention. If your only research questions pertain to the feasibility of intervention delivery, it would not be necessary to conduct a six-month follow-up similar to the trial you are planning.

Some things to consider in designing pilot or feasibility studies

- *Criteria for success*: Just as hypothesis testing requires a clearly defined hypothesis and alternative or null hypothesis, feasibility or pilot studies should have clearly defined 'criteria for success' a priori (Thabane *et al.*, 2010). One cannot ask 'Is it feasible?' or 'Will our plan for the trial be a success?' in an unbiased way without having a predefined idea of what feasibility or success is. Feasibility goals, or criteria for success, should be balanced between what is ideal and what is realistic, and the outcome may be: (1) not feasible; (2) feasible with modification or monitoring; or (3) feasible as is. Similarly, for a pilot study that is testing the success of protocol elements in the context of a trial, the outcome might be to decide whether the trial or certain elements are not possible, possible with modifications to the protocol or close monitoring, or possible as is, based on the results relative to the criteria for success. *Example*: Our planned study requires 240 people to be recruited in one year, so it will be possible to reach the target for the full trial if we can recruit ≥20 people per month for three months to participate in the pilot. After the pilot study, it was discovered that ~15 people per month were recruited, so the team modified the recruitment timeline to 18 months to ensure the main trial targets could be reached.
- *Similarity of the design with the main trial*: A pilot study can be a randomized controlled trial, but doesn't have to be. If a pilot study includes an assessment of the primary outcome used in the main trial, and the protocols for the pilot study and the main trial do not differ to the extent that the assessment of the primary outcome might be affected, it is possible that the data collected can be used in the final analysis – this is referred to as an internal pilot (Wittes and Brittain, 1990), or sometimes informally as 'rolling' the pilot into the full trial.
- *Target population and sample size*: The population studied in a pilot or feasibility study should be representative of the study population or the population about which you wish to make inferences. For example, a pilot study should have the same inclusion/exclusion criteria as the main trial. A feasibility study should include participants that are representative of those about which you wish to make inferences. So for example, if the feasibility of intervention delivery and associated fidelity is to be tested, the participants could be those that receive the intervention *and* those that deliver it: the feasibility study should employ the people that will actually deliver the intervention, and it should be tested on individuals with characteristics similar to the target population. The sample size for a pilot or feasibility study should be large enough to provide useful information about the aspects being assessed. Another strategy might be to use a 95 per cent confidence interval approach to estimate sample size (Thabane *et al.*, 2010).
- *Funding*: Granting agencies may fund a pilot or feasibility study if a case can be made for the need for the pilot or feasibility study and the importance of the main trial.

Examples of feasibility or pilot studies and their applications in complex interventions

By their nature, trials of complex interventions present additional complexity in design and overall processes when compared to the trial of a sole pharmaceutical intervention, so pilot or feasibility studies can be very valuable. Examples of areas where pilot or feasibility studies can be used to inform trials of complex interventions can be clinical, procedural or methodological, such as:

Clinical

- A pilot study could test the willingness of health care providers to contribute to the research or adhere to study protocols.
- Feasibility studies could be used to inform the development of the intervention, e.g. how and what to administer, who to deliver, what setting, documentation, standardization, how to introduce a complex intervention into a setting, how to maintain intervention fidelity (i.e. ensuring it is reproduced accurately and contains essential components), acceptability of intervention to patients, health care providers or other stakeholders.

Procedural

- A pilot study could evaluate the potential for recruitment, or the time and resources required for recruitment, retention and follow-up for a trial, or cluster randomized trial, which may be needed if the health care provider or setting is the unit of randomization (see example in Table 13.1 where recruitment of both family medicine groups and the individual physicians was evaluated).
- A feasibility study could evaluate the time and resources required for the delivery of complex interventions (which often involve multiple people or steps) or comparators.

Methodological

- Feasibility or pilot studies could be used to evaluate the responsiveness of outcomes, or feasibility of assessing outcomes, especially those that are subjective but important to patients, health care providers or researchers (e.g. satisfaction with intervention), or the amount of missing data.
- Feasibility studies could assess the preliminary safety of an intervention, or provide estimates of effect and associated variability in the effect. They could also assess the technical performance of new devices (e.g. biomedical) in practice.

We have outlined a few examples of published pilot or feasibility studies in Table 13.1. In all cases, the pilot or feasibility study identified areas where the plans for the main trial could be refined to improve the chances of success, or

TABLE 13.1 Examples of pilot studies involving complex interventions

Intervention (and comparator) (ref)	Feasibility/pilot outcomes	Area	Key findings
Single-arm feasibility studies – no randomization			
Diagnostic and treatment algorithms to optimize the use of antibiotics in nursing homes (no comparator) (Loeb, 2002)	✓ Staff adherence to algorithms ✓ Intervention usability/feasibility ✓ Barriers to completing the study	Clinical Procedural	✓ Poor adherence to algorithms → training revised, training videos, adherence logs, on-site visits added ✓ Algorithms were user-friendly and feasible in long-term care
Decision aid for individuals with stage IV non-small cell lung cancer, or NSCLC (no comparator) (Leighl et al., 2008)	✓ Decision aid acceptability/feasibility from patient perspective: amount, length, clarity of information, usefulness, patient anxiety, patient knowledge	Clinical Procedural	✓ Decision aid reports as useful, knowledge improved ✓ Despite clear statements that there were no curative therapies, patients reported that NSCLC was curable ✓ Prognostic information was upsetting, patients said that need to maintain/promote hope is essential ✓ Challenge to protect hope without being misleading remains
A wearable haemodialysis device for patients with end-stage renal failure (no comparator) (Davenport et al., 2008)	✓ Safety (e.g. adverse changes in cardiovascular variables, electrolytes) ✓ Efficiency (e.g. flow rates, urea and creatinine clearance)	Methodological	✓ Fluid removal successful, blood and dialysate flow rates lower than conventional ✓ No adverse cardiovascular changes or changes in electrolytes, bubbles noted in dialysate compartment ✓ Clotting occurred in patients not receiving adequate anticoagulants, one instance of dislodged needle → safety mechanisms successfully engaged ✓ Reported recovery time less than conventional

Randomized controlled pilot trials

Study			
DECISION+ continuing medical education programme to optimize antibiotic use in primary care – three interactive workshops, reminders and feedback (compared with delayed intervention) (LeBlanc et al., 2011)	✓ Recruitment of: family medicine groups, individual physicians ✓ Satisfaction of participants ✓ Amount of missing data	Procedural Methodological	✓ Some, but not all criteria for success were reached ✓ Areas for improving future trials in this area were identified, e.g. more realistic expectations for response rates, expand inclusion criteria, less demand on physicians' time
Effect of skin-to-skin care on the initiation and duration of breast feeding (compared with routine care) (Carfoot, 2004)	✓ Successes and challenges in processes ✓ Recruitment rates ✓ Response of outcomes to intervention ✓ Time required for on-call	Clinical Procedural Methodological	✓ Higher than anticipated consent rate ✓ Several participants not randomized → change procedures ✓ Success rate for routine care higher than anticipated → inform sample size calculation ✓ Loss to follow-up was 13% ✓ Confirmed required number of research assistants and required duration of trial

TABLE 13.2 Some useful resources

Reference	Utility
Thabane *et al.* (2010) http://www.ncbi.nlm.nih.gov/pmc/articles/PMC2824145/	Definitions of pilot studies, proof-of-concept, adaptive designs, reasons for conducting pilots, challenges and misconceptions, sample size, criteria for success, frequently asked questions, ethical aspects, recommendations for reporting
The CONSORT Statement and extensions http://www.consort-statement.org/	Provides guidance on reporting of clinical trials, including checklists and templates for flow diagrams
The SPIRIT Statement and resources http://www.spirit-statement.org/	Provides guidance on the design and reporting of clinical trial protocols, including checklists and templates for summary tables
Arain *et al.* (2010) http://www.biomedcentral.com/1471–2288/10/67	Definitions of pilot and feasibility studies, types of outcomes, examples
Wittes and Brittain (1990)	Information on internal pilots
Tickle-Degnen (2013) http://www.ncbi.nlm.nih.gov/pmc/articles/PMC3722658/	Pilot studies in a rehabilitation context, definitions, typology, process, resource, management and scientific assessment when planning an RCT

conduct the trial more efficiently. An additional benefit of pilot or feasibility studies of complex interventions is the opportunity to engage knowledge users in the research process – to participate in integrated knowledge translation. By engaging the knowledge users early in determining the feasibility of the research, as well as the feasibility of implementing the complex intervention, there is increasing chance that the research will actually inform a change in practice.

Reporting the findings of pilot or feasibility studies

Researchers can and should choose to publish the results of a pilot or feasibility study. Given the work that goes into conducting clinical trials, publishing a pilot or feasibility study serves the researcher well because they can be productive during the pilot/feasibility phase, and it serves the scientific community well because they can learn from the team's mistakes and successes.

To ensure thorough and transparent reporting, guidelines for reporting exist for clinical trials developed by the Consolidated Standards of Reporting Trials (CONSORT) working group (http://www.consort-statement.org/). There is a need for consensus on reporting guidelines specific to pilot/feasibility studies; a CONSORT working group to develop an extension for pilot studies has been established, but the reporting guidelines were not available at the time this book chapter was being written. We have previously published a detailed overview of pilot studies, their interpretation and guidance on their conduct and reporting (Thabane *et al.*, 2010), which is the first on the list of useful resources in Table 13.2.

Conclusions

In summary, pilot or feasibility studies can improve the chances that a large, expensive study will successfully achieve its objectives so that valid inferences can be made from the research. Pilot or feasibility studies may help engage the knowledge users in the creation of knowledge, which may not only increase the chance that the research objectives are met, but also may lead to successful implementation in practice.

14

HOW TO USE FEASIBILITY AND PILOT TRIALS TO TEST ALTERNATIVE METHODOLOGIES AND METHODOLOGICAL PROCEDURES PRIOR TO FULL-SCALE TRIALS

Rod S. Taylor, Obioha C. Ukoumunne and Fiona C. Warren

Introduction

Feasibility and pilot studies play a key role in health research in providing information for the planning of full-scale randomized controlled trials (RCTs). The UK Medical Research Council (MRC) guidance states that pilot and feasibility studies are essential in the development and testing of an intervention prior to a large-scale evaluation (Medical Research Council, 2008). Before committing investment in costly and time-consuming full-scale trials, funding bodies increasingly demand that investigators provide evidence from pilot/feasibility studies addressing the question: 'Can this full-scale trial be done?'

As described in other chapters in this section on pilot studies, there are many uncertainties that can be addressed in a feasibility/pilot study in order to answer the question of whether a full-scale trial scale trial can be done (or not). Often these are issues to do with the intervention itself, e.g. whether a newly developed intervention package has been appropriately assembled, whether the intervention is acceptable to trial participants and clinicians, or whether the intervention can be implemented in the setting of the main trial setting. In this chapter we seek to focus on uncertainties in methodology and methodological procedures that need to be addressed before preceding to a full-scale trial, e.g. whether the proposed battery of outcome assessments and tests will be acceptable to trial participants or whether the assessment of the primary outcome can be blinded.

Learning objectives

*   To identify the common methodological uncertainties in the design and execution of full-scale trials.

- To review approaches to testing these methodological uncertainties in feasibility/pilot studies.
- To discuss the design and selection of feasibility and pilot studies to best address these uncertainties.

These objectives are illustrated by reference to two recent feasibility/pilot studies (Boxes 14.1 and 14.2).

BOX 14.1 THE DOCTOR-DELIVERED PHYSICAL ACTIVITY INTERVENTION (DDELPHI) FEASIBILITY STUDY (WARREN *ET AL.*, 2014)

The DDELPHI feasibility study aimed to inform the design and conduct of full-scale trials to assess the clinical effectiveness of delivering two interventions (brief advice from GP or brief advice from GP plus a pedometer to self-monitor physical activity), to promote physical activity in inactive individuals identified in primary care compared with control (written advice alone). The starting point of this study was that 29 per cent of UK trials in primary care recruited as planned, with 50 per cent requiring longer than planned. Delays in participant recruitment can occur at the level of the practice or the individual trial participant. For example, GPs may delay recruitment if they were randomizing individually as this is more demanding for them than clustering, i.e. they give the same intervention to all patients. Therefore, the feasibility study set out to examine whether recruitment and loss to follow-up could be influenced by controlling two methodological factors: (i) recruitment strategy (opportunistic: approaching patients attending their GP surgery; or systematic: approaching patients selected from practice lists by letter); and (ii) randomization method (individual or cluster (by general practice)). In addition to randomizing participants to one of the two intervention groups or control, this feasibility RCT study employed a factorial design, randomizing practices to one of the two recruitment and participant randomization methods (Figures 14.1a, 14.1b).

The DDELPHI investigators found that opportunistic recruitment was associated with less time to target recruitment compared with systematic (mean difference 55 days, 95 per cent confidence interval 6 to 104) but was also associated with a greater loss to follow-up (28.8 per cent vs. 6.9 per cent). There appeared to be no difference in participant recruitment time between cluster and individual randomization methods. The difference in proportions lost to follow-up between the two randomization methods was smaller than that between recruitment methods, and not statistically significant. The authors concluded that the interventions and an RCT design were feasible and acceptable to primary care staff and patients, and appropriate for evaluation in a

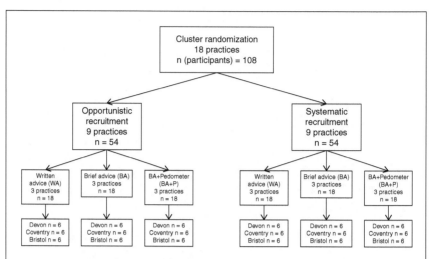

FIGURE 14.1a Cluster randomization and two different recruitment strategies

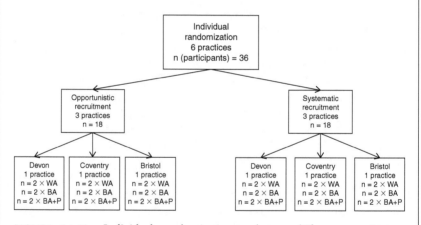

FIGURE 14.1b Individual randomization and two different recruitment strategies

full-scale trial. In designing a full-scale trial, randomization should be undertaken at the individual patient level as this is most efficient in terms of sample size and was not associated with any losses either in recruitment time or to follow-up. A full trial would need to consider the trade off between time to full participant recruitment and loss to follow-up in choosing an opportunistic or systematic recruitment strategy.

What are the common methodological uncertainties prior to full-scale trials and how are these addressed by feasibility and pilot studies?

Three reviews have empirically assessed the use of feasibility and pilot studies published over the last ten years (Arain *et al.*, 2010; Lancaster *et al.*, 2004; Shanyinde *et al.*, 2011). Two reviews were based on studies published across different time periods in high-impact general medical journals (including *British Medical Journal*, *JAMA*, *The Lancet* and the *NEJM*); one review included 90 pilot studies published in 2000 and 2001 (Lancaster *et al.*, 2004) while the second included 54 feasibility and pilot studies published in 2007 and 2008 (Arain *et al.*, 2010). The third review included 50 feasibility and pilot studies published between 2000 and 2009, randomly selected from 3,652 trial publications identified by searching MEDLINE and EMBASE (Shanyinde *et al.*, 2011). Across these three reviews, the common areas of methodological uncertainty tested in feasibility/pilot studies were: (i) recruitment; (ii) randomization; (iii) retention/drop out; (iv) blinding; and (v) data collection/outcome assessment. Table 14.1 shows examples of the methods for monitoring for each of these five methodological issues and the possible outcomes for each of these issues. Progression from pilot/feasibility study to a full-scale trial should be based on explicit criteria set out in advance (Thabane *et al.*, 2010). For example, the case study of the pilot trial of computerized cognitive behavioural therapy for the treatment of depression in people with multiple sclerosis observed much lower recruitment rates than predicted (Box 14.2). Although the investigators of this pilot trial did not explicitly state progression criteria, they did conclude that these recruitment findings compromised the feasibility of taking a definitive trial forward. Table 14.2 shows an example from a recent funding application of the rules for progression from the internal pilot to full trial dependent on three different scenarios for potential recruitment rate and intervention engagement outcomes.

BOX 14.2 COMPUTERIZED COGNITIVE BEHAVIOURAL THERAPY FOR THE TREATMENT OF DEPRESSION IN PEOPLE WITH MULTIPLE SCLEROSIS (MS) (COOPER *ET AL.*, 2011)

This external pilot trial of computerized cognitive behavioural therapy (CCBT) for the treatment of depression in people with MS was conducted to test the feasibility of undertaking a full trial. Before undertaking a full RCT, the investigators were concerned with the following uncertainties: (i) recruitment rates and practicalities of recruitment; (ii) withdrawal and loss to follow-up rates during treatment phase; and (iii) feasibility and acceptability of the proposed outcome measures. Following baseline outcome assessment, a total of 24 participants with relapsing remitting or secondary progressive MS were randomized 1:1 either to CCBT or to usual care. Outcomes were assessed pre-randomization and at 8 and 21 weeks post-randomization. Qualitative data were collected on all participants regarding how they felt about the processes of recruitment and randomization, reasons for withdrawal and burden of outcomes. The pilot trial achieved its target sample size, showing CCBT was well accepted by participants, and the intervention appeared to lead to larger reductions in depression symptoms than control. However, the pilot trial revealed a number of problems that impacted on the design and deliverability of a definitive RCT. Recruitment yield (4.1 per cent consented of all screened) was relatively low and the observed rate of recruitment (1.5 participants/month) was much slower than expected (7.1 participants/month). Participants expressed concern about the face validity of one of the self-report depression measures (Beck Depression Inventory II) and instead recommended an alternative (Multiple Sclerosis Impact Scale). The recruitment findings led the investigators to question the feasibility and practicality of undertaking a definitive trial as proposed and concluded that such a study would require participants recruited from 13 MS centres, and expansion of eligibility criteria to include either other neurological conditions or people with more severe depression.

TABLE 14.1 Methodological issues commonly tested by feasibility and pilot studies (from Arain *et al.*, 2010; Lancaster *et al.*, 2004; Shanyinde *et al.*, 2011) – examples of approaches to assessment and outcomes

Issue	Example approaches to assessment	Example outcomes
Recruitment	Monitor flow of participants with proposed recruitment strategy; compare participant flow across different recruitment strategies	Recalculate sample size; revise trial duration/ number of recruitment centres; revise trial costing; select most effective recruitment strategy
Randomization	Check fidelity of procedure (sequence generation and concealment); check acceptability of randomization to participants; check accuracy of stratification variables; check practicality of conducting proposed allocation method in trial setting; monitor number of participants who refuse participation because of randomized design	Refine randomization procedures, e.g. change the stratification variables or switch from telephone- to web-based allocation; provide further training on participant allocation for research staff

Issue	Example approaches to assessment	Example outcomes
Retention/dropout	Monitor number of participants at each follow-up point, i.e. assess withdrawal/ loss to follow-up; monitor differential withdrawal/ loss to follow-up across trial arms; seek participant reasons for withdrawal	Recalculate sample size; refine trial procedures to reduce dropout rates, e.g. provide opportunity for telephone/postal follow-ups for participants who find it difficult to attend face-to-face assessment visits
Blinding	Check whether assessors can determine individual participant allocations; check whether unblinded researchers can keep outcome assessors blinded	Refine blinding procedures within trial, e.g. emphasize to participants not to disclose their group allocation at assessment visits
Data collection/ outcome assessment methods	Assess adherence to interview schedule, questionnaire/ test completion; elicit views of participants on burden of assessment; monitor occurrence of missing data; review time duration of participants completing assessment; review choice of the primary outcome	Refine assessment protocol to reduce participant burden; revisit selection of primary outcome and update sample size calculation

Another issue that often arises in the design of trials of complex interventions is the choice of random allocation either at the individual participant or cluster level. Advantages of cluster RCTs over individually randomized trials include the ability to study interventions that cannot be directed towards selected individuals (e.g. the implementation of a new clinical guideline in a general practice) and the ability to avoid 'contamination' across individuals (e.g. an intervention to change the eating habits of school children may also influence the behaviours of their peers in the control group within the same school). However, cluster randomized trials have important disadvantages. They are more complex to analyse compared with individually randomized trials and usually require more participants to achieve the same statistical power. The DDELPHI feasibility study (Box 14.1) sought to address the question of whether it was practically more efficient to implement an intervention aimed at enhancing the physical activity of participants recruited through their general practice using cluster (by practice) or individual randization. This feasibility study assessed this question using the outcomes of the time to recruit participants and the level of outcome attrition.

TABLE 14.2 Example of rules of progression from internal pilot to full trial

Criteria	Scenario 1	Scenario 2	Scenario 3
Percentage of internal pilot sample size target (180 patients) recruited	<65%	65–79%	≥80%
Intervention engagement (percentage who access intervention at least once)	<65%	65–79%	≥80%
Proposed action	No progression to full trial	Discuss with Trial Steering Committee and funders about progression and resources needed to achieve target	Proceed to full trial

Selecting between feasibility and pilot studies to address methodological uncertainties prior to full trial

Although definitions in the literature of what constitutes a feasibility study versus a pilot study vary (see Chapter 13 by Giangregorio and Thabane), feasibility studies are typically described as having flexible designs and can encompass a variety of pieces of research to inform the design and conduct of the main trial. Feasibility studies for a full RCT are therefore often not randomized. In contrast, pilot studies are usually defined as 'miniature versions of the main study', and therefore help to inform the design and conduct of a full RCT and usually employ randomization (Arain *et al.*, 2010; Lancaster *et al.*, 2004; Medical Research Council, 2008; Shanyinde *et al.*, 2011).

A question that often arises in designing a study to address methodological uncertainties prior to full trial is whether the pilot/feasibility study requires a randomized controlled design. Single-arm non-RCT designs can have a number of particular advantages, e.g. larger numbers would be available that may include the collection of routine data; single-arm studies are generally easier to conduct, and it may be possible to undertake a more detailed qualitative study if all participants are receiving the intervention. Clearly, some issues cannot be satisfactorily addressed other than in the context of an RCT, e.g. the percentage consenting to randomization, attrition in intervention and control groups, the fidelity of the blinding process, and whether all components of the protocol work together. Given the burden of research governance concerning RCTs, it would seem sensible to evaluate specific methodological issues of a protocol using simpler studies wherever possible. Table 14.3 summarizes those methodological issues that require piloting in the context of an RCT and those that would be adequately addressed by a non-RCT feasibility study.

TABLE 14.3 Methodological issues requiring evaluation in the context of a pilot randomized controlled trial design

Issue	Need for pilot randomized controlled trial (RCT) design	Comments
Recruitment	Uncertain	Referrals may depend on the trial context
		If more than one candidate recruitment strategy, consider random comparison of strategies
Randomization procedure	Yes	By definition, testing randomization procedures requires an RCT design
Cluster vs. individual	Yes	Consider random comparison of cluster vs. individual allocation
Retention/attrition	Yes	Rates of retention/attrition often asymmetric across the intervention and control arms of an RCT and depend on participant preference
Blinding	Yes	By definition, assessment of fidelity of blinding (participants, clinicians and outcome assessors) requires a two-group design
Outcome assessment		
Data collection	Uncertain	Willingness/incentive to provide outcomes may vary across intervention and control arms of an RCT
Outcome burden	No	Can often be assessed by qualitative methods (e.g. individual patient interviews) in a single-arm study
Selection of most appropriate outcomes	No	Can often be assessed by qualitative methods (e.g. individual patient interviews) in a single-arm study

An issue of feasibility or pilot study trial design in assessing methodological issues that appears to have been infrequently applied in the literature is the 'stratified-by-method' approach. For example, if investigators are uncertain about which of two methods of recruitment (strategy A or strategy B) is the more efficient, a pilot study could include two levels of randomization: (i) randomization of half the trial centres to recruitment strategy A and the other half of the centres to recruitment strategy B followed by (ii) randomization of participants to intervention to control. The substantive advantage of this stratified-by-method randomized design is that the impact of a particular methodological issue can be quantified in a less biased manner than simply comparing those centres that are non-randomly allocated to the two recruitment strategies. This method is not limited to pilot RCTs but could also be used in a single-arm (intervention) feasibility study where, for example, participants (all receiving the intervention) could be randomly allocated (before baseline outcome assessment) to complete their outcome questionnaires by paper by mail or online. The stratified-by-method approach is illustrated by the DDELPHI feasibility study, an RCT with a factorial design specifically aimed to address two methodological uncertainties (Box 14.2).

Summary

In addition to assessing issues such as intervention acceptability, pilot and feasibility studies provide an important opportunity to test alternative methodologies and methodological procedures prior to full-scale trials. Although pilot trials often default to a randomized controlled design, some methodological uncertainties (such as outcome burden) can be addressed using a single-arm approach. When needing to compare two or more methodological options (e.g. recruitment or randomization methods) for a full trial, investigators should consider designing the study using randomization to allocate these options across study units, such as trial centres.

Further reading

Lancaster, G. A., Dodd, S. and Williamson, P. R. 2004. Design and analysis of pilot studies: recommendations for good practice. *Journal of Evaluation in Clinical Practice,* 10: 307–12.

Shanyinde, M., Pickering, R. M. and Weatherall, M. 2011. Questions asked and answered in pilot and feasibility randomized controlled trials. *BMC Medical Research Methodology,* 11: 117.

Thabane, L., Ma, J., Chu, R., Cheng, J., Ismaila, A., Rios, L. P., Robson, R., Thabane, M., Giangregorio, L. and Goldsmith, C. H. 2010. A tutorial on pilot studies: the what, why and how. *BMC Medical Research Methodology,* 10: 1.

15

HOW TO USE FEASIBILITY STUDIES TO DERIVE PARAMETER ESTIMATES IN ORDER TO POWER A FULL TRIAL

Obioha C. Ukoumunne, Fiona C. Warren, Rod S. Taylor and Paul Ewings

Introduction

Feasibility studies are used to assess the practicality of definitive randomized controlled trials for evaluating health and health care interventions and to obtain information that is used to design those trials (Arain *et al.*, 2010). They play a major role in the development and evaluation of complex interventions (Craig *et al.*, 2008). One of the common objectives of feasibility studies is to obtain estimates of the parameters that are used to calculate the sample size for definitive trials.

Learning objectives

- To gain an overview of how quantitative data from feasibility studies can be used to estimate parameters that inform sample size calculation for definitive randomized controlled trials.
- To learn how to calculate the number of participants required in a feasibility study to estimate sample size parameters.
- To learn how to quantify precision in parameter estimates from feasibility studies.

This chapter describes how to obtain estimates of the parameters related to recruitment and retention that can be used to calculate the sample size for definitive trials. These are:

- number of subjects who are eligible for a trial;
- percentage of eligible subjects that participate;
- percentage of participants that provide data at follow-up,

and also parameters related to the outcome:

*   prevalence of binary outcomes in the control arm;
*   standard deviation of continuous outcomes;
*   correlation between baseline (pre) and follow-up (post) scores on continuous outcomes.

Subsections in this chapter are devoted to these parameters. They address how to calculate the sample size required in a feasibility study to estimate the parameters with a specified level of precision and how to quantify the precision in the parameter estimates. The focus is on the use of quantitative information from feasibility studies to inform the design of definitive trials, complementing the more qualitative approach described elsewhere. To illustrate our discussion we describe examples of two studies, a feasibility study (Box 15.1) and an external pilot study (Box 15.2), used to obtain information to plan definitive trials.

Recruitment and retention parameters

Several chapters in this book have discussed how qualitative data can be used to learn about parameters central to planning definitive randomized controlled trials, such as barriers to recruitment and retention. In this section a quantitative framework is used to show how data from feasibility studies can inform decisions relating to these aspects.

Number of eligible subjects

The number of eligible subjects identifiable from a given source (e.g. hospital inpatients, practice list) can be estimated from the feasibility study and used to inform the likely number of sites and/or recruitment duration that is required for the main trial. One might want to know, for example, the number of eligible subjects on a general practice database or the number of new eligible subjects that present at a hospital clinic during a pre-specified period. In the context of the STEPS study (Box 15.1), we would want to know the number of adults that have been newly referred for treatment from IAPT services during the recruitment period who also satisfy the eligibility criteria. In the DIAT study (Box 15.2), information is required regarding the number of eligible diabetic patients with a scheduled inpatient appointment during the recruitment period.

BOX 15.1 STEPS STUDY

Project STEPS was a mixed-methods feasibility study conducted to obtain information required to design a fully powered definitive randomized controlled

---

trial of the clinical and cost effectiveness of stepped care (intervention) versus high-intensity psychological therapy (control) for patients with depression. The participants were adults diagnosed with major depressive disorder, referred from Improving Access to Psychological Therapies (IAPT) services and awaiting psychological therapy in the county of Devon, UK. All patients referred by two IAPT teams over a nine-month period were approached via written invitation to participate in the study. It was anticipated that 1,500 patients would be invited to take part. Recruited participants had a baseline assessment prior to randomization. The main outcomes (which included the Beck Depression Inventory) were measured at baseline and six-month follow-up. The study sought to estimate the percentage of eligible subjects recruited, the percentage of participants followed up at six months, the standard deviation of the continuous outcomes at follow-up and the correlation between baseline and six-month follow-up scores for each continuous outcome.

To quantify the precision of the estimate of the number of eligible subjects it is appropriate to assume it follows a Poisson distribution. Where there are at least around 100 eligible subjects (Armitage *et al.*, 2002), we can use the Normal approximation to the Poisson distribution to construct a 95 per cent confidence interval for the parameter:

$$n - (1.96 \times \sqrt{n}) \text{ to } n + (1.96 \times \sqrt{n})$$

where n is the number of eligible subjects identified in the feasibility study. To demonstrate the calculations, assume the STEPS feasibility study finds that 1,500 eligible referrals have been made by the two IAPT teams during the nine-month recruitment period. Using the above formula, the 95 per cent confidence interval is 1,424 to 1,576 (i.e. $1500 \pm 1.96\sqrt{1500}$). Based on these figures we can extrapolate that the mean number of referrals made by a single IAPT team in a month is around 79 to 88.

Percentage of eligible subjects that participate

The number of eligible subjects and the percentage of these that consent to participate determine the number recruited to the trial. A sufficient number of eligible subjects needs to be approached in the feasibility study to estimate the participation percentage with a specified level of certainty. A precision-based sample size calculation is appropriate where one calculates the number of eligible subjects required to estimate the participation percentage with some pre-specified margin of error that is considered tolerable. For example, the investigators may want to be reasonably sure that the estimated participation percentage is no more than 10 percentage points away from the true value. The number of eligible subjects that we need to approach in the feasibility study (n) to estimate the participation percentage depends on both the true (unknown) participation percentage and the required margin of error:

$$n = \frac{15.37 \times p(100 - p)}{w^2}$$

where p is the assumed percentage that will be recruited in the feasibility study and w is the desired width of the 95 per cent confidence interval for the estimated percentage. The formula is based on the Normal approximation to the Binomial distribution, appropriate for making inferences about percentages (Kirkwood and Sterne, 2003). Greater numbers of eligible subjects are required the closer the true participation percentage is to 50, based on the Binomial distribution. In calculating the number of eligible subjects that need to be approached, one should conservatively err towards assuming the closest plausible value of the participation percentage to 50 per cent – for example, if certain that the recruitment percentage is at least 70 then assume this value in the calculation. As a guide, one could specify w as double the size of the margin of error (i.e. the maximum error) that is tolerable. The smaller the desired margin of error (i.e. the greater the precision) is for estimating the participation percentage the greater the required number of eligible subjects. Using the above equation, 97 eligible referrals are required to estimate a participation percentage of 50 per cent with margin of error ±10 per cent (i.e. $w = 20$).

We can quantify the margin of error with which the participation percentage has been estimated in the feasibility study by constructing a 95 per cent confidence interval:

$$p - \left(1.96 \times \sqrt{\frac{p \times (100 - p)}{n}} \right) \text{ to } p + \left(1.96 \times \sqrt{\frac{p \times (100 - p)}{n}} \right)$$

where p is the percentage of eligible subjects recruited to the feasibility study and n is the number of eligible subjects that were approached to participate. The formula used to calculate the required sample size is a rearrangement of this. Provided there are at least five subjects that participate and five that do not participate, the use of the formula is valid (Brown *et al.*, 2001). If the participation percentage in the STEPS feasibility study was estimated to be 5 based on recruiting 75 of the 1,500 eligible referred subjects, the 95 per cent confidence interval would be 3.9 to 6.1 per cent, calculated by substituting into the formula

$$5 - \left(1.96 \times \sqrt{\frac{5 \times (100 - 5)}{1500}} \right) \text{ to } 5 + \left(1.96 \times \sqrt{\frac{5 \times (100 - 5)}{1500}} \right)$$

Follow-up percentage

The follow-up percentage is a parameter of interest when planning definitive trials because, together with the number recruited, it determines the number of participants that will be assessed on the main outcomes used to evaluate the intervention. We can calculate the number of participants (n) that need to be recruited to a feasibility study in order to estimate the follow-up percentage with a specified level of precision using

$$n = \frac{15.37 \times p(100 - p)}{w^2}$$

where p is the assumed percentage that will be followed up in the feasibility study and w is the desired width of the 95 per cent confidence interval for the estimated percentage. Percentages that are closer to 50 will be estimated with poorer precision for a given sample size, so a conservative approach in using this formula to estimate the number of required study participants is to err towards the plausible value that is closest to 50 per cent. In the DIAT study (Box 15.2), the 120 participants the investigators planned to recruit is large enough to estimate a follow-up of 50 per cent with margin of error ±9 per cent (w = 18) based on the 95 per cent confidence interval.

BOX 15.2 DIAT STUDY

Project DIAT was an external pilot randomized controlled trial of a pre-clinic intervention (PACE-D) to help diabetic patients identify an agenda for their impending clinic appointment (Frost *et al.*, 2013). The study, conducted in two centres in Devon, was designed to provide the necessary information for the planning of a future definitive trial to assess the clinical and cost effectiveness of PACE-D. It was planned that the pilot study would recruit 120 patients with Type 1 or Type 2 diabetes mellitus who were due to attend for hospital outpatient appointment with a diabetologist. Participants were randomized to receive the PACE-D intervention immediately prior to their appointment (intervention arm) or to usual clinical care (control arm). Participants were followed up for six months, with data collected on HbA1c levels and patient-reported outcomes at baseline and three- and six-month follow-up. One of the main aims of the pilot study was to collect data to inform the estimation of the required sample size for a definitive trial. The study sought to estimate the percentage of eligible subjects that consented to participate, the percentage of participants followed up at six months and the standard deviation of the continuous outcomes.

Having estimated the follow-up percentage in a feasibility study, confidence intervals are constructed for the parameter using

$$p - \left(1.96 \times \sqrt{\frac{p \times (100 - p)}{n}} \right) \text{ to } p + \left(1.96 \times \sqrt{\frac{p \times (100 - p)}{n}} \right)$$

where p is the estimated percentage that is followed up and n is the number of recruited participants.

Outcome parameters

Prevalence of binary outcomes in the control arm

Sample size calculations for evaluating health care interventions in definitive randomized trials require quantification of variability in the study outcomes. For binary outcomes this variability is effectively quantified by the percentage of participants with the disease or health status of interest (prevalence) in the control arm; this is an important parameter to know and may be estimated in feasibility studies with a control arm. We use

$$n = \frac{15.37 \times p(100 - p)}{w^2}$$

to calculate the number of participants required to be followed up in the control arm (n) of the feasibility study in order to estimate the prevalence, where p is the assumed prevalence and w is the desired width of the 95 per cent confidence interval. Again, given the uncertainty in the true prevalence one should err towards the closest plausible value to 50 per cent for the calculation. In practice, the number of participants recruited and followed up in a feasibility study will often be too small to estimate the prevalence of the outcome with the level of precision that would be desired to inform the sample size calculation for a definitive trial.

Confidence intervals are constructed for the control arm prevalence using

$$p - \left(1.96 \times \sqrt{\frac{p \times (100 - p)}{n}} \right) \text{ to } p + \left(1.96 \times \sqrt{\frac{p \times (100 - p)}{n}} \right)$$

where p is the estimated prevalence expressed as a percentage and n is the number of participants in the control arm at follow-up.

Standard deviation for continuous outcomes

The standard deviation is used to quantify variability for a continuous outcome, and knowledge of this is required to calculate the sample size to detect differences in such outcomes in definitive randomized controlled trials. The sample size required

TABLE 15.1 Sample size required to estimate the standard deviation of a continuous variable to within a specified percentage of its true value based on the upper bound of the 95 per cent confidence interval for the parameter

% of true standard deviation	Sample size
5	850
10	234
15	114
20	70
25	49

at follow-up in a feasibility study to estimate the standard deviation to within some specified percentage of its true value is presented in Table 15.1 for different scenarios. In the DIAT study, the investigators anticipated that 60 participants would be followed up at six months. This would be large enough to estimate the standard deviation for a continuous outcome to within 22 per cent of its true value.

The formula used to calculate the sample size required to estimate the standard deviation in the feasibility study is based on rearranging the formula for the 95 per cent confidence interval for the parameter

$$\sqrt{\frac{(n-1)s^2}{\chi^2_{0.025,n-1}}} \text{ to } \sqrt{\frac{(n-1)s^2}{\chi^2_{0.975,n-1}}}$$

where s is the estimated standard deviation, n is the sample size used to calculate the standard deviation and $\chi^2_{0.025,n-1}$ and $\chi^2_{0.975,n-1}$ are the 2.5th and 97.5th quantiles, respectively, of the Chi-squared distribution with $n - 1$ degrees of freedom (Armitage *et al.*, 2002). These quantiles can be obtained from books of statistical tables and standard statistical software, such as Stata. The resulting confidence interval for the standard deviation is asymmetric, with a greater difference between the upper bound and the point estimate than there is between the lower bound and the point estimate.

In feasibility studies with two or more trial arms, the pooled standard deviation across the trial arms can be estimated. It is possible, however, that the interventions increase or decrease the variability in the continuous outcome, in which case one would ideally want to know the standard deviation in each arm. The sample size in the feasibility study may not be large enough to identify a clear difference in variability between arms. Furthermore, the standard deviation for each arm would be estimated with less precision as based on only half the participants in a two-arm trial if allocation is made on a 1:1 ratio, so a pooled estimate may generally be preferable.

TABLE 15.2 Sample size required to estimate the correlation between the baseline (pre) and follow-up (post) measurements on a continuous outcome with specified margin of error based on the lower bound of the 95 per cent confidence interval for the parameter

Correlation coefficient	Margin of error	Sample size
0.3	0.05	1316
	0.1	340
0.4	0.05	1137
	0.1	298
0.5	0.05	924
	0.1	247
0.6	0.05	691
	0.1	189
0.7	0.05	457
	0.1	130
0.8	0.05	247
	0.1	75
0.9	0.05	86
	0.1	31

Correlation between baseline and follow-up scores for continuous outcomes

In trials with a continuous outcome, a more precise estimate of the mean difference at follow-up between trial arms is obtained by adjusting this comparison for baseline imbalance on the measure (Vickers and Altman, 2001). This additional precision resulting from adjusting for baseline score can be factored into the sample size calculation for the definitive trial, resulting in fewer participants required in each arm. The calculation requires knowledge of the correlation between the baseline (pre) and follow-up (post) scores on the outcome, which may be obtained from feasibility studies that have followed up participants for a similar duration to the planned definitive trial. In Table 15.2 we present the sample size required at follow-up in a feasibility study to estimate the correlation coefficient with a specified margin of error, covering a range of hypothetical scenarios. For example, 130 participants would need to be followed up in the feasibility study to estimate a correlation coefficient of 0.7 with margin of error 0.1, based on the lower bound of the 95 per cent confidence interval for the parameter. The table shows that the margin of error is greater for smaller values of the correlation coefficient, so if using such a table to guide sample size determination in the feasibility study one should, conservatively, assume lower values for the correlation; precision can then be presented assuming the worst-case scenario. The sample size required to estimate a low correlation with a small margin of error, however, will often be unattainable in feasibility studies. The figures in Table 15.2 were calculated based on formulae for constructing confidence intervals for correlation coefficients (Altman and Gardner, 2000). The confidence interval for the parameter is asymmetric, with a greater difference between the lower bound and the point estimate than there is between the upper bound and the point estimate.

Discussion

This chapter has described how feasibility studies can be used to estimate the parameters required for calculating the sample size in definitive randomized controlled trials. Focus has been on methods for calculating the sample size that is required in the feasibility study itself and quantifying the uncertainty in the estimates of the parameters of interest. The quantitative approach used in this chapter complements the more qualitative approach described elsewhere regarding the recruitment and retention parameters. Taken together these chapters demonstrate the utility of using a mixed-methods approach to assessing feasibility.

Traditionally, sample size calculations have not played a role in the design of feasibility studies as these are not designed to evaluate the intervention, rather to obtain information for making decisions on the design of the definitive trial (Leon *et al.*, 2011). The need to obtain precise estimates of sample size parameters for use in definitive trials motivates the use of explicit criteria for calculating the required sample size of the feasibility studies. As there will often be several parameters of interest, a sufficient number of potential participants need to be invited to take part in the study to estimate all parameters with the required level of precision. In situations where the sample size for the feasibility study is less strongly dictated by practical limitations, one must make a judgement about the desired level of precision. The basis for this could be an assessment of how uncertainty in the estimated parameters translates into uncertainty in the resulting sample size calculation for the definitive trial. In other words, the more sensitive the definitive trial sample size is to a given parameter, the greater the precision with which that parameter needs to be estimated in the feasibility study.

Confidence intervals should be calculated for all parameter estimates as the size of feasibility studies is generally small (Browne, 1995). When subsequently using the estimates to design the definitive trial, their uncertainty should be formally recognized by carrying out sensitivity calculations in which different parameter values within a plausible range (informed by the confidence interval) are assumed to assess how sensitive the required sample size is to these (Kraemer *et al.*, 2006). In the context of continuous outcomes, it has been shown that using the point estimate of the outcome standard deviation from previous studies to calculate the sample size for new studies results in lower than nominal statistical power (Shieh, 2013). It may, therefore, be appropriate to use parameter values that result in larger sample sizes for the definitive trial than those using point estimate.

Whilst feasibility studies provide the opportunity to estimate sample size parameters, given the small size of such studies, ideally data from relevant routine sources, where available, will often be preferable. The estimates from the feasibility study would then be used to provide greater confidence in the routine data and to check that the setting and context in which the trial is based are not markedly different from those that provided the routine data used to inform the sample size calculation for the definitive trial. This issue is particularly relevant for cluster randomized trials where entire clusters (e.g. general practices) are randomized but outcomes are measured on individuals within those clusters (Eldridge and Kerry, 2012). This design is commonly used to evaluate the effectiveness of complex interventions. The intra-cluster correlation coefficient (ICC) (Eldridge *et al.*, 2009) for the outcome, which quantifies the similarity between participant responses from the same cluster, is a key parameter for sample size calculation for such studies. Because the sample size in feasibility studies is generally small, both in terms of the number of participants and the number of clusters, it is likely that the ICC will be estimated so imprecisely that the point estimate and confidence interval will be of little value in a sample size calculation for the definitive trial. An ICC calculated from a large relevant routine data set or the distribution of several previously published ICCs for similar outcomes at the same level of clustering would generally be more informative than a single ICC estimated from a small feasibility study (Adams *et al.*, 2004; Turner *et al.*, 2005).

We do not advocate the use of estimates of the intervention effect from feasibility studies to plan the sample size for definitive randomized controlled trials. The sample size in definitive trials should be calculated based on the smallest difference between the trial arms that is worth detecting (Leon *et al.*, 2011); this is informed by knowledge of the topic area. In rare cases confidence intervals for the effect size in feasibility studies may provide useful data, for example, on the plausibility that the intervention effect is of some specified size, but generally these small studies yield little information on the true intervention effect.

Notwithstanding efforts to quantify the uncertainty with which sample size parameters are estimated in feasibility studies, estimates of participation and follow-up may indicate an over-optimistic situation in feasibility studies, given the relative ease of conducting studies in smaller numbers of sites and the fact that host institutions may tend to be more enthusiastic than centres in the wider pool in regard to be used in the definitive trial. Trialists should be mindful that estimates from a feasibility study can potentially mislead the design of the definitive trial through imprecise estimation or changing contexts between those phases (Thabane *et al.*, 2010).

Further reading

Everitt, B. 2006. *Medical Statistics from A to Z: A Guide for Clinicians and Medical Students.* Cambridge: Cambridge University Press.

Ryan, T. P. 2013. *Methods of Determining Sample Size: Sample Size Determination and Power.* Hoboken, NJ: John Wiley.

16

ADDRESSING ISSUES IN RECRUITMENT AND RETENTION USING FEASIBILITY AND PILOT TRIALS

Shaun Treweek

Introduction

Recruiting and retaining trial participants, be they patients or health care professionals, can be extremely difficult. Many trials do not meet their recruitment targets, or do so only after extending the duration of the trial. Retention problems mean participants are lost to the trial and contribute little or no outcome data. These issues have important consequences: they may result in an underpowered trial which, in turn, may lead to non-significant results that nevertheless do not rule out the possibility of important benefits. This increases the risk that an effective intervention will be abandoned before its true value is appreciated, or leads to delay in demonstrating the benefits of an intervention while further trials are done. Ineffective interventions may remain in use longer than they should.

This chapter outlines what is known about barriers to effective recruitment and retention, strategies that can be used to address them and how to use feasibility and pilot work to predict and avoid future recruitment and retention problems.

Learning objectives

- To learn about the problems in recruiting to time and on target in clinical trials.
- To understand what is known about barriers to recruitment and retention.
- To gain an overview of strategies known to improve recruitment and retention.
- To learn how to test recruitment and retention strategies in feasibility and pilot work.

Background

Problems with recruitment and retention keep trialists awake at night. Among 180 National Cancer Institute (NCI) Cancer Evaluation Program-sponsored CTs started between 2000 and 2004 and closed to recruitment, 36 per cent of early-stage trials testing efficacy (called phase 2 trials) and 62 per cent of final efficacy and safety trials (called phase 3 trials) did not attain their recruitment goals (Cheng et al., 2010). A study looking at recruitment to 78 primary care studies done in the Netherlands, including trials, found that almost 40 per cent of them had to extend their recruitment periods by at least 50 per cent (van der Wouden et al., 2007). A recent survey of the 48 directors of UK Clinical Trials Units (CTUs), units set up to provide expertise in trial design, conduct and analysis, rated recruitment as the top priority for methodology research (Smith et al., 2014). Retention came joint second with outcomes. This is understandable: a trial with no participants will fail regardless of how good the rest of the trial is.

Studies of recruitment suggest that around 50 per cent of RCTs fail to achieve their recruitment targets (McDonald et al., 2006; Sully et al., 2013; van der Wouden et al., 2007). In the UK, those with CTU support do better and about 65 per cent recruit to target (Sully et al., 2013). Around half of trials received an extension of some kind though many of these still failed to recruit to target (McDonald et al., 2006; Sully et al., 2013;). In many cases, trials may have to close prematurely due to recruitment problems (Foy et al., 2003). Once participants are in a trial, keeping them (i.e. retaining them) is essential given the challenges of recruiting them in the first place. It is generally accepted that a trial that loses more than 20 per cent of its participants will have its validity compromised (Schulz and Grimes, 2002), although Hewitt and colleagues (Hewitt et al., 2010) did not find evidence of bias in a small sample of trials with up to 28 per cent retention loss. More recent work suggests that losses of much less than 20 per cent can in some situations substantially reduce confidence in the reported treatment effect (Walsh, 2014). Bias is clearly introduced when retention losses are not random across the trial, such as when participants drop out at different rates depending on which treatment they received (called differential loss to follow-up), or where dropout rates are similar for each treatment but the reasons for dropping out are different. Poor retention also has a recruitment cost because trials routinely inflate the recruitment target to compensate for losing participants along the way (see, for example, Abbott et al., 2009; Craigie et al., 2011).

The reasons behind recruitment and retention challenges are not a complete mystery. A large review by Prescott and colleagues (1999) looked at the barriers to trial participation for both patients and health professionals. Key barriers for patients included:

* lack of time and the additional demands of the trial;
* patient preferences for one treatment or another;
* worries about uncertainty regarding treatment effect;

- worries about trial information (both too much and too little);
- information provided during the consent process put people off.

For health professionals barriers included:

- lack of time, both the pressures of normal clinical practice and of trial demands;
- perceived lack of importance of the trial;
- lack of staff and research experience;
- the difficulty of admitting to patients that they did not know which treatment was best;
- incompatibility of the trial protocol with normal practice.

It is worth noting that many of these barriers are practical (e.g. lack of time) or linked to information provision (e.g. the consent process) and therefore within the control of trial teams. Others have highlighted problems such as inaccurate estimates of eligible participants (van der Wouden *et al.*, 2007), the proportion of potential participants who agree to take part (Treweek *et al.*, 2014) and the ability of trial sites to actually start up and recruit participants (Dal-Ré *et al.*, 2011; Treweek *et al.*, 2014; Warden *et al.*, 2012). A meta-ethnography of qualitative work investigating people's reasons for taking part in trials (McCann, 2007) found that personal circumstances at the time of being invited to participate were salient to participation decisions, and that being able to perceive some personal benefit from trial participation was clearly associated with willingness to take part. Participation is not only, or even mainly, about altruism (McCann *et al.*, 2010).

Are there things we can do to improve recruitment and retention?

There are Cochrane systematic reviews of interventions to improve recruitment (Treweek *et al.*, 2010, 2013) and retention (Brueton *et al.*, 2013). Recruitment interventions have also been the subject of other reviews (Caldwell *et al.*, 2010; Fletcher *et al.*, 2012; Watson and Torgerson, 2006). Some interventions are effective in increasing recruitment (e.g. telephone reminders to non-respondents and use of opt-out, rather than opt-in, procedures for contacting potential trial participants). Financial incentives also look promising although these come with potential ethical problems. The effect of many other interventions (e.g. less information, video presentations, different types of people doing recruitment) is much less certain. A single-page summary of the effect of 40 recruitment interventions from Treweek *et al.* (2013) is shown in Figure 16.1. The retention review identified studies evaluating measures to increase response rates, which are relevant because many trial outcome data are collected on questionnaires returned by participants. Financial incentives were effective, and shorter, rather than longer, questionnaires seem promising but

Recruitment intervention [Reference ID]	Increase	Decrease	Little impact	Inconclusive
Trial design				
Open design[16, 32]	●			
Placebo*[59]		⊙		
Patient preference design[18]			⊙	
Zelen design†[25]		⊙		
Internet-based data capture†[42]		⊙		
Obtaining consent				
Process – opt-out approach[55]	⊙			
Process – consent to experimental treatment*[48, 50]			●	
Process – consent to standard treatment*[48, 50]			●	
Process – refuser chooses treatment option*[50]			⊙	
Process – physician modified chance of experimental*[48]			⊙	
Process – participant modified chance of experimental*[48]			⊙	
Form – researcher read aloud[56]			⊙	
Form – altered readability level†[19]			⊙	
Approach to participants				
Delivery – video presentation*†[28, 35]			●	
Delivery – video presentation plus written information[60]	⊙			
Delivery – audiovisual overview of trials[21–22, 33]			●	
Delivery – interactive computer presentation*[36, 44]				●
Delivery – verbal education session[45]	⊙			
Supplementing info – booklet on clinical trials*[23, 34]			●	
Supplementing info – study-relevant questionnaire[31, 37]			●	
Supplementing info – newspaper article[51]			⊙	
Framing – treatment as faster*[52]	⊙			
Framing – treatment as new*[38]		⊙		
Framing – emphasis on pain or risk*[54]		⊙		
Framing – positively or negatively*[43]			⊙	
Content – more detailed info (inc. total disclosure)*[27, 53]			●	
Content – financial disclosure of investigator interest*†[57–58]		●		
Telephone reminders[31, 49]	●			
SMS messages[26]	⊙			
Eligibility screening – face-to-face*[24, 29]				●
Eligibility screening – telephone*[20]	⊙			

FIGURE 16.1 Recruitment interventions and effect on participation

Eligibility screening – electronic self-complete*[29]		⊙	
Screening personnel[46]		⊙	
Financial incentives			
Cash incentive with invitation[26]	⊙		
Paid participation*†[17,30]	●		
Level of trial risk*†[17,30]			●
Training for recruiters			
Training lay advocates†[40]	⊙		
Education sessions†[39]		⊙	
Trial co-ordination			
On-site visits†[41]		⊙	
Additional communication†[47]		⊙	

Key: ● Multiple studies; ⊙ Single study
*Includes recruitment to hypothetical trial(s); †Includes result reported by study authors only (effect size not calculated).

FIGURE 16.1 *(cont.)*

much uncertainty remains (Brueton *et al.*, 2013). There were no studies evaluating methods to support participants' attendance at face-to-face visits, for example, despite these being a feature of practically all trials.

Avoiding recruitment and retention problems in your trial

Given the above, what's the best way to avoid recruitment and retention problems in complex intervention trials? In its framework for the evaluation of complex interventions, the UK Medical Research Council (MRC) strongly recommended that trialists do feasibility and pilot work prior to running a full-scale trial (Craig *et al.*, 2008). This is indeed where many future problems can be avoided. There is a stage before this though, which is when the intervention is designed.

Improving recruitment and retention through better design

It is important to remember that the nature of the complex intervention itself will have an effect on recruitment and retention. The more the intervention requires health professionals and patients to do, the more difficult it will be to recruit and retain participants. This is not rocket science: imagine having to choose between a single 20-minute phone call or a 12-week course of one-hour sessions at a location ten miles from your home. Which would be the easier to commit to? This is particularly important where trial participants are very ill, frail and/or elderly, children, or come from vulnerable groups such as people with mental disabilities. For these groups, repeated visits and measurements are almost certainly a substantial burden; for a frail elderly person, having to get in and out of a taxi twice a week may be more than enough to cause that person to decide against participation, irrespective of any other aspect of the trial, including the importance of the research question. Trialists should design their intervention to be as simple and unobtrusive as possible because, among other things, this will make recruitment and retention easier. It is useful to ask the following questions:

- How much time (especially direct contact time) will the intervention require from health professionals and patients?
- Is the intervention very different from current practice?
- Will the patient have to travel more, and more often, than would be expected in current practice?

If the answer to these questions is 'lots' then expect recruitment and retention problems. Trialists will either need to design away some of the problem (e.g. does the intervention *really* need five face-to-face sessions rather than, say, three to generate its effect?) or reduce the problem for participants (e.g. by providing free transport to face-to-face sessions, or by developing targeted help to support vulnerable groups and those considered most likely to struggle with participation). Similarly, anything that requires health professionals to do extra work is likely to be a potential problem; remember that providing clinical care is their top priority, not the trial. If taking part in a trial actually reduces their workload, so much the better (see Box 16.1). A useful toolkit for assessing the impact a proposed intervention might have on health professionals and patients, particularly the way they interact with each other, is available at http://www.normalizationprocess.org. This toolkit is based on Normalization Process Theory (May and Finch, 2009; Murray *et al.*, 2010), which is concerned with explaining what people do in their work and can be a good way of sensitizing a trial team to potential problems not only with regard to recruitment and retention but trial implementation more generally (see Chapter 30). As Donovan and colleagues found (Donovan, 2014), many recruitment difficulties arise because of issues among recruiters in terms of knowledge and views about evidence, equipoise, trial design, role conflicts, specialty interests and particular personal preferences. It would clearly be sensible to deal with these issues before the trial starts.

BOX 16.1 THE SCOTTISH BELL'S PALSY TRIAL

The Scottish Bell's palsy trial was a factorial trial of prednisolone, acyclovir, both agents or placebo for the early treatment of Bell's palsy (Sullivan *et al.*, 2007). The trial needed to recruit 472 patients, mainly through general practitioners. Bell's palsy is relatively rare and it was unlikely that an individual general practitioner (GP) would be involved more than once in the trial. It was essential that their role should be clear and relatively simple to carry out if recruitment was not to be a problem.

> Things were kept simple: recruiting GPs made the initial diagnosis and confirmed that the patient was interested in taking part in the trial. The patient was then referred to an on-call otolaryngology specialist. Taking part in the trial actually *reduced* the work GPs had to do because outside the trial they would normally follow up patients without support from hospital colleagues. Moreover, the patient got immediate specialist assessment which was not normal in usual care. Together, these two features made trial participation attractive to both GP and patient.

Feasibility and pilot testing

Having fine-tuned the intervention, trialists need to reassure themselves that their recruitment and retention strategies will be effective and that there still isn't something about either the intervention, the comparator or the trial procedures that will deter potential participants. This is what feasibility and pilot testing are for, although the two have different purposes. While feasibility testing of recruitment and retention strategies is always likely to be necessary, pilot testing, effectively a mini-version of the trial, may not be needed unless there are doubts about how the trial protocol as a whole works. General guidance about feasibility and pilot testing (and the difference between them) is given by Shanyinde (2011) and Arain (2010) and in the chapters by Giangregorio and Thabane (Chapter 13), Ukoumunne *et al.* (Chapter 15) and Taylor *et al.* (Chapter 14) in this section of the book.

Table 16.1 gives some example recruitment and retention research questions together with methods that could be used to address them. Some of these questions are best addressed as part of feasibility work but prior to actually trying to recruit any participants. An obvious example is finding out how many potentially eligible participants there actually are. This is more of a problem than might be thought. Indeed, optimism about this number is so common it has a name – *Lasagna's Law* (van der Wouden *et al.*, 2007) – and unfounded optimism about the number of eligible participants can easily threaten the feasibility of a trial. It is best to know early that a trial will need more sites, need to run for longer, or both, since doing this once the trial has started is time consuming and costly. Other questions in Table 16.1 can only be answered through actually trying to recruit participants, for example by evaluating alternative recruitment strategies. Some strategies may work but require a lot of effort and the trial team needs to use judgement as to whether that effort is worth it. Telephone reminders to non-responders, for example, are effective (Treweek *et al.*, 2010, 2013) but can be very time-consuming. Other strategies may recruit modest numbers but be so simple as to be worth doing anyway so long as they do no harm (e.g. constantly emailing people is easy and cheap but recipients might start to get irritated after a while). The comparison of strategies does not need to be randomized unless you are making a formal, methodological

TABLE 16.1 Example recruitment and retention questions for feasibility and pilot work

Focus	Example research question	Research methods that could be applied	Best juncture to collect data
Recruitment	How many potentially eligible participants are there per month?	Retrospective documentation/medical record check applying trial eligibility criteria at potential clinical sites. Best done very early in trial planning/feasibility work to plan how many sites will be needed and how long trial will need to recruit	Prior to active recruitment
	How engaged are staff with your intervention and trial?	Focus groups/interviews with key staff involved in recruitment chain, e.g. research nurse, doctor, receptionist	Prior to active recruitment
	What are the barriers to participants taking part?	Focus groups with individuals like those you intend to recruit to investigate potential problems and barriers to taking part	Prior to active recruitment
	What do potential participants think about the participant information materials and the consent form?	Focus groups with individuals like those you intend to recruit to investigate understanding of, and reaction to, your trial materials	Probably prior to active recruitment but could also be during it
	Are sites able to start recruitment?	Checking site's history of recruitment to trials. Monitoring of how long it takes for a site to start recruiting. Interviews with key staff to discuss any delays	Probably during active recruitment but could also be prior to it
	How many eligible participants are approached and invited to participate?	Qualitative analysis of observational data collected at potential sites, together with interview data from key individuals involved in recruitment chain, e.g. research nurse, clinical staff, reception staff, patients	During active recruitment

	How many potentially eligible participants agree to take part?	Compare number of eligible to number of consented participants. Qualitative analysis of interview data with recruiters and patients	During active recruitment
	Who agrees to take part?	Qualitative comparison of recruited and non-recruited individuals. Comparison across sites is also likely to be useful	During active recruitment
	Which recruitment strategy is most effective?	Quantitative comparison of the number of participants recruited through various routes. Also consider the resources involved (e.g. time, cost) per recruit	During active recruitment
Retention	How long does it take participants to complete your trial data collection forms?	Observation of participants completing forms/ interviews	Probably during active recruitment but could also be prior to it
	How many participants withdraw or fail to provide outcome data?	Quantitative evaluation of returns. May also interview individuals who failed to provide outcome data, or ask those withdrawing if willing to say why. Perhaps those who withdraw misunderstood some aspect of the trial	During active recruitment
	Are there differences in retention between sites?	Quantitative evaluation of retention rates. Interviews with key staff to discuss any delays	During active recruitment

comparison of two methods (see Graffy *et al.*, 2010; Treweek *et al.*, 2012); the judgement of the trial team, combined with some quantitative data about number of recruits and effort per recruit per method, is generally sufficient.

It is also worth thinking about retention during feasibility work. Almost all trials inflate the recruitment target to allow for loss to follow-up, sometimes by as much as 30 per cent. A trial with a sample size of 100 then needs to actually recruit 130 so that there are still 100 people providing primary outcome data at the end of the trial. An obvious way to reduce the recruitment challenge is therefore to increase retention, which is also sensible for validity reasons (Schulz and Grimes, 2002). One problem with retention testing may be that the main trial outcome is long-term (e.g. two years) but the feasibility work cannot run for this length of time because, for example, a funder is unwilling to fund such a long feasibility study. Retention data then become approximate and judgement is again required when extrapolating this to the full-term retention in a full-length trial. That said, if even short-term retention is poor, it is pretty safe to assume the trial has a problem. Finally, the research methods used for feasibility work are largely qualitative. Green and Thorogood (2004) is a good introduction as is Chapter 17 by Feeley and Cossette in this section of the book.

Feasibility studies of recruitment and retention strategies do not inevitably need to be randomized, and many of the research questions listed in Table 16.1 do not require it. For example, there is no need to randomize staff to be able to assess their attitudes to the intervention and trial procedures; what is essential here is that the sample is representative, not random. Randomization would only be essential if there was doubt as to whether randomization *itself* might affect the feasibility of the trial. This is most likely because of uncertainty around potential participants' willingness to have their treatment allocated by chance, which may be important if, for example, there are already strong preferences among potential participants for particular treatments. Pilots, mini-versions of the trial, will be randomized because they test the full version of the protocol.

How many participants are needed?

Feasibility and pilot work does not generally use formal sample size calculations to determine how many people need to be involved because these are studying process, not treatment effect, although it is possible to power studies on process outcomes (see Chapter 15 by Ukoumunne and colleagues). For recruitment and retention, what is needed are enough people to give the trial team confidence that the conclusions drawn from the data are sound. A target of around 60 is what trialists generally decide is enough, large enough to give meaningful results but not so large that the study becomes large, long and costly. It is also important to have a clear idea of what recruitment and retention results need to be achieved in the feasibility and pilot work before moving to a full-scale trial. For example, a trial team might decide that the following requirements must be met before moving to a full-scale trial:

- We are able to identify at least 100 eligible participants across two centres in a three-month period.
- Of these, at least 90 per cent are invited to take part in the study by staff, either face-to-face, or by mailed, SMS or telephone invitation.
- Of those invited, at least 50 per cent agree to take part.
- Of those recruited, at least 90 per cent complete the final three-month outcome measure (the full-scale trial would use a six-month outcome so this is a proxy).

The trial team will need to think about the thresholds; the above are examples, not gold standards. If achieved though, they need to lead to a feasible full-scale trial and the lower they are, the longer the full-scale trial will take. Some degree of pragmatism is required (e.g. what happens if the consent rate is 49 per cent?) and the requirements need to be taken together, not as individual 'all or nothing' criteria. Failure to meet many of the preset recruitment and retention targets though would mean the trial team would have to carefully consider whether going to a full-scale trial is sensible; sometimes the answer is no.

Conclusion

Recruitment and retention plans rarely survive contact with actual participants. It is best to make use of existing systematic reviews, other literature and local knowledge when drawing up your recruitment and retention plans and then to try them out in feasibility and pilot work prior to a full-scale trial. Recruitment and retention are challenging but much of that challenge is within triallists' control: an important research question and simple and efficient trial design will make recruitment and retention easier.

Further reading

Donovan, J. L., Paramasivan, S., deSalis, I. and Toerien, M. 2014. Clear obstacles and hidden challenges: understanding recruiter perspectives in six pragmatic randomised controlled trials. *Trials*, 15: 5.

Prescott, R. J., Counsell, C. E., Gillespie, W. J., Grant, A. M., Russell, I. T., Kiauka, S., Colthart, I. R., Ross, S., Shepherd, S. M. and Russell, D. 1999. Factors that limit the quality, number and progress of randomised controlled trials. *Health Technology Assessment*, 3: 1–143.

Treweek, S., Lockhart, P., Pitkethly, M., Cook, J. A., Kjeldstrøm, M., Johansen, M., Taskila, T. K., Sullivan, F., Wilson, S., Jackson, C., Jones, R. and Mitchell, E. 2013. Methods to improve recruitment to randomised controlled trials: Cochrane systematic review and meta-analysis. *British Medical Journal Open*, 3: e002360.

17

TESTING THE WATERS

Piloting a complex intervention

Nancy Feeley and Sylvie Cossette

Introduction

A feasibility or pilot study preceding an evaluation study or a clinical trial has two main purposes (Feeley *et al.*, 2009). The first is to examine the feasibility and acceptability of the design and procedures of the evaluation study. The second purpose is to examine the feasibility and acceptability of the intervention that will be tested in the evaluation study. This chapter discusses the assessment of the intervention. Assessment of feasibility is concerned with determining whether the intervention can be provided as planned, while an assessment of acceptability considers the appropriateness and relevance of the intervention for the intended recipients, the intervention providers or health care professionals involved in participants' clinical care (Feeley *et al.*, 2009).

Learning objectives

- To describe the goals of feasibility studies in the development and evaluation of complex interventions.
- To identify means to evaluate feasibility and acceptability issues in feasibility studies.

Background

A feasibility study is an essential step in the development and evaluation of complex interventions that should not be omitted. Evaluation studies are expensive from a cost and time perspective. Many funding agencies are hesitant to fund such studies without pilot work. Furthermore, assessing the feasibility and acceptability of the intervention is essential to optimize the intervention in preparation for testing efficacy. Serious challenges encountered in evaluation studies can be avoided if pilot work is undertaken. For example, an intervention program to prepare people for discharge from the emergency room sought to deal with patients' specific concerns about discharge to optimize their ability to manage these concerns, and thus prevent return visits to the emergency room. However, in the clinical trial to evaluate the intervention's efficacy, most participants wanted to go home immediately upon learning of their discharge, and were not interested in receiving the first session of intervention (Cossette *et al.*, 2013). This led to a decision early in the trial to adapt the intervention so that the pre-discharge intervention was very brief. Eventually, the findings of the trial indicated that this intervention was not effective in preventing return emergency room visits. Issues related to timing and dose may have contributed to this result, and could have been addressed earlier if a feasibility study had been conducted.

Major decisions about the features of the intervention, such as the content, timing and dose, are made during development phase. These major decisions arise from a review of relevant theory, available evidence and clinical experience (Campbell *et al.*, 2000). Ideally, inductive approaches such as case studies, focus groups, interviews or surveys with the recipients and providers are used as well to develop an intervention that will be acceptable to recipients. At the completion of the development phase, the intervention design has been determined and the next step is to test feasibility and acceptability. An intervention is considered acceptable to recipients if it is appropriate to address the problem, easily adopted and adhered to, effective in managing the problem, and the associated risks acceptable (Sidani and Braden, 2011). Thus, at the feasibility stage of the process the main research questions are: Can the intervention be provided as planned? Is the intervention acceptable to participants?

Examining intervention features in a feasibility study

In a feasibility study, the feasibility and acceptability of many of the key intervention features can be examined. Certain features will be more important to scrutinize than others. This will depend on the particular challenges that the researcher anticipates, and the questions that remain at the end of the intervention development phase. Examples of the key intervention features that might be examined and the associated study questions are provided in Table 17.1.

Who will be the focus of the intervention? Who will provide the intervention?

While some interventions target an individual, others are designed to be provided to the individual and their significant other(s). It is important to ascertain whether

TABLE 17.1 Feasibility study questions

Intervention feature	Possible questions
Who?	
Recipient	Can the intervention be provided to the intended recipients?
Provider	Who should provide the intervention (i.e. considering expertise, cost and transferability issues)?
	Which provider is more acceptable for the recipients?
What?	
Content	Is all the necessary content included in the intervention? Is it feasible to provide the content? Is the content acceptable to the recipients?
Sequence	Is the sequence of the intervention components appropriate, feasible and acceptable?
Dose	Can the dose of the intervention be provided as intended? Is the dose sufficient to bring about desired change? What is acceptable to the recipients?
Tailoring	Is tailoring of the intervention feasible? Which aspects of the intervention should be tailored (e.g. content, timing)?
When?	
Timing	Is the timing of the intervention feasible and acceptable?
Where?	
Setting	Is it feasible and acceptable to provide the intervention in the setting chosen?
How?	
Mode of delivery	Is the mode of providing the intervention (e.g. face-to-face, group or one-on-one, e-tech) feasible and acceptable?
Equipment or material for delivery	Is it feasible and acceptable to utilize the equipment needed to provide the intervention? Are the intervention materials (e.g. brochures, DVDs) acceptable?

it is possible to provide the intervention to the intended recipient(s). In a pilot study with acute coronary syndrome patients, one aim was to examine whether the patient's care-giver would also agree to participate in the intervention to modify the patient's cardiac risk factors (Cossette *et al.*, 2009). Participation of the significant other was not a requirement, but considered advantageous to increase the effects of the intervention. The percentage of caregivers who agreed to participate was documented. These data indicated that only a small proportion of patients had a significant other who agreed. It was not feasible to require another person to participate, so this requirement was omitted for the evaluation study (Cossette *et al.*, 2012).

A feasibility study could explore who should provide the intervention, comparing providers with different professional preparation, levels of education or experience to determine which provider might be most acceptable to participants. The issue of the transferability of the intervention into clinical practice should also be considered. Choosing a highly qualified provider may decrease the likelihood that the intervention would be adopted into clinical practice.

What will be the content, sequence, dose, intensity and duration of the intervention?

In many feasibility studies, the content of the intervention is scrutinized to ensure that all the necessary elements have been included. Intervention logs and a list of modifications made to the intervention manual can be helpful tools to track necessary content changes. Regular meetings with the providers during the course of the feasibility study, and interviews with providers and/or recipients during and after the intervention, can also identify gaps in content as well as determine the acceptability of the intervention.

Other aspects of the structure of the intervention might also be examined including the sequence of the components, dose (e.g. number of sessions), intensity (i.e. frequency of sessions) and duration of each session (e.g. hours). For example, an intervention for mothers of preterm newborns requiring neonatal intensive care consisted of two components (Feeley *et al.*, 2008). The first component aimed to reduce mothers' anxiety. A second component was designed to help mothers learn how to interact with their infant. Anxiety reduction was deemed a necessary first step to enable mothers in subsequent sessions to learn about their infant's interactive behavior. Based on the providers' observations of participants' responses during the pilot study recorded in the intervention logs, it was concluded that this sequence was appropriate.

In another case, while developing an intervention program for patients after a myocardial infarction, a needs assessment and clinical experience suggested that three major topics needed to be addressed: safety issues such as bleeding, symptom management and return to activities of daily living, and modification of cardiac risk factors such as diet and smoking. The plan was to include the content on safety in the first encounter while the patient was in hospital. The topics of symptom management and activities of daily living would be presented in the second encounter shortly after patients returned home. Risk factors were to be discussed in the third encounter after the other issues had been addressed, if participants had not raised this topic in previous encounters. Pilot work examined whether this sequence coincided with patients' needs (Cossette *et al.*, 2009). Findings indicated that the sequence was acceptable and feasible for the provider, and acceptable to patients as well. The sequence was retained for the clinical trial with excellent adherence (Cossette *et al.*, 2012).

The dose of the intervention is a critical intervention design decision. A balance must be achieved between providing an adequate dose of the intervention to effect the desired change, and minimizing the burden and costs to both the participant and the health care system. Treatment adherence is a challenge in the care of heart failure patients. An intervention was developed to address adherence, and the plan was for the intervention to be provided to patients and their caregivers in one hour during hospitalization to ensure transferability into practice (Belaid *et al.*, 2011). The pilot study indicated that this was feasible and acceptable, and this dose will be utilized for the forthcoming evaluation study.

An intervention was developed to decrease patients' anxiety and increase their acceptance of an implantable defibrillator to prevent sudden death, as a review of the literature showed that patients are highly anxious and have difficulty accepting the device. Patients were to receive the intervention just prior to discharge home. The acceptability of the timing of this intervention was assessed in a feasibility study (Charchalis *et al.*, 2013). The investigators found that soon after the procedure a large proportion of participants were not anxious, and were relieved to have the device. It was concluded that the intervention might be more relevant if it was provided after discharge when participants were no longer in the safe hospital environment and they had perhaps experienced an episode of being 'shocked' by the defibrillator.

An intervention can be standardized across participants, or tailored to the needs of each individual participant. If the intervention is tailored, an assessment of the feasibility of doing so is important. An intervention to promote care-givers' participation in the management of their family members' postoperative delirium in the intensive care unit after cardiac surgery was created (Mailhot *et al.*, 2013). Caregivers were offered a menu of possible strategies they could use while visiting their family member to orient them to time and place. Care-givers were also able to suggest other strategies that might help based on their personal knowledge of the patient. However, any strategies they suggested had to be feasible in the intensive care unit environment and acceptable to hospital staff. A feasibility study is underway, and shows that most care-givers select strategies from the menu. Very few proposed other activities, and only one of the proposed activities needed to be discussed with the staff to ensure acceptability. Thus, this approach to tailoring the intervention by care-givers seems feasible.

Where should the intervention be provided?

It is important to ascertain that it is feasible to provide the intervention in the setting where it is meant to be provided. The setting should be acceptable to both the recipients and their care-givers if applicable. The plan for the intervention program for mothers of preterm newborns was to provide the program to mothers at their infant's bedside in the neonatal intensive care unit (NICU), as some of the learning activities required mothers to observe their infant's behavior. However, in the pilot study it became apparent early on that in the open ward unit where the study was conducted there were many distractions and interruptions that made it difficult for the provider and the mother to have a discussion, and for mothers to observe their infants. Based on these findings, it was decided not to provide sessions at the bedside but rather in a private location (Feeley *et al.*, 2008).

How should the intervention be provided?

The feasibility and acceptability of the mode of provision of the intervention was examined in a pilot study for a web-based intervention program (Côté *et al.*, 2012). The program was aimed at helping people living with HIV manage their daily therapy. It involved a series of interactive, tailored sessions provided by a virtual nurse during sessions at a computer. The researchers found that participants liked interacting with the virtual nurse, and appreciated the practical advice they acquired. Nonetheless, some participants found that the first session took too much time because of difficulties registering to begin the intervention. Adjustments were required to streamline the registration process so that it was easier for participants with little computer experience.

A feasibility study is particularly critical when the use of equipment is required for the provision of the intervention. An intervention to reduce exposure to noise in children requiring pediatric intensive care hospitalization involved having school-age children and adolescents wear noise reduction headphones for one hour each afternoon (Rennick *et al.*, 2014). In their pilot work, the researchers soon discovered that although the headphones chosen were very effective in reducing noise, they were unacceptable to participants. Children reported that the headphones were uncomfortable and made them feel hot. Parents and staff complained that the headphones were too bulky to allow children to change position in bed or to lie on their side. None of the children wore the headphones for more than 20 minutes. The investigators eventually replaced the headphones with a soft headband that was acceptable to children, parents and staff.

Methods to evaluate the feasibility and acceptability of the intervention

In feasibility studies, mixed methods can be useful. Quantitative methods can contribute to an assessment of the intervention's feasibility and acceptability. Qualitative methods can also help to gain an in-depth understanding of participants' perceptions of the intervention and its specific features, as well as challenges implementing the intervention. Consider, for example, how to examine the acceptability of the intervention. What is the best approach to measure acceptability? Multiple types of data from multiple sources should be collected. Two possible indicators of intervention acceptability are the rate of enrollment of eligible participants, and the rate of retention. However, many other factors may also influence these rates aside from the acceptability of the intervention. Intervention logs are an invaluable tool to assess acceptability. Intervention logs document the details of intervention delivery to each study participant, and can be completed by the intervention providers, participants or others. These data can be analyzed to quantify the percentage of sessions provided as planned. Problems that arise and if and how these were resolved, participants' responses to the intervention, and reasons for withdrawal during the intervention can also be documented in intervention logs and content analyzed. There are also self-report questionnaires that measure intervention acceptability (Sidani and Braden, 2011). Although some information can be gleaned from such measures, most participants report that the intervention and its features are for the most part acceptable.

Qualitative interviews can be more informative to fine-tune the intervention for the evaluation study. Participants should be asked to share their impressions of all the intervention features (e.g. content, sequence, dose, tailoring, timing, setting and mode of delivery), as well as their perceptions of the intervention providers. Suggestions for modifications should be solicited. Participants who completed the intervention can be asked why they persisted. Moreover, whenever possible brief interviews with those who do not complete the intervention, to explore why they did not complete the intervention, can be enlightening. Data from all these sources are synthesized to arrive at an understanding of what aspects of the intervention require modification and how these should be altered to enhance acceptability.

Other questions to examine

If applicable, possible contamination and co-intervention should be examined in a feasibility study. Both contamination and co-intervention can pose threats to the validity of the evaluation study findings. Thus, it is important to determine whether these problems arise, and how they might be addressed before the evaluation study. Contamination occurs when participants in the control group inadvertently obtain the intervention, or part of it (Cochrane Collaboration, 2005). Contamination is a serious problem as it can spuriously reduce the intervention effect. Control group participants can obtain the intervention when experimental group participants or others share intervention information or materials with them. Contamination between groups can also occur when study participants are in contact with one another for extended periods, such as in waiting rooms or intensive care units.

Participants in both the experimental and the control group may be exposed to a co-intervention. Co-intervention occurs when participants in either the experimental or the control group receive additional therapeutic interventions (Cochrane Collaboration, 2005). For the experimental group, participants may receive additional interventions outside of the study other than those planned in the protocol. In this case, co-intervention may spuriously increase the treatment effect. Co-intervention in the control group occurs when they receive the intervention, or a similar intervention, outside the study. This may decrease differences between the two groups.

In the pilot study with mothers of NICU infants, we assessed contamination by asking experimental group mothers when they had finished the intervention whether they shared any information they acquired during the intervention with any other mothers, and if so who. We then examined whether these other mothers were in the study control group. To assess co-intervention, we asked all participants whether they had received services from a psychologist, psychiatrist, social worker or other counsellor during the intervention, and if yes how often, to determine whether they had received help for their emotional distress from other sources. Findings indicated that neither was problematic. Nonetheless, these same data were collected in the evaluation study as well, to ensure that contamination or co-intervention were not occurring. If the feasibility study indicates there is a problem, then strategies to eliminate or minimize this require consideration. For example, one strategy to reduce co-intervention is to add an exclusion criterion to exclude those who planned to receive another form of intervention during the study period.

To determine whether an intervention is efficacious it is essential that the intervention be provided reliably and competently by the intervention providers. This is referred to as intervention fidelity (Stein *et al.*, 2007). Methods to assess intervention fidelity can be determined and piloted during the feasibility phase. A variety of different methods can be employed. However, audio or videotaping of the intervention sessions, and an assessment of the extent to which the essential elements of the intervention are implemented in the way these are intended to be provided, is considered to be the most rigorous approach. This assessment is undertaken using a checklist or tool developed explicitly for this purpose. Participants can also be asked to provide feedback on the quality of the provision of the intervention. Other methods for assessing fidelity include having the intervention provider complete a checklist, rating the extent to which they were able to implement the required elements of the intervention soon after a session, or live observations of intervention sessions (Sidani and Braden, 2011).

The next step

Most feasibility studies discover that there are feasibility and acceptability issues to address, and the intervention is revised accordingly. Common problems are excessive participant burden; complicated intervention materials; the need to front-load key intervention content or components when attention and attendance is greatest; contamination; and training of the intervention providers (Polit and Tatano Beck, 2012). A crucial question to contemplate once pilot work is completed is: How much can an intervention be modified before another pilot is indicated to establish feasibility and acceptability? There are currently no guidelines to assist investigators in determining whether the intervention is feasible and acceptable, or whether further piloting is required before proceeding to the evaluation study. The development of a systematic approach to guide decision-making at this point in the process of intervention development and evaluation is warranted.

Conclusion

The effective implementation of a complex intervention in an evaluation study is critical to conducting an assessment of the intervention's efficacy. A feasibility or pilot study is a precious opportunity to identify feasibility and acceptability challenges, and to fine-tune the intervention content and its delivery through feedback from the participants and others to optimize implementation in an evaluation study.

Further reading

Bellg, A. J., Borrelli, B., Resnick, B., Hecht, J., Minicucci, D. S., Ory, M., Ogedegbe, G., Orwig, D. and Ernst, D. 2004. Enhancing treatment fidelity in health behavior change studies: best practices and recommendations from the NIH behavior change consortium. *Health Psychology*, 23: 443–51.

Conn, V. S., Cooper, P. S., Ruppar, T. M. and Russell, C. L. 2008. Searching for the intervention in intervention research reports. *Journal of Nursing Scholarship*, 40: 52–9.

Sidani, S. and Braden, C. J. 2011. *Design, Evaluation, and Translation of Nursing Interventions*. Chichester: Wiley-Blackwell.

18

FEASIBILITY IN PRACTICE

Undertaking a feasibility study to answer procedural, methodological and clinical questions prior to a full-scale evaluation

David A. Richards

This section of the handbook has described how feasibility and pilot trials can be used to address procedural, methodological and clinical uncertainties. By addressing such uncertainties directly, we can shine a light on these uncertainties. We are then able to proceed to a full-scale evaluation with greater confidence that we can design the intervention, procedures and methods to give us the best chance of optimizing both the performance of the intervention and the methodological conditions with which to conduct a fair test.

So far, we have seen examples in previous chapters of how feasibility and pilot trials can be used to address individual uncertainties. But in many cases we will be faced with the full range of uncertainties, for none of which can we make a confident decision. In this situation we need to construct a feasibility or pilot trial that can address multiple uncertainties. The example described in this chapter shows how one research team was able to use a modest amount of research funding to prepare the ground for a full-scale evaluation. To do so, we had to design a mixed-methods study that explicitly asked questions of procedure, method and intervention design.

Learning objectives

- To describe a real-world feasibility case study using a mixed-methods design.
- To demonstrate how a single mixed-methods study can address multiple feasibility research questions.
- To appreciate how a novel trial design and a concurrent qualitative study can inform the design of a full-scale evaluation.

Background

Depression is known to be one of the most disabling health care problems – physical or mental – with a very large emotional, behavioural and economic impact on sufferers, their families and wider society. Responsibility for sufferers' treatment often falls between generalist primary care practitioners and specialists, although the majority of people receive their treatment from primary care. Lack of coordination and poor management has been recognized as a major factor in this continuing misery.

Although both pharmacological and psychological treatments exist, many patients receive neither, or inadequate treatment provision. During the 1990s, a system of organizing depression management was developed in the United States, referred to as 'collaborative care'. Collaborative care generally includes (1) a multi-professional approach to patient care often provided by a case manager. These case managers work with the primary care medical staff whilst receiving weekly supervision from specialist mental health clinicians; (2) a structured management plan including support for medication and brief psychological therapy; (3) scheduled patient follow-ups where case managers attempt to actively maintain contact with patients; and (4) enhanced patient-specific inter-professional communication between case managers and primary care clinicians. When the Enhanced Care for Depression team started work, systematic reviews had shown that collaborative care was effective in the United States, but its effects were not known elsewhere. This was important because research into organizational systems is heavily contextually influenced, with no guarantee that positive findings in one health system will transfer to another.

In preparation for a full-scale evaluation, our team had adopted the existing UK Medical Research Council's recommendations for researching complex interventions (Medical Research Council, 2000). In our prior development phase we had both reviewed the existing literature and conducted in-depth qualitative research with patients and clinicians. We had undertaken both these studies to identify the ingredients likely to be important for good clinical outcomes. Our meta-regression analysis of published trials (Bower *et al.*, 2006) had identified that trials using case managers specifically trained with mental health skills and who were supervised by expert mental health clinicians using a scheduled programme of supervision achieved better outcomes. When we undertook innovative qualitative research in which people with previous experience of depression, primary care clinicians and mental health workers were asked to comment on a video of a collaborative care, we found that whilst all concerned generally supported the theory of collaborative care we needed to make some initial adaptations to the structure and content of our proposed clinical protocol (Richards *et al.*, 2006).

Our clinical protocol consisted of an initial face-to-face appointment followed by telephone case management from a qualified mental health worker in primary care, supervised by expert psychological and psychiatric practitioners. Case managers supported patients with managing their medication and brief behavioural activation – a psychological treatment for depression. They recorded patients' symptoms each time they made contact, using the Patient Health Questionnaire-9

(Kroenke *et al.*, 2001), a standardized depression questionnaire. Finally, they communicated regularly with the patients' family doctors to advise on medication issues or further specialist referral. At this stage we were ready to start the feasibility and piloting stage of our research programme.

Uncertainties

Despite the extensive development work that had been undertaken, there were a number of critical uncertainties that prevented us moving immediately to a fully powered clinical trial.

1   Firstly, although we had synthesized outcome data in our systematic reviews, we did not have a good idea of how collaborative care would perform in our UK context. As described above, we had had to adapt the US principles of collaborative care during the development stage. We needed an estimate of the likely effect size of our adapted intervention in order to determine the sample size for our full evaluation.

2   Secondly, because collaborative care is at least in part an organizational intervention, we were concerned that there would be contamination between the intervention arm of our planned trial and our intended usual care comparator. Contamination of this nature can occur in individually randomized trials when clinicians implement an experimental intervention that relies on their skills and behaviours. If these same clinicians are also treating participants in the usual care comparator group, there is a danger that some of their experimental treatment behaviours will 'spill over' and become part of how they treat control participants. Furthermore, an organizational intervention by its very nature alters the context within which individual patient-directed interventions in a trial are being delivered, another source of contamination. Complex interventions such as collaborative care may actually have both an individual patient level *and* an organizational level intervention.

3   Thirdly, we were unsure whether we would be able to recruit sufficient participants to the trial. Indeed, we did not know which would be the most productive strategy to do so.

4   Finally, our previous qualitative work had been theoretical. We wanted to find out what actual participants receiving the collaborative care intervention, and clinicians delivering it, really thought about it, specifically whether further adaptations were required.

Design

We chose to answer these procedural, methodological and clinical uncertainties in a feasibility study using a mixed-methods design including a novel randomized controlled trial and a qualitative study. We embedded a patient-randomized trial within a cluster-randomized trial, represented in Figure 18.1.

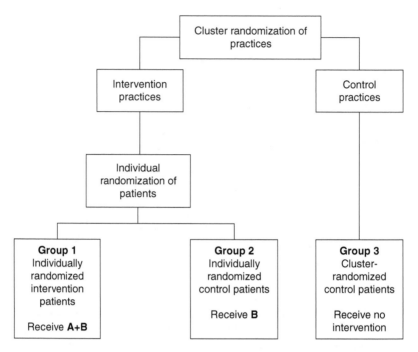

FIGURE 18.1   Design of the Enhanced Care for Depression feasibility trial

Given our concerns about contamination or 'spillover' of the intervention from experimental to control groups, we chose an initial cluster randomized design to guard against this happening. Therefore, we randomized clusters of clinicians – in this case primary care practices – to intervention or control (usual care) arms. We recruited patient participants from both these arms to be included in the study. Those in the cluster control group received usual care.

However, before we allocated treatment to participants in the cluster-randomized intervention arm, we conducted a further patient-level randomization. Half of these participants were randomized to the collaborative care intervention, the other half to receive usual care. As can be seen from Figure 18.1, these procedures resulted in three randomized groups, two of which apparently received usual care (groups 2 and 3) and one that received the intervention (group 1). However, it would be truer to say that group 1 received both the individual- *and* the organizational-level intervention components (in that their usual care was being delivered in a primary care practice which had been *potentially* influenced by the presence of case managers collaborating with the primary health care team); group 2 were exposed to just the organizational component and group 3 neither.

This design allowed us to empirically test for the magnitude of effect between the full intervention – comprising the individual- and organizational-level components – and a true control group that received neither component. The presence of group 2, being exposed to organizational elements of the intervention only, allowed us to test whether this element had an effect independent of the individual component. If this was the case, we might be forced to conclude that the true magnitude of collaborative care would be diluted if tested in a patient-randomized trial through leakage of elements of the protocol into the participant group treated by usual care.

Whilst this design addressed two of our uncertainties (prediction of effect size and most appropriate randomized design), we had to include other procedures for assessing the best recruitment method and determining the acceptability of the clinical protocol. Whilst we did not experimentally manipulate recruitment methods, we used three different ones – referral by primary care doctors, primary care case note screening and screening of patients in the waiting room prior to attending a primary care consultation – and carefully measured the yield of each one. We also undertook qualitative interviews with case managers and patients to gather information in order to further refine the clinical protocol.

Results

Effect size and contamination: we recruited 24 primary care practices, of which 19 recruited individual participants – 41 to the intervention group, 38 to the patient-randomized control group and 35 to the cluster-randomized control group (Richards *et al.*, 2008). We found that collaborative care was significantly effective in reducing depression symptoms when comparing group 1 to group 3 (the cluster comparison of 'uncontaminated' arms). Interestingly, when we compared group 1 to group 2 (individual patient-randomized comparison) we found the between-group effect was somewhat less than that observed in the cluster comparison, an effect which was no longer significant. We were led to conclude, therefore, that there was a potential for contamination between randomized arms of any future patient-randomized controlled trial. This is represented graphically in Figure 18.2.

Given that this was a small and underpowered feasibility trial and we had no intention of making definitive claims for the effectiveness of collaborative care, the significance of the findings was less important for us than the differential effect between the two comparisons. From these data, we were able to estimate the degree of clustering (i.e. the extent to which individual data were not independent) by calculating the intra-cluster correlation coefficient. We could also use the effect size itself, although subject to considerable uncertainties due to the wide confidence intervals around it, to estimate the likely effect of collaborative care if tested in a full trial. Together, these two figures allowed us to calculate the sample size needed to adequately power the full evaluation.

Recruitment yield: we found that the highest-yielding recruitment method was screening of primary care case records. Of the 309 patients who were identified as potentially eligible for the study, almost 20 per cent returned a form consenting to be interviewed of which 80 per cent were eligible for the study and agreed to participate. We found that GPs handed out 11 per cent of recruitment packs which

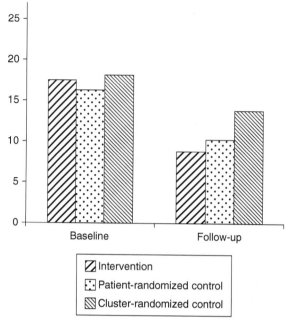

FIGURE 18.2 Effect of intervention compared to control conditions on depression, measured by the Patient Health Questionnaire-9

we provided for them, with 84 per cent of those consenting to be interviewed being eligible. Waiting room screening was a very research labour-intensive strategy which yielded a very small recruited population. In total, 15.5 per cent of potentially eligible patients were recruited through case note screening, 9.2 per cent through GP referral and 2.2 per cent through waiting room screening.

There was thus no advantage in the GP presenting the trial invitation and patient information sheet to patients directly. Indeed, keeping GPs interested in the trial had a considerable impact on researcher time. For waiting room screening, aside from the need to station research workers in waiting rooms, there were many subsequent problems contacting patients by telephone in order to establish possible eligibility. In contrast, case note screening was a largely automated process conducted by practice administration staff which did not rely on the enthusiasm of individual GPs or a large time commitment from researchers.

Views on collaborative care: our qualitative results showed that there was a remarkable similarity between the views of patients and those of case managers. The provision of accurate and easy-to-read information was particularly appreciated by patients, as was the telephone delivery, but they suggested a greater degree of flexibility, including the opportunity to vary face-to-face and telephone working so that a working alliance could be maintained, adapted according to psychological need and clinical progress. Case managers made suggestions as to how the protocol could be improved, but wished to retain the central aspects of telephone-delivered support to psychological and pharmacological treatment. Like patients, they made suggestions to incorporate materials for treating co-morbid anxiety disorders and relapse prevention into the protocol. They asked for specific training in telephone working and suggested that full-time case managers employed specifically to deliver collaborative care might be a more appropriate means of testing collaborative care in a phase III trial.

Next steps

The information that we gathered in this mixed-methods feasibility study addressed important procedural, methodological and clinical uncertainties. We used these findings to design and implement a fully powered randomized controlled trial of collaborative care in the UK (Richards *et al.*, 2009). Given the findings from the feasibility stage, we felt it prudent to undertake a cluster-randomized trial, which we powered to detect an inter-group effect size of 0.4 at 90 per cent power (alpha 0.05), requiring us to recruit 550 participants. This figure was inflated above the 264 participants required for a patient-randomized trial to account for a design effect of 1.65 caused by clustering and a 20 per cent enlargement to insure us against loss to follow-up. We chose to recruit participants through case note screening in primary care. We were able to calculate the number of primary care practices required and the frequency of searches needed by extrapolating from the findings of our feasibility recruitment exercise. We amended our clinical protocol to allow greater flexibility in delivery and content, and recruited case managers who could allocate at least 50 per cent of their working week to the trial. Our fully powered trial results were subsequently published (Richards *et al.*, 2013) and we showed that collaborative care was effective in the UK, with effects that persisted to at least 12 months after baseline and at a cost which was within commonly accepted thresholds of health care provider ability to pay.

Conclusion

This chapter has illustrated how the practical application of feasibility and pilot methods can address multiple procedural, methodological and clinical factors that might make investigators uncertain about proceeding to a fully powered randomized controlled trial, or worse, might make that trial fail if it went ahead without addressing these issues first. Feasibility and pilots are essential for addressing these uncertainties and can ensure that investigators design, plan and implement fully powered trials that are both a fair test of an intervention and can be completed on time and to target.

Further reading

Bowling, A. and Ebrahim, S. 2005. *Handbook of Health Research Methods: Investigation, Measurement and Analysis.* Maidenhead: Open University Press.

Creswell, J. W. and PlanoClark, V. L. 2007. *Designing and Conducting Mixed Methods Research*. Thousand Oaks, CA: Sage.

Medical Research Council. 2008. *Developing and Evaluating Complex Interventions: New Guidance*. London: Medical Research Council.

Teddlie, C. and Tashakkori, A. 2009. *Foundations of Mixed Method Research: Integrating Quantitative and Qualitative Approaches in the Social and Behavioral Sciences*. Thousand Oaks, CA: Sage.

SECTION 3

Evaluation of complex interventions

Introduction to Section 3

Ingalill Rahm Hallberg

This section focuses on evaluating the effect and efficiency of a complex intervention in order to be able to state whether this specific way of intervening in a certain situation is more effective than the interventions that are already in place, or whether it is an improvement compared with any other interventions addressing the same problem.

There are many challenges and pitfalls in setting up a study to evaluate the effect of an intervention and to be able to claim external validity and generalizability. This is even more challenging when we want to prove categorically the effect of an intervention that is complex and when parts of the intervention cannot be separated from each other in terms of effect. It has been claimed that most interventions are complex and that may be true, but the complexity may differ greatly between a trial of a drug and a trial which tries to establish the effect of a psychosocial intervention in cases of depression (Richards *et al.*, 2013) or the effectiveness of triage in emergency care (Richards *et al.*, 2002), or other such studies.

Ioannidis (2005) discussed and listed problems that we have to be aware of when setting up an intervention study. These include the studies being too small, the expected effects too small to have any impact in practice or the possibility that there may be alternative hypotheses not investigated or taken into account when trying to explain the results or when setting up the study. From the previous sections, readers have hopefully gained inspiration and sufficient knowledge concerning the preparatory work that needs to be done before entering into a major study. The investigator has to systematically go through the relevant literature, pertaining both to the intervention and the context in which is meant to be tested, its possible effects and any contextual issues, and they also have to construct tentative theories about the intervention, the context and the expected outcome. Feasibility and pilot studies have to be carried out (Sections 2 and 3) to ensure that the major study will be feasible. The MRC guidance (2008) is not meant to be interpreted linearly and thus the preparatory work entails going back and forth until the investigator feels satisfied with the way the major study is set up. Once the effect of an intervention is established the research needs to continue, perhaps to refine the intervention, to study alternative hypotheses or to move forward to implement it in practice, on a broad or narrow scale (see Section 4).

Just as there are alternative hypotheses to draw on in setting up and evaluating a specific intervention and its effect, there are also alternative ways of designing an intervention study, alternative concepts that are applicable and the definitions of which may differ. There are also different ways of modelling the intervention, the implementation process of the intervention under study, measuring the outcome and possible confounding variables. In this section we have focused on different possible designs: randomized and cluster-randomized trials; the stepped wedge design, natural experiments and interrupted time series analysis; non-standard and preference designs; and single-subject designs. In addition we have chosen to provide chapters addressing: intervention fidelity; qualitative process evaluation; and economic evaluation. Introducing and implementing the intervention to be studied in the clinical setting where it is to be tested has been covered in previous sections, and also in the section about implementation of established knowledge found to fulfil the criteria for effectiveness.

As always not everything has been covered and the last word or the ultimate method for setting up and studying a complex intervention has yet to be presented. This section has perhaps not addressed the ethical aspects of carrying out such a study in sufficient detail. This is mainly due to the fact that regulations/laws and organizations responsible for ethical reviews and protecting participants' interests and health differ from country to country. The Helsinki Declaration, however, is applicable worldwide (http://www.wma.net/en/30publications/10policies/b3/index.html) and should be followed. It was developed for the medical profession but is applicable to all health care research. The researcher needs to be conversant with and conform to the country's latest regulations/laws and organizations responsible for safeguarding participants' interest. The researcher also needs to be conversant with and conform to standards within the current international research community, by being aware of the agreements made among editors of medical journals (http://www.icmje.org) concerning such aspects as ethics, design and reporting to ensure that all the steps needed for publication in the best journals are taken. CONSORT (Consolidated Standards of Reporting Trials, http://www.consort-statement.org) is a site that provides updated information about what to bear in mind when setting up and reporting an intervention study of this kind. Before the intervention study is started it also has to be reported on one of the accepted sites for intervention trials, for instance http://www.trial.gov. This is to ensure that the design and the protocol are followed and made public before the main study starts, and are not subsequently changed. All these steps are to ensure that the study follows ethical and good practice routines. Among other ethical issues to consider is that it is unethical to carry out a study that is underpowered or designed in a manner that prevents the investigator from drawing firm conclusions. Thus the ethical reflections should not only take into account the aspects of informed consent, the presentation of proper and transparent information and risks to the study participants, but should also ensure that the design, the process and the methods are thought through carefully and that to the best of the investigator's knowledge the study will be able to answer the research question.

One very important movement not addressed in any of the chapters has taken place in many countries, and that is the movement towards involving patients/consumers and the public in the entire research process. The attitude to patient/consumer involvement is more developed in some countries and, for instance, is acknowledged by funding bodies as a requirement that should be met when applying for funding. In other countries it is less developed but under way. The intention is not to establish an advisory group only but to recognize the fact that those experienced in the field can make a positive contribution to the setting up and carrying out of an intervention study (see Richards, Chapter 4 for a more thorough discussion).

There are many choices to be made in setting up an intervention trial; one is selecting an appropriate design that will potentially elicit the best response (in terms of external validity) to the research question. The first chapter in this section, written by Sallie Lamb and Douglas Altman, is about randomized and cluster randomized trials. They cover the entire research process specific to these designs. They also raise an issue that is relevant irrespective of design – the importance of setting up a research protocol that illustrates the plan from random allocation to analyses. Establishing a research protocol and a document describing all amendments or problems that arise during the process is crucial for verifying how the research project was initially planned and how it unfolded during the process. The protocol should preferably be made public early on in the process so that those interested in the project can trust that there has been no tampering with the project. Firm conclusions cannot be drawn from one study alone, and thus the protocol and the documentation of changes or challenges are helpful if someone else wants to replicate the study.

When traditional randomized trials are not applicable, the stepped wedge design, natural experiments and interrupted time series analysis as described in the chapter by Professor Yan Hu are available. The chapter is illustrated by practical examples for the sake of clarity to the reader. Natural experiments frequently take place in society and in the area of health care, but often as researchers we fail to make use of social or nature's experiments even though the consequences of any changes may impact greatly on health, recovery, prevention, etc. Researching the outcome of such changes could perhaps teach us more about prevention and health.

Later in this section there is a chapter about non-standard and preference designs written by Louise von Essen. In this chapter the author deals with the problem that participants for potential inclusion in a study may have preferences and these preferences will probably have an impact on the outcome. In some cases this can result in a situation that is more true to real-life circumstances than the random assignment of people equally to either the control or the experimental situation. In real life the treatment offered to the patient (depending on its type) is chosen to fit the patient's situation and preferences. In this chapter the author presents various ways of setting up studies taking preferences into account and thus strengthening the validity of the outcome.

Single-subject designs are presented by Lena Nilsson-Wikmar and Karin Harms-Ringdahl. These designs are well suited, for instance, to research where limited numbers of subjects are available, or where the investigator needs to follow the individuals closely or before setting up a larger randomized study. Repeated measurements characterize single-subject designs and many ways to set up the study are described in the chapter. Researchers have to consider and deal with the challenging issues of external validity and generalizability when presenting the findings of such a study.

Research methodology is constantly under development and it is with great pleasure that we have been able to include very new material on process evaluation. Graham Moore and colleagues have compiled a summary of new guidance for process evaluation launched by the Medical Research Council. The chapter covers key functions of process evaluation and takes the reader through the research process from planning, resourcing, designing and conducting the process evaluation, research questions, methods, sampling and so on, all the way to reporting the findings of a process evaluation. Recommendations are provided for the entire process and readers who want to go further can now turn to the newly published MRC process evaluation guidance.

In the next chapter, fidelity as a part of process evaluation is elaborated further, thus investigating one aspect of the previous chapter in depth. The chapter is written by Henna Hasson and deals with an aspect of complex interventions research that is extremely important for ensuring that the outcomes of the intervention study really reflect the intervention implementation. There are several risks that an intervention will not be applied at all or as it is meant to be applied, and thus it is unclear what the outcome really reflects. Both the content of an intervention and its form can be amended by those applying the intervention, who are expected to follow the established protocol. These changes may not be documented if there are no means of establishing the fidelity in place. The chapter presents various ways with which to establish intervention fidelity including observations, logbooks, interviews, etc. The investigator needs to balance the methods and the data collection so that the results will not be biased by the data collection itself. It may be fair to say that awareness of the risk that the intervention may not be applied properly and the means for ensuring fidelity have been rare in research so far, but nowadays it is expected that this is remedied in some way.

Process evaluation is also addressed more in detail in the chapter by Atkins and co-workers. The uniqueness of this chapter lies in the use of qualitative methods not only to ensure fidelity but also to deepen the understanding of the intervention or the data collection process. It is common to claim that qualitative methods have no place in intervention studies for manifold reasons. Development has now changed direction and today many researchers recognize that the information obtained from a traditional intervention study does not reveal very much about the mechanisms involved in the effect or lack of effect. The addition of qualitative methods, however, can tell us more than is already known about moderators or mediators, contextual factors that may increase or reduce the effect as well as intervention fidelity. Thus a mixed-methods approach is suggested as providing more information about the intervention and its effect and efficiency. The authors of this chapter point out the need to be transparent in presenting all parts of the data collection, the sampling and the design, and that this is relevant for any design and can be achieved by publishing the protocol and all the data collected in the study.

In order to be able to present a case in discussions with health care managers or decision-makers it is necessary also to evaluate the intervention from an economic perspective. Decisions about implementing a new intervention have to be made in relation not only to the fact that it has an effect but also in relation to its costs. The chapter by Katherine Payne and Alexander Thompson addresses concepts related to economic evaluation, the principles to be included in the design and methods allowing economic analysis of an intervention. This chapter also highlights the fact that an intervention study needs expertise of various kinds in order to ensure that the design, methods and analysis are properly addressed. A research group responsible for any study of this kind needs to have a variety of scientific competence. Researchers may be more or less closely related to the research group but they have to be involved in all the planning and analysis of the outcome of the intervention to be studied.

It goes without saying that there are other ways and other designs, apart from those covered here, which can deliver results that tell the reader about the effect and efficiency of an intervention aimed at improving the health and recovery of patients or consumers. Development of research and research designs is, moreover, an ongoing process and as researchers we should also involve ourselves in developing designs and methods. Deciding how a study may best be set up is as an ongoing process, just like any knowledge development strategy, and today's truth may not be valid tomorrow.

19

INDIVIDUALLY AND CLUSTER-RANDOMIZED TRIALS

Sallie Lamb and Douglas G. Altman

Introduction

A randomized trial is a planned experiment that is designed to compare two or more forms of intervention where allocation of participants to an intervention arm is 'by chance'. Although used in many disciplines, randomized clinical trials pose particular problems in design, analysis and interpretation, and ethical problems. While there are many aspects to the quality of a trial, the most important are those relating to steps taken to avoid bias, such as randomization and blinding. Empirical evidence is accumulating that failure to use such methods leads to bias (Moher *et al.*, 2010).

Learning objectives

- The concepts and procedures needed to deliver a high-quality randomized controlled trial.
- The particular benefits and difficulties of using randomized controlled trials for the evaluation of complex interventions.
- The features of individually and cluster-randomized controlled trials.
- Practitioner cluster effects, learning curves, choice of comparator.

The key idea of a randomized controlled trial is that we compare groups of participants who differ only with respect to their intervention. The study must be prospective because biases are easily incurred when comparing groups treated at different times and possibly under different conditions. It must be comparative (controlled) because we cannot assume what will happen to the participants in the absence of any therapy. The most common trial design is a comparison of two interventions, often labelled experimental and control, although some trials compare more than two interventions. *Outcome measures* are collected at key points in the follow-up of the trial and used to quantify the differences between the groups, in terms of both intended and unintended effects of the interventions.

There are several books devoted to clinical trials, of which those by Pocock (1983), Matthews (2000), Eldridge and Kerry (2012) and Wang and Bakhai (2006) are particularly recommended. Further commentary on the role of randomized controlled trials in the development and evaluation of complex interventions is given in the MRC Complex Interventions Framework (Campbell *et al.*, 2007).

Firstly, we will discuss trials in which individual participants are randomly assigned to receive one of two or more different intervention regimens.

Trial design

Protocol

Clinical trials are complex and require considerable care in planning. It is essential to develop a detailed trial protocol that explains the rationale for the trial, and describes in detail the methods to be used. It serves as the foundation for all aspects of study planning, conduct and reporting. In particular the section on trial design should specify the participants (eligibility criteria), intervention of primary interest, comparison intervention (control), and outcomes to be assessed (collectively known as PICO), including how and when they will be assessed. The protocol should also specify how the data will be analysed. Recent guidelines detail what to include in a clinical trial protocol (Chan *et al.*, 2013). The main features of a trial protocol are shown in Table 19.1. A detailed protocol must accompany an application for a grant for a trial, and the research *ethics committee* (or the equivalent) will also require most of the above information. As well as aiding the conduct of a trial, a protocol makes the reporting of the results much easier as the introduction and methods section of the paper should be substantially the same as the methods sections in the protocol.

Random allocation

A vital issue in design is to ensure that, as far as is possible, the groups of participants receiving the different interventions are similar with regard to their characteristics that may affect how well they do. These features are usually assessed within the trial. The usual way to avoid bias is to use *random allocation* to determine which intervention each participant gets. With randomization, which is a chance process, variation among trial participants in characteristics that might affect their response to intervention (such as age or disease severity) will on average be the same in the different groups. In other words, randomization ensures that there is no bias in the way the interventions are allocated. However, there is no guarantee that randomization will lead to the groups being similar in a particular trial. Any differences that

TABLE 19.1 The main features of a trial protocol (Chan *et al.*, 2013)

Background and rationale
Objectives
Trial design
Participants
Interventions
Outcomes
Study setting
Eligibility criteria
Interventions
Outcomes
Sample size
Recruitment
Assignment of interventions
Blinding (masking)
Data collection methods
Data management
Statistical methods
Data monitoring

arise by chance can be at least inconvenient, and may lead to doubts being cast on the interpretation of the trial results.

While the results can be adjusted to take account of differences between the groups at the start of the trial, major imbalance can be prevented at the design stage using *stratified randomization*. In essence, this involves separate randomization of sub-groups of participants, such as those with mild or severe disease. If you know in advance that a few key variables are strongly related to outcome, these can be incorporated into a stratified randomization scheme. It is preferable to limit the number of strata to simplify the randomization process. There may be other important variables that we cannot measure or have not identified, and we rely on randomization to balance them.

It is essential that stratified randomization uses *blocking*, otherwise it gives no benefit over simple randomization. With blocking, allocations to each treatment are balanced within each consecutive series, or block, of patients within each stratum. For example, blocks of a size of six will each include three patients on each of two interventions ordered randomly within the block. This strategy helps in smoothing the staff commitment and resources needed to deliver complex interventions over the entire course of the trial. Investigators should consider using a *random block length* that reduces the ability of study personnel to be able to predict future allocations.

While randomization is necessary it is not a sufficient safeguard against bias (conscious or subconscious) when participants are recruited. The treatment allocation system must be set up so that the person entering participants does not know in advance which intervention the next person will get (known as *allocation concealment*). One method of concealing allocations is to use a series of sequentially numbered, sealed, opaque envelopes, each containing an intervention specification. For stratified randomization, two or more sets of envelopes are needed. Generally, however, the optimal methods of randomization are by using a telephone- or web-based system.

Blinding

The key to a successful clinical trial is to avoid any biases in the comparison of the groups. Randomization deals with possible bias at the treatment allocation, but bias can also creep in while the study is being run. Both participants and formal care-givers may be affected in the way they respond and observe by knowledge of which treatment was given. For this reason, ideally neither the participant nor their care-giver should know which intervention was given. Such a trial is called *double blind (investigator and patient blind)*. If only the patient is unaware, the trial is called *single blind (patient blind)*. Blinding can be difficult to achieve in trials of complex interventions because participants will have had to take an active role in the intervention (for example to exercise or undergo a specific psychological therapy). In nearly all circumstances, however, it will be possible to ensure that researchers measuring the outcome, or handling follow-up data, are blind to the intervention allocation (*outcome assessor blind*). A variety of methods can be used, such as anonymized postal follow-up or masking of scars or other indicators of intervention received.

When there is no standard effective intervention, it is reasonable *not* to give the control group any active intervention. However, it is often better to give the control group participants either usual care, or an inert or placebo intervention. The act of receiving an intervention may itself have some benefit to the participant, so that part of any benefit observed in the intervention group could be due to the knowledge or belief that they have had an intervention. For a study to be double blind, the two interventions should be indistinguishable, and this often represents an insurmountable challenge for complex intervention trials.

Sample size and power

At the most simple level, the calculation of sample size is based on either comparing means (*t*-test) or proportions (Chi-squared test). Most trials set out to estimate the superiority of one intervention over another, and sample size calculations are based on the idea that the trial should be large enough to have a high probability (called 'power', and usually set at 80–90 per cent) of getting a statistically significant difference if the true difference between the treatments is of a given size.

Unfortunately, specifying this target *true difference* or *effect size* is not easy. For common diseases, such as heart disease, small benefits are worthwhile. One way of thinking here is to identify the smallest difference that would be clinically important, and thus might impact on clinical practice. A common fault is to overestimate the potential effect of an intervention, without considering the implication of real-world factors such as adherence and loss to follow-up. Detecting small effects requires large trials. For example, a trial designed to have a high probability of detecting a reduction of mortality from 30 to 25 per cent would need at least 1,250 patients per group.

There are many different types of randomized design, and sample size estimation varies according to design.

Type I errors

At the end of a randomized controlled trial, we want to be able to draw a conclusion about the benefit, or otherwise, of a treatment. A *Type I error* occurs when we conclude that there is an intervention effect, when in fact none exists (i.e. the trial yields a false positive finding). In the sample size calculation, by setting the probability threshold (alpha) at 0.05 or less, the chance of such an error is kept to 5 per cent or less.

In most clinical trials, many outcomes are assessed, sometimes on more than one occasion. There is a temptation to analyse each of these outcomes and see which differences between intervention groups are significant. This approach leads to misleading results, because multiple testing will increase the chance of a Type I error. A *pre-specified statistical analysis plan* is considered good practice, and helps to protect against issues relating to Type I error. Just presenting the most significant results as if these were the only analyses performed is scientific misconduct, so authors are strongly encouraged to report all analyses performed.

Researchers are recommended to decide in advance of the analysis which outcome measure is of major interest and to focus attention on this variable when the data are analysed. Other data can and should be analysed too, but these variables should be considered to be of secondary importance. Any interesting findings among the secondary variables should be interpreted rather cautiously, more as ideas for further research than as definitive results. Adverse effects of treatment should usually be treated in this way. The trial protocol should thus specify the primary outcome, including when it will be assessed (occasionally there may be more than one primary outcome). Secondary outcomes should be clearly identified as such.

Type II errors

A *Type II error* occurs when we conclude there is no intervention effect, when in fact one does exist (i.e. the trial yields a false-negative finding). Generally studies are set up with a power of 80 or 90 per cent to minimize the chances of this happening, but studies that overestimate the effect size in the sample size calculation, or fail to achieve the target recruitment, will be too small to detect the target effect size reliably.

Ethical issues

One of the main ethical issues is the importance of providing adequate information about the trial and the interventions to potential participants. In general the trial is explained including what the alternative treatments are and what assessments will be made. Participants are then invited to be enrolled in the trial, although they will not know which intervention they will get. They can decline, in which case they will receive the standard treatment. In a few cases it is not possible to gain informed consent from a participant at the point of study entry/randomization, for example if they are unconscious. Most countries have specific laws to deal with research ethics and these situations.

Trials should only be initiated in situations where *we do not know which treatment is better*. This is sometimes called the *uncertainty principle*.

The methodological quality of a trial is also an ethical issue. A trial that uses inadequate methods, such as failing to randomize, and thus fails to prevent bias may be seen as unethical. Likewise, having an adequate sample size is also often considered to be an ethical matter (Altman, 1980).

Alternative designs

The simplest and most frequently used design for a clinical trial is the *parallel group design*, in which two (or more) interventions are evaluated simultaneously, with each participant's treatment being randomly assigned as they are enrolled in the trial. The most common alternative in the field of complex interventions is the *cluster-randomized design* in which groups of patients, health providers or organizations (called clusters) are randomized. Clusters may also be families, general practices, schools, hospitals, hospital departments, communities or geographical areas. Here the cluster is the unit of randomization rather than the individual, and all individuals within a cluster receive the same intervention. Special considerations are necessary in the design and analysis of such trials. The most important of these is to ensure that, as far as is possible, the clusters are assembled prior to randomization, and that the sample size has adequately considered the degree to which individuals within a cluster might behave in a similar fashion or share certain characteristics. These issues are described by Donner and Klar (2000) and Eldridge and Kerry (2012). Cluster designs require larger sample sizes than individually randomized trials. Their particular benefit is in situations where there might be 'contamination' between the intervention groups if participants were randomized individually (e.g. inpatients in the same ward).

A variation of the parallel group trial is the *group sequential trial*, in which the data are analysed at planned times as the data accumulate, typically at three to five time points. This design is suitable for trials that recruit and follow up participants over several years. It allows the trial to be stopped early if a clear treatment difference is seen, if adverse effects are unacceptable, or if it is obvious that no difference will be found. Adjustment must be made to significance tests to allow for multiple analyses of the data.

One further type of design is the *factorial design*, in which two active treatments, A and B, are simultaneously compared to each other and to a control. Participants are randomized into four groups, who receive either A only, B only, both A and B, or neither. This design is effectively two trials in one, for example comparing A vs. placebo and, separately, B vs. placebo. The design assumes that there is no interaction (or synergy) of the effects of A and B, but occasionally the interaction is the main point of interest. Factorial designs can be difficult to implement for some complex interventions, because one arm of the trial will require participants to commit to two packages of treatment. If the two packages of treatment require face-to-face attendance, the overall volume of attendance required can be too challenging for participants (for example, UK BEAM Trial, 2004).

Analysis

Comparison of intervention groups

Randomization does not guarantee that the characteristics of the different groups are similar. The first analysis should be a summary of the baseline characteristics of the participants in the two groups. This information is important to show the characteristics of the trial participants and also to demonstrate that the groups were similar with respect to variables that may affect the participant's response.

If the randomization is performed fairly we know that any differences between the two intervention groups *must* be due to chance, and hence a hypothesis test makes no sense except as a test of whether the trial was indeed randomized (Knol *et al.*, 2012). The question at issue is whether the groups differ in a way that might affect their response to treatment. That question is clearly one of clinical importance rather than statistical significance. If we suspect that the observed differences (imbalance) between the groups may have affected the outcome we can take account of the imbalance in the analysis, using regression methods. A particular example is when the trial assesses the change in the outcome (e.g. pain score) between the start and end of the trial. In this situation the regression method is called analysis of covariance. When techniques such as stratified randomization have been used, the stratifying variables should be adjusted for in the analysis (although the impact of so doing tends to be minimal). Such analyses should be pre-specified in the protocol.

Incomplete data

Data may be incomplete for several reasons. It is important to use all the data available and to report how many observations are missing. Also, some information may simply not have been recorded. It may seem reasonable to assume that a particular symptom was not present if it was not recorded, but such inferences are in general unsafe and should be made only after careful consideration of the circumstances.

The most important problem with missing information in trials relates to patients who do not complete the study and so their outcome is unknown. Some participants may be withdrawn, perhaps because of side effects. Others may move to another area or just fail to return for assessment. Efforts should be made to obtain at least some information regarding the status of these participants at the end of the trial, but some data are still likely to be missing. If there are many more withdrawals in one treatment group the results of the trial will be compromised, as it is likely that the withdrawals are treatment related.

A further difficulty is when some participants have not followed the protocol, either deliberately or accidentally. Included here are participants who actually receive the wrong intervention (in other words, not the one allocated) and participants who do not take up or participate in their treatment, known as *non-compliers*. Also, sometimes it may be discovered after the trial has begun that a participant was not in fact eligible for the trial.

The only safe way to deal with all of these situations is to keep all randomized participants in the trial. The analysis is thus based on the groups as randomized, and is known as an *intention-to-treat analysis*. Any other policy towards protocol violations will depart from the randomization, which is the basis for the trial. Also, excluding some participants involves subjective decisions and thus creates an opportunity for bias. In practice, participants who are lost to follow-up and thus have no recorded outcomes will need to be excluded, but all other participants should be included.

Missing outcomes for some participants causes major difficulties in both analysis and interpretation (Lachin, 2000). It is important to try to design and conduct a trial so as to minimize missing data; Little *et al.* (2012) discuss various strategies. Modern statistical methods, especially multiple imputation, are becoming more popular as a means of dealing with missing outcomes (Sterne *et al.*, 2009). Such analyses are usually performed as sensitivity analyses, to evaluate the impact on the results.

Interpretation of results

Generalizability

Inference from a sample to a population relies on the assumption that the trial participants represent all such patients. In most trials, however, participants are selected to meet certain eligibility criteria, so extrapolation of results beyond such participants may be unsafe. For example, trials of antihypertensive agents, such as beta-blocking drugs, are mainly conducted on middle-aged men. Is it reasonable to assume that the results also apply to women, or to older men? It is common to infer wider applicability of results, but the possibility that different groups would respond differently should be borne in mind. This issue is discussed by Rothwell (2005).

Compliance with treatment

Compliance with treatment is an issue in many randomized trials, but particularly in trials of complex interventions. Collecting data on important aspects of treatment delivery, for example attendance at sessions, provides valuable data to understand the mechanisms of treatment failure or success. Complier Averaged Causal Effect analysis can be used to assess and adjust for the role of compliance (for example, Knox *et al.*, 2014).

Reporting the results of clinical trials

As hinted above, not all trials are done well. In addition, inadequate reporting of trials is widespread. The CONSORT statement gives guidance for reporting clinical trial results, in the form of a checklist and diagram showing the flow of participants through the trials (Moher *et al.*, 2010). CONSORT is a widely accepted standard for reporting trials, and hundreds of medical journals expect authors to follow these recommendations. Full reporting of trials assists in the assessment of the quality of the methodology used in a trial, and thus helps the reader judge the reliability of the results. The TIDieR guidelines provide essential added guidance on reporting complex interventions (Hoffmann *et al.*, 2014).

Further reading

Chan, A. W., Tetzlaff, J., Gøtzsche, P. C., Altman, D. G., Mann, H., Berlin, J. A., Dickersin, K., Hróbjartsson, A., Schulz, K. F., Parulekar, W. R., Krleža-Jerić, K., Laupacis, A. and Moher, D. 2013. SPIRIT 2013 explanation and elaboration: guidance for protocols of clinical trials. *British Medical Journal*, 346: e7586.

Hoffmann, T. C., Glasziou, P. P., Boutron, I., Milne, R., Perera, R., Moher, D., Altman, D. G., Barbour, V., Macdonald, H., Johnston, M., Lamb, S. E., Dixon-Woods, M., McCulloch, P., Wyatt, J. C., Chan, A. W. and Michie, S. 2014. Better reporting of interventions: template for intervention description and replication (TIDieR) checklist and guide. *British Medical Journal*, 348: g1687.

Matthews, J. N. S. 2000. An Introduction to Randomized Trials. London: Arnold.

Moher, D., Hopewell, S., Schulz, K. F., Montori, V., Gøtzsche, P. C., Devereaux, P. J., Elbourne, D., Egger, M. and Altman, D. G. 2010. CONSORT 2010 explanation and elaboration: updated guidelines for reporting parallel group randomised trials. *British Medical Journal*, 340: c869.

20

STEPPED WEDGE, NATURAL EXPERIMENTS AND INTERRUPTED TIME SERIES ANALYSIS DESIGNS

Yan Hu

Introduction

As recommended by the UK Medical Research Council (MRC), when conventional randomized parallel group designs are not appropriate, alternative designs can be chosen (Medical Research Council, 2008). Stepped wedge, natural experiments and interrupted time series analysis designs are among the alternatives. This chapter will address these three types of design and provide research examples.

Learning objectives

After studying this chapter, readers are expected to be able to:

- State the characteristics of stepped wedge, natural experiments and interrupted time series designs.
- Understand research examples applying stepped wedge, natural experiments and interrupted time series designs.
- Differentiate between studies adopting stepped wedge, natural experiments and interrupted time series designs.

The Stepped wedge design

The stepped wedge is a type of randomized cross-over design in which different clusters cross over at different time points (Hussey and Hughes, 2007). The intervention is rolled out sequentially to a cluster of study participants over a number of time periods (Brown and Lilford, 2006). More than one cluster may start the intervention at any time point, but the time at which a cluster begins the intervention

Clusters (random allocation)

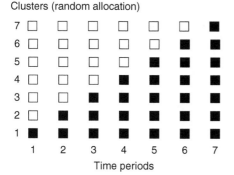

Time periods

Note: Each cell represents a data collection point, in which black cells represent intervention periods, white cells represent control periods.

FIGURE 20.1   An example of a stepped wedge design

is randomized. As a result, the stepped wedge design allows the researcher to implement the intervention in a smaller fraction of the clusters at each time point. All clusters eventually receive the intervention and the intervention is never removed once it has been implemented, which may alleviate ethical concerns (Brown and Lilford, 2006). For population-based trials that have already been shown to do more good than harm (such as Ciliberto *et al.*, 2005, a malnutrition study), a stepped wedge design may provide a solution to the ethical and practical problems of evaluating an intervention, especially when it is difficult to introduce the intervention to the whole group at once due to resource constraints. However, stepped wedge designs have some drawbacks such as greater complexity and longer trial duration than parallel group studies (Medical Research Council, 2008).

An example of a stepped wedge design with seven steps is shown in Figure 20.1. Data analysis to determine the overall effectiveness of the intervention subsequently involves comparison of the data points in the control section of the wedge with those in the intervention section.

A study with a stepped wedge design

Ciliberto *et al.* (2005) adapted a stepped wedge design with seven steps to compare the recovery rates of home-based therapy vs. standard inpatient therapy with ready-to-use therapeutic food (RUTF) among Malawi children with moderate and severe malnutrition. In this study, 1,178 malnourished children receiving treatment in Nutritional Rehabilitation Units (NRUs) were included and systematically allocated to either eight-week standard inpatient therapy (186 children) or eight-week home-based therapy (992 children) with RUTF. Children receiving standard therapy were recruited at six of the seven NRUs during the first three weeks of center participation, during which home-based therapy with RUTF was not offered. The seventh participating NRU was offered home-based therapy with RUTF at the onset of the study. After the first center began participation in December, an additional NRU began participating every three weeks thereafter. After three weeks of enrollment of children receiving only standard therapy, home-based therapy with RUTF was offered to all eligible children for eight weeks. Thus, children receiving standard therapy were enrolled throughout the duration of the study, but in fewer numbers. The stepped wedge design was used to control any bias that might be introduced by seasonal variations in the severity or type of childhood malnutrition in southern Malawi, where the prevalence of childhood malnutrition is high in the pre-harvest season from December to April each year.

Care providers and children returned to the clinic for reassessment of the children's weight, length and mid-upper arm circumference every two weeks. If the child was receiving home-based therapy with RUTF, an additional two-week supply of RUTF was distributed at each visit. Children receiving standard therapy either continued to receive feeding in the hospital or received additional cereal-legume supplements for use at home.

Recovery was defined by reaching a specific weight-for-height z score (WHZ). Relapse or death were the primary outcomes. The rate of weight gain and the prevalence of fever, cough and diarrhea were the secondary outcomes. Linear and logistic regression modeling were used to account for the effect of covariates on the comparisons. Time-event analysis was used to compare rates of reaching the desired WHZ over the eight-week study period. The study result indicated that home-based therapy with RUTF is associated with better outcomes for childhood malnutrition than standard therapy.

Natural experiments

A natural experiment is a study taking place in a real situation or community when deliberate manipulation of the independent variable is not possible. It works best in circumstances where a relatively large population is affected by a substantial change in a well-understood environmental exposure, and where exposures and outcomes can be captured through routine data sources, such as environmental monitoring and mortality records (Medical Research Council, 2008). It is useful when offering opportunities for non-randomized evaluations of complex interventions. A combination of multiple methodologies may be used in answering research questions in natural experiments.

Morgan (2013) differentiated 'natural experiments' from 'nature's or society's experiments' in that the former emerge as the retro-fitting by social scientists of events that have happened in the social world into the traditional forms of field or randomized trial experiments. Researchers reconstruct the normal events of life into natural experiments by post hoc 'reverse designing' the natural/social situation in its environment into an experimental one. In contrast, nature's experiments are natural situations displaying the characteristics of experiments; they are events in the world that happen in circumstances that are already sufficiently controlled to be open for direct analysis without reconstruction work. These controls are not naturally present but have to be added retrospectively by the researchers to establish the natural experimental site. Morgan (2013) stressed that the distinction between these two forms needs to be maintained because nature's experiments cannot necessarily be reduced to natural experiments.

A study with a natural experiment design

Yu et al.'s (2012) study on the pattern of hand, foot and mouth disease (HFMD) incidence in China is an example of a natural experiment investigating the reconstruction of complex social events into a natural experiment. This study analyzed changes in the incidence of HFMD during the declining incidence periods of 2008–10 in China after the Chinese National Guidelines for Diagnosis and Treatment of HFMD were introduced on May 2, 2008. Reported HFMD cases over a period of 25 months were extracted from the National Disease Reporting System (NDRS) and analyzed. A total of 3.58 million individual cases were reported to the NDRS system during the study period. An interrupted time series (ITS) technique was used to detect changes in HFMD incidence rates in terms of level and slope by a regression analysis between declining incidence periods in the three years. Data were aggregated monthly, and monthly HFMD incidence rates were calculated and expressed as number of cases per 10,000 people. Graphs were used to present and evaluate patterns in HFMD incidence rates from May 1, 2008 to May 31, 2011.

To control for the different effects of 'interventions' in different provinces, the incidence rate data were reanalyzed using the ITS technique with the variable of 'province' with 31 dummy variables in the model.

The results of the ITS analysis demonstrated a significant decrease in incidence rate level (p <0.0001) when comparing the current period to the previous. There were significant changes in declining slopes when comparing 2010 to 2009, and 2010 to 2008 (all p <0.005), but not 2009 to 2008.

Incremental changes in the incidence rate level during the declining incidence periods of 2009 and 2010 can be potentially attributed to factors such as more case reporting, silent infections in the previous year, the peak of an epidemic cycle in 2009 to 2010, and neonates being added to the sensitive pool. The steeper declining slope in 2010 may be ascribed to more effective interventions and preventive strategies or to abrupt changes in risk factors associated with HFMD such as air temperature humidity level and socio-economic indicators.

Interrupted time series

The randomized controlled trial is perceived as the gold standard by which effectiveness is measured in a study. However, alternative types of quasi-experimental designs – controlled before and after studies and ITS studies – are recognized as practical approaches for improving the quality of information for decision-makers in the real world. Interrupted time series designs use routine monitoring data collected at equally spaced intervals of time before and after an intervention, with the period before intervention serving as a control group (Grimshaw *et al.*, 2003). ITS can be used to assess change of behavior, practices or outcomes over time. This design can be particularly applied to routine surveillance data that have no obvious control group. The ITS design is a much more practical option in many settings, even though the allocation of subjects is not randomized. Therefore, when experimental study is not possible, an ITS study can provide a robust method of measuring the effect of an intervention (Grimshaw *et al.*, 2003). The ITS approach has been used to assess the effectiveness of a variety of interventions in various fields such as in environmental, financial and health sciences.

Behaviors and practices can be repeatedly measured. The result is a 'repeated time series' that enables investigation into the pattern of change over time. Parameters of such a time series include its mean level, its slope and numerous more complex, non-linear changes in the shape of the time series. Once there is a repeated measure of the process of interest, one can assess the effects of any independent variable in terms of its impact on the average level of the slope of the measured process. The judgement that the independent variable affects the process is based on how much change its introduction produces in either or both the level and slope of the measured process (Biglan *et al.*, 2000).

A study with an interrupted time series design

Richards *et al.* (2002) adopted an ITS design to compare the workloads of general practitioners and nurses, and the costs of patient care for nurse telephone triage and standard management of requests for same-day appointments (SDA) in routine primary care. Standard management meant that patients requesting an SDA were fitted into extra general practitioner appointments at the end of each surgery by receptionists. In contrast, the triage system involved receptionists passing on requests for SDA to experienced practice nurses, supported by computerized management protocols developed by the practice.

This study took place in a large general practice in York in the UK. Three out of five surgery sites participated, with a total population of 20,800. A multiple interrupted time series design was chosen to detect differences between the two systems in routine practice. All consecutive patients requesting SDA were entered into the study using the broadest possible inclusion criteria. To control for threats to internal validity (such as increasing professional expertise) or continuous and discrete historical events (such as undefined health trends or defined events such as influenza epidemics), three repeated measurement points were initiated to establish stable baselines at each site during standard management. Sequential introduction of triage into multiple sites controlled for any interaction between the intervention, time and different settings. At each site, all patients requesting SDA entered the trial

Month	1	2	3	4	5	6	7	8	9	10	11	12	13	14	15	16	17	18
Surgery A n patients	Standard Management			Triage System														
	130	130	115	141	117	122	135	127	127	102	140	118						
Surgery B n patients				Standard Management			Triage System											
				151	157	134	129	135	135	150	124	171	121	134	126			
Surgery B n patients							Standard Management			Triage System								
							151	141	155	137	143	134	109	128	114	130	104	134

FIGURE 20.2 An example of an interrupted time series design in three units (from Richards *et al.*, 2002)

and were managed by the standard management system. The triage system was then continuously introduced, with data being collected on patients for one week in each of the next nine months. Surgery sites entered the study sequentially at three monthly intervals. The multiple measurement points allowed the researchers to use autocorrelation analyses to assess for any trends caused by confounding effects of associations between data points over time, unrelated to the intervention. Type of consultation (telephone, appointment or visit), the time taken for the consultation, up to three presenting complaints per patient, and up to three clinical decisions made during the consultation were recorded. All costs for the same-day appointment activity and one-month follow-up care were calculated. Time series analyses of the mean total, general practitioner and nurse times per patient, checking for autocorrelations or seasonal effects for the complete sample and individual practices were applied. The design and flow chart of a multiple interrupted time series design is shown in Figure 20.2.

The results indicated that the triage system reduced appointments with general practitioners by 29–44 per cent. Compared with standard management, the triage system had a relative risk of 0.85 for home visits, 2.41 for telephone care and 3.79 for nurse care. Mean overall time in the triage system was 1.70 minutes longer, but mean general practitioner time was reduced by 2.45 minutes. It was concluded that triage reduced the number of same-day appointments with general practitioners but resulted in busier routine surgeries, increased nursing time and a small but significant increase in out-of-hour and accident and emergency attendance. In addition, triage did not reduce overall costs per patient for managing same-day appointments.

Summary

Although interventions happening in society have several interacting factors that make it difficult to standardize the design and deliver the intervention, alternative designs such as the stepped wedge, natural experiments and interrupted time series can contribute to the adoption of appropriate and flexible methods. The advantage of these alternative designs is that they provide a means to reconstruct missing *ceteris paribus* (i.e. all other things being equal or held constant) controls to turn a social event into a trial, that is, make uncontrolled social events tractable for study. However, researchers should pay attention to the limitations of these alternative designs when they are used, as they are either non-randomized or have no standardized control. Thus findings from these studies should be interpreted and presented with caution. Wherever possible, evidence should be combined from different sources that do not share the same weaknesses (Craig *et al.*, 2008). These methods are still in the process of improvement to reach consensus for better practice.

Further reading

Anderson, R. 2008. New MRC guidance on evaluating complex interventions. *British Medical Journal*, 337: a1937.

Doghety, E., HarrisonM. B., Baker, C. and Graham, L. D. 2012. Following a natural experiment of guideline adaptation and early implementation: a mixed methods study of facilitation. *Implementation Science*, 7: 9.

Grimshaw, J., Alderson, P., Bero, L., Grilli, R., Oxman, A. and Zwarenstein, M. 2003. Study designs accepted for inclusion in EPOC reviews. *EPOC Newsletter*, March. Cochrane Effective Practice and Organization of Care Review Group. http://epoc.cochrane.org/newsletters.

Liu, M., Hong, Z. H. and Zhan, S.Y. 2010. Development and evaluation of complex intervention. *Chinese Journal of Epidemiology*, 31: 1410–13.

Ramsay, C. R., Matowe, L., Grilli, R., Grimshaw, J. M. and Thomas, R. E. 2003. Interrupted time series designs in health technology assessment: lessons from two systematic reviews of behavior change strategies. *International Journal of Technology Assessment in Health Care*, 19: 613–23.

21

NON-STANDARD AND PREFERENCE DESIGNS

Louise von Essen

Introduction

Randomized controlled trials (RCT) are accepted as the 'gold standard' design for evaluating the effectiveness of a single intervention such as a drug. Within the health sector there are a range of complex interventions that involve an intervention with interacting components. RCT designs evaluating these interventions have shortcomings with regard to recruitment, ethics and preferences. The majority of RCTs have difficulty recruiting sufficient numbers of participants (McDonald *et al.*, 2006) and trial populations are often unrepresentative of the population 'with need'. Additionally, in routine real-world health care, patients are rarely told of interventions that they cannot be provided, or that these may be decided by chance, yet this is regarded as an ethical requirement for clinical trials. For trials with a usual care comparator, where usual care is available outside the trial, the only incentive to participate is to receive the new intervention. Individuals who do not receive their preferred intervention may drop out or comply poorly, which may lead to worse outcomes either directly through poor adherence or indirectly through a negative placebo-like effect (Janevic *et al.*, 2003). On the other hand, individuals receiving their preferred intervention may comply better than average and exaggerate the effectiveness of the intervention. This is particularly challenging when variables such as quality of life and well-being rather than objective measures are a major outcome. Additionally, individuals with strong preferences for an intervention often do not get into a trial because randomization does not guarantee that they will get what they want (King *et al.*, 2005). It can be argued that the best way of dealing with preferences for interventions is to take account of these within an RCT (Howard and Thornicroft, 2006). An option is to take preferences for interventions into consideration in the trial design, not assuming that an intervention is equal for everyone.

Recruitment to clinical trials may be affected by the choice of intervention that participants might make, if they were allowed to choose, and by whether they actually receive their preferred intervention. These effects cannot be estimated in the randomized controlled trial design.

Learning objectives

This chapter is written to enable the reader to:

*   Understand advantages and challenges of using non-standard and preference designs.
*   Use research designs taking preferences for interventions into consideration.

Non-standard and preference designs

With the comprehensive cohort design (CCD) (Olschewski and Scheurlen, 1985), participants with strong preferences are offered their preferred intervention while the others are randomized in the usual way. The design is ideal when it is likely that many will refuse randomization because of strong preferences for an intervention. The design allows for most eligible participants to be followed up under RCT conditions, comparisons of outcomes between preference and randomized participants, and an analysis of the effect of intervention preference on outcome. However, important baseline differences between preference and randomized participants may compromise the value of this comparison. The design does not necessarily solve failure to recruit participants with strong preferences or attrition. See Box 21.1 for a summary of the internal and external validity and study administration of the design. The design was used by Leiva-Fernández and co-workers (2012) to investigate the effect of written information about inhalation techniques vs. written information plus training by an instructor on performance of correct inhalation technique among patients with chronic obstructive pulmonary disease.

Another alternative to deal with preferences is the pre-randomized Zelen single consent design in which potential participants are randomized to intervention and control groups; thereafter consent is requested from those in the intervention group (Zelen, 1979). This design aims to remove rather than account for preferences and is relevant when awareness of allocation among controls might lead to contamination, or when recruitment and consent constitutes a partial intervention. In the double consent variant, consent to intervention is sought from both groups and those who decline the allocated intervention receive the other (Zelen, 1990). The single consent design has been subject to ethical criticisms because of lack of information regarding study intervention(s) to all participants, and scientific criticisms because of the dilution of effect due to 'cross-over' of participants to the non-randomized intervention. However, the design may be ethically preferable to a conventional design where it would be intolerable to the control group to know that a potentially effective intervention is denied through randomization (Torgerson and Roland, 1998). See Box 21.1 for a summary of the internal and external validity and study administration of the design. In a variant of the method, Campbell *et al.* (2005) sought consent among patients with painful patello-femoral osteoarthritis of the knee joint to a one-year observational study. Participants were subsequently randomized into intervention and control groups. Those randomized to the intervention group were asked whether they were willing to participate in a study involving regular sessions with a physiotherapist. Those in the control group were not told about this, but were followed up as agreed.

Many competing interventions for the same condition have not been compared or compared inaccurately, which is a waste of information and money. Relton *et al.* (2010) proposed an approach, the cohort multiple randomized controlled trial (cmRCT), offering a solution to this problem. This design does not allow estimates of preferences but tries to minimize dropout due to preferences. The design is relevant for chronic conditions where many pragmatic RCTs will be conducted of interventions in comparison with treatment as usual (Relton *et al.*, 2010). An observational cohort with the condition of interest consenting to provide data to be used to look at the benefit of treatments for this condition is recruited and their outcomes are regularly measured. Then, participants eligible for a certain RCT are identified in the cohort and some are randomly selected and offered the trial intervention. Consent is only sought from those offered the intervention replicating the process of obtaining consent in real-world health care. The outcomes of the randomly selected persons are compared to the outcomes of eligible individuals not randomly selected. The process can be repeated for further RCTs. The capacity for multiple RCTs over time using individuals from the same cohort is unique to this design, and the informed consent approach offers a solution to the ethical criticisms of the Zelen design. When researching interventions available in routine health care, it is necessary to identify and monitor which individuals use or have used interventions offered in routine health care (Relton *et al.*, 2010). See Box 21.1 for a summary of the internal and external validity and study administration of the design. In a pilot study (Relton *et al.*, 2012), a cohort of women with hot flushes who consented to provide observational data were recruited. The cohort was screened in order to identify patients eligible for a pragmatic RCT of the offer of treatment by a homoeopath, and a proportion of these patients was randomly selected to be offered the treatment and asked about consent. The outcomes of these patients were compared to the outcomes of eligible patients not randomly selected.

A further design taking preferences into account is the two-stage randomized design, the so-called Rücker or Wennberg design (Rücker, 1989; Wennberg *et al.*, 1993). The design is useful to estimate direct intervention effects, as well as preference and selection effects. Participants are initially randomized to two groups to reduce baseline imbalances between randomized and preference groups. One group is then offered a choice of intervention in the same way as the preference groups in a comprehensive cohort design. The other group is randomized as in an RCT. In the Rücker design, participants randomized to the preference group in the first randomization and who do not have a strong preference for an intervention are randomized a second time to an intervention. These designs offer a more powerful method of determining the influence of preference on outcome than the CCD, in which preferences are not evenly distributed between groups within the preference arm because participants are free to choose which group they will join. The design overcomes the ethical problem created by the Zelen design in that consent is achieved prior to randomization. However, the design does not circumvent the difficulty of recruiting those who have such strong preferences that they are not prepared to risk the first randomization. See Box 21.1 for a summary of the internal and external validity and study administration of the design. McCafferey and colleagues (2011) used the Rücker method to understand the effect of patient choice on patient outcomes in a trial of management strategies for women with atypical cells of undetermined significance detected at routine cervical screening. Women were randomized to either an informed choice of human papillomavirus triage testing or to repeat pap testing or to no choice with random allocation to management by either option.

BOX 21.1 INTERNAL AND EXTERNAL VALIDITY AND STUDY ADMINISTRATION FOR THE COMPREHENSIVE COHORT DESIGN, PRE-RANDOMIZED DESIGN, COHORT MULTIPLE RANDOMIZED CONTROLLED TRIAL, AND TWO-STAGE RANDOMIZED DESIGNS

Comprehensive cohort design

Participants with strong preferences are offered their treatment of choice, while those without strong preferences are randomized in the conventional fashion.

Internal validity: preference effects (e.g. randomization vs. preference) are confounded, although can be controlled.

External validity: almost all eligible potential participants enter the study allowing examination of characteristics of participants with all strength of preferences.

Study administration: potentially costly if large numbers express a preference and not feasible if very few have a preference.

Pre-randomized design

Individuals eligible for inclusion are randomized before consent to participate.

Internal validity: all potential participants are randomized but, depending on consent process, uneven dropout may occur between intervention and control arms.

External validity: all eligible potential participants enter the study; ethical objections exist for the single consent design over lack of fully informed consent.

Study administration: potentially low cost as all eligible potential participants enter the study but, depending on later consent process, dropout or switching between arms may make increased recruitment necessary.

The cohort multiple randomized controlled trial

Internal validity: increased as data are collected on patients before they accept or refuse the intervention and as the design allows collection of information about why patients refuse an intervention and why certain patients are unable to complete an assigned intervention.

External validity: increased by the approach to provide information and consent.

Study administration: the recruitment process is less likely to screen out non-accepters prior to random selection, and the intention to treat analysis runs the risk of a Type II error (Relton *et al.*, 2012). Some non-compliance can be avoided by presenting the cohort with a list of possible interventions at enrolment and asking which they would consider agreeing to use if offered.

Two-stage randomized designs

In the Wennberg design, participants are initially randomized to two groups; in one group they are offered a choice of treatment while in the other they are randomized to treatment. The Rücker design is similar but participants randomized to preference in the first randomization and who do not have a strong preference for a treatment are randomized a second time to a treatment.

Internal validity: all potential participants are randomized, increasing internal validity. However, comparisons between randomization and preference groups are subject to confounding because participant characteristics may determine choice of treatment.

External validity: reduced because only potential participants accepting randomization enter the study.

Study administration: people with strong preferences may refuse randomization.

Advantages and challenges with non-standard and preference designs

The RCT runs counter to the current emphasis on patient choice, which is the cornerstone of many governments' current health strategies. Where preferences or ethical objections to an RCT exist, alternatives that replicate more closely the behaviours in real-world health care rather than conform to standard trial design should be considered. Citizen participation in research is advocated by governments, research councils and other funding bodies and as the public, patients and significant others become more involved in research activities they may be unwilling to be passive participants of a research randomization process. Although patients and others have a choice to enter RCTs, it is often forgotten that they also have preferences about the interventions on offer. Non-standard and preference designs go some way towards addressing the problem of non-implementation of results of clinical research. However, incorporating preferences into a design evaluating an intervention in a meaningful way presents challenges. First, a preference effect cannot be disentangled from possible confounding arising from differences with regard to, for example, intervention history, social class and education. Second, preference designs are connected with an increased demand for sample size based on stratification by preference being incorporated into the design.

Summary of advantages of non-standard and preference designs

- With the comprehensive cohort design almost all eligible participants enter the study, allowing examination of participants' characteristics with all strengths of preferences.
- There are circumstances in which the pre-randomized design may be preferred on ethical grounds; however, it should be used with caution because of added complexity and the incomplete consent process.
- The cohort multiple randomized controlled trial offers a unique possibility for multiple RCTs over time using patients from the same cohort, comparing interventions for the same condition.
- The two-stage randomization designs can provide unbiased estimates of the selection and preference effects, and the direct effect of treatment. The method can be used to illuminate the impact of choice on participant outcomes.

Further reading

Hewitt, C. E., Torgerson D. J. and Miles, J. V. N. 2006. Is there another way to take account of noncompliance in randomized controlled trials? *Canadian Medical Association Journal,* 175: 347.

King, M., Nazareth, I., Lampe, F., Bower, P., Chandler, M., Morou, M., Sibbald, B. and Lai, R. 2005. Conceptual framework and systematic review of the effects of participants' and professionals' preferences in randomized controlled trials. *Health Technology Assessment,* 9: 1–186.

Walter, S. D., Turner, R. M., Macaskill, P., McCaffery, K. J. and Irwing, L. 2012. Optimal allocation of participants for the estimation of selection, preference and treatment effects in the two-stage randomized trial design. *Statistics in Medicine,* 31: 1307–22.

22

SINGLE-SUBJECT DESIGNS

Lena Nilsson-Wikmar and Karin Harms-Ringdahl

Introduction

In a clinical situation it can be difficult to design a randomized clinical trial (RCT) with enough power. Therefore an alternative could be to use a single-subject design to put focus on the individual in order to recall the common clinical setting, where patients/clients or persons are treated individually in order to obtain optimal effect.

Learning objectives

After study of this chapter, readers are expected to:

- Know how to use single-subject designs such as a basic design, withdrawal designs, multiple baseline design and alternating treatment design for treatment outcome evaluations in a clinical setting.
- State the characteristics of different designs.
- Understand how to evaluate outcome measures using different designs.
- Understand research examples using different designs.

Single-subject designs enable an experimental investigation for evaluation of outcome measurements when only a few individuals with similar conditions are expected to participate. It has been frequently used within educational and behavioral sciences. The designs are prospective, experimental, and involve repeated measurements in a baseline phase as well as in an intervention or treatment phase. A limitation of the design is the external validity because of the number of subjects being restricted to one. This can, however, be solved with a replication of the same set-up in more subjects in different clinical settings. Frequently collected measurements that make it possible to follow trend, levels and variability over time for more than one outcome measurement considered to be important for assessing improvement are also used as an indication of the external validity, if they follow similar patterns for the different subjects. Careful patient description and a controlled starting time point for intervention are also of importance. Other names used in the literature are single-subject experimental design (SSED), single-subject research design and single-system design. It is important not to compare the single-subject designs to clinical case reports and clinical case studies, since those are non-experimental.

The overall components in the single-subject designs are repeated measurements in two phases – baseline, i.e. the A-phase defined as no intervention or treatment, and the B-phase with an intervention or treatment. The two phases are combined in different ways in the different designs, as discussed later in this chapter.

The single-subject designs begin with defining the baseline phase or A-phase by frequent measurements of the variable that is expected to change with the intervention or treatment (B-phase), the dependent variable. The aim is to predict how the patients will behave without any treatment and therefore it is important that the data are stable and characterized by the absence of a trend/slope and with little variability. The trend is defined as a decrease or increase over time and the variability to the fluctuation of the measured variable. To predict the level, trend/slope and variability of no treatment or intervention at least three measurements are required. The more data points that are used a more proper baseline will be defined and the control of the internal validity will be more secure. Figure 22.1 illustrates different patterns for the baseline in relation to pain ratings on a visual analogue scale (VAS).

The B-phase is the intervention or treatment phase and is defined by frequent measurements of the same variable as in the A-phase during the treatment period.

The number of measurement points needed in different phases is dependent mainly on the variability and trend shown and how soon a change is going to happen. If, for example, there is time dependence in pain over the 24 hours or during the week, this needs to be captured, and also needs to be reflected in the measurements during the next phase. If there is a debilitating trend during the A-phase, an effective treatment is supposed to change this trend and improve the condition. However, if the trend shows that the condition is already improving by itself during the A-phase, no matter how many measurements you collect, it will be very difficult to show that the intervention is improving the condition in a more rapid way. If statistical methods for result analysis are used, as described later, more data points entail higher measurement precision.

There is a strength to identifying a few outcome variables that are supposed to (approximately) follow each other, even if for practical reasons it will not be possible to measure them both with the same frequency. Maybe the expected change is

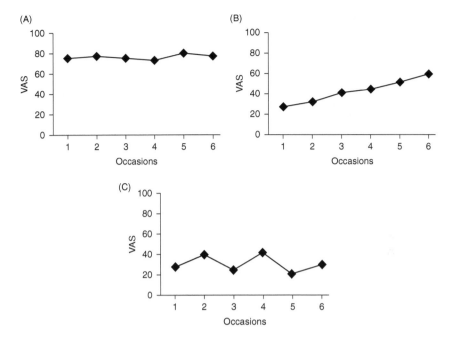

FIGURE 22.1 Examples of different patterns of a baseline (A-phase) regarding pain rating using a visual analogue scale (VAS) on six occasions during the A-phase, a stable baseline (A), an increased trend (B), and a baseline with variability (C)

also supposed to happen at a different rate, as is the case, for example, with assessed pain intensity and functioning.

There are different designs used depending on the question asked. The designs most used will be presented below: basic design, withdrawal designs, multiple baseline design and alternating treatment design.

Designs

Basic design

The A-B design is a basic single-subject design answering the questions, 'Does this treatment work?' and 'How well does it work?' It includes a baseline phase with repeated measurements of the dependent variable and an intervention or treatment phase continuing the measurement of the dependent variable (Figure 22.2). The A-B design is suitable to describe the pattern of the clinical change, but cannot demonstrate a causal inference between the change in the outcome variable and a specific intervention. To solve that, a withdrawal design can be used.

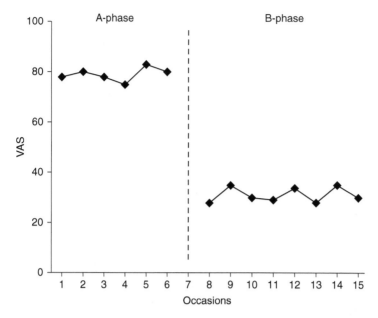

FIGURE 22.2 Example of an A-B design with pain ratings using a visual analogue scale (VAS) six times during the A-phase and eight times during the B-phase

Withdrawal designs

A withdrawal design is characterized by stopping the intervention or treatment for a period of time. There are two main designs. In the A-B-A design the treatment is followed up by frequent measurements of the outcome variable in order to track the long-term effect of the treatment. Depending on the duration of the follow-up period it may be possible to determine the length of time the effect persists. This design therefore answers the question, 'Does the effect of the intervention persist beyond the period in which treatment is performed?' (Figure 22.3). In the second design – the A-B-A-B design – a second baseline phase is followed with a second treatment or intervention phase.

Multiple baseline design

A multiple baseline design is a series of A-B designs that are implemented at the same time in more subjects, but with different lengths of both the baseline and intervention phases in order to control for external outcome a cross the subjects.

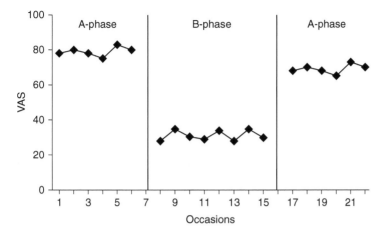

FIGURE 22.3 Example of an A-B-A design with rating of pain on a visual analogue scale (VAS) six times during the first A-phase, eight times during the B-phase and six times during the second A-phase

The second and third subjects act as a control for external events in the first case, and the third case acts as a control for the second subject (Figure 22.4). The design can be modified across subjects through a non-concurrent multiple baseline design if patients do not start at the same time point. It can also be modified across outcomes with a stepwise change of the intervention and across settings using different settings.

The number of patients needed in order to draw a conclusion about the potential treatment effects depends on the persistence of the outcome among the patients. Using an approach from the statistical Sign Test, there should be an effect in the same direction in eight out of ten patients. However, the design can also be used simply in order to test the suitability of an intervention in a certain patient subpopulation, the instruments of the outcome measurements with regard to variability, and possible floor and ceiling effects, before planning an RCT. This design is also suitable for development work in order to improve practice and treatment quality in a clinical situation where the patients are followed more carefully with regard to intervention and outcome.

Changing intensity and alternating treatment designs

Changing intensity and alternating treatment designs evaluate the effect of two or more different treatments across periods of time in a random order (Table 22.1).

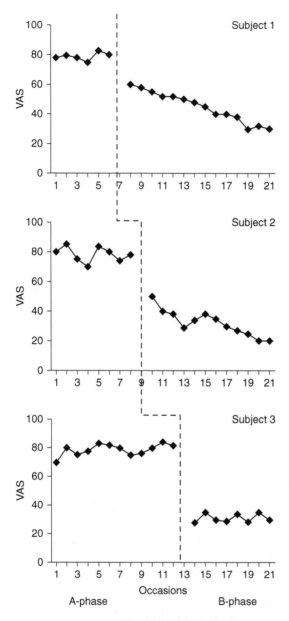

FIGURE 22.4 Example of a multiple baseline design with pain ratings using a visual analogue scale (VAS) from three subjects with different durations of A and B-phases

TABLE 22.1 Description of changing intensity and alternating treatment designs, respectively, regarding combinations of phases (A denotes baseline phase, and B and C intervention phases)

Changing intensity	A-B^1-B^2-B^3 (e.g. type, intensity, duration)
Alternating treatments	A-B-C; A-C-B; A-B-A-C; A-B-A-C-A; A-C-A-B-A
	Consider intervention order effects (i.e. use different order for different patients). Evaluate consistency of data patterns.

Data analysis

There are two main methods for data analysis: visual and statistical. In both methods a graphical presentation is crucial.

Visual method

The visual method is the traditional one where the level, trend/slope and variability are analysed. Visual analysis works well if there is a clear treatment effect (Figure 22.5).

Statistical method

In statistical analysis the mean and the two standard deviation bands are calculated from the measurements collected during the baseline phase. A horizontal line is drawn for the mean from the baseline data across all phases, as well as horizontal lines from calculations of the two standard deviations. The area between the two standard deviations is the 'two standard deviation (2-SD)' band. A statistically significant effect is achieved when at least two consecutive measuring points are outside the 2-SD band, indicating a difference ($p = <0.05$) between two phases. With no effect the points are within the 2-SD band. The advantage of using statistical analysis is that small effects of the treatment can also be detected and statistical significance is not dependent on who is analysing the data (Figure 22.6).

Examples

Two studies will be described as examples. In a study by Marklund and Klässbo (2006), an A–B design was used in order to investigate possible effects on constraint-induced movement therapy for the lower extremity during two weeks with training six hours per day in five patients post-stroke, and the measurements were followed up three and six months later. Motor function in the lower extremity, mobility, dynamic balance, weight-bearing symmetry and walking ability were assessed on six occasions during a two-week period during the A-phase and at similar frequency during the two-week training period – the B-phase. Different

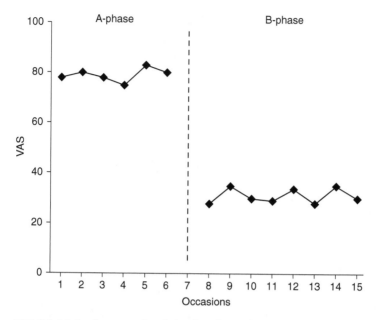

FIGURE 22.5 An example of visual analysis of the effect of treatment with the aim of reducing pain (a clear reduction in pain intensity level is denoted by the absence of trend/slope and little variability)

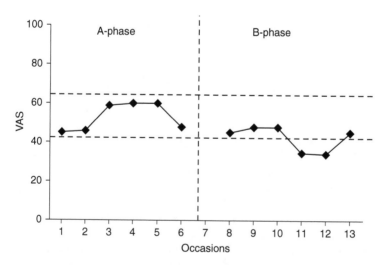

FIGURE 22.6 An example of analysis of a 2-SD band with a statistically significant decrease in pain intensity in the B-phase

outcome measurements were used such as Fugl–Meyer assessment, the Timed up-and-go, the Step test, the Timed Walking test and the Six-Minute Walk test. In this study the intensive training programme was seen as a treatment package where several proxies for mobility and walking ability showed concurrent improvement. The result showed a either positive change or statistical improvement in motor function, mobility, dynamic balance and walking ability in four out of the five patients. The effects persisted after three and six months in almost all variables measured for the four patients.

In a study by Gustafsson and Nilsson-Wikmar (2008) using an A–B–A design, the aim was to test the influence of specific trunk muscle training on pain, activity limitation and kinesiophobia in 10 subjects with back pain postpartum. Whereas pain intensity is expected to vary over the day, assessments need to be performed at the same time point on each occasion. Activity limitation include the ability to perform commonly performed tasks, and can be assessed by, for example, the Disability Rating Index (DRI), a self-reported instrument. As pain and the DRI are supposed to correlate with each other, they were used together to strengthen the design. However, according to the scientific literature, the relation between pain intensity and activity limitation is unclear since other factors may influence the relation. The Tampa Scale for Kinesiophobia measures the individual's fear of being physically active despite pain symptoms, and kinesiophobia is also supposed to influence assessments of activity limitation. Pain and disability data were collected at similar intervals during the three phases but kinesiophobia measurement only twice, once before and once after treatment. In the present study the visual analysis showed a trend towards reduced pain and activity limitation for all 10 subjects. The statistical analysis showed a mixed result. All subjects reported kinesiophobia both before and after treatment.

Conclusion

In conclusion, the single-subject design covers different designs in order to focus on the individual patient. It is characterized by a good description of both the patient's characteristics and the intervention. There is an experimental design with regard to starting and stopping the intervention, conducted where the frequent measurement points are plotted during the baseline and the intervention period, sometimes also during a follow-up period. Outcome measures are analysed with regard to level, trend/slope and variability using visual inspection or statistical analyses. The same intervention can be conducted and results compared between patients in order to strengthen external validity.

23

PROCESS EVALUATION OF COMPLEX INTERVENTIONS

A summary of Medical Research Council guidance

Graham Moore, Suzanne Audrey, Mary Barker, Lyndal Bond, Chris Bonell, Wendy Hardeman, Laurence Moore, Alicia O'Cathain, Tannaze Tinati, Daniel E. Wight and Janis Baird

Introduction

The updated UK Medical Research Council's (MRC) guidance on complex interventions reflected a shift away from a paradigm focused solely on effectiveness, towards recognition of the need to understand how complex interventions are implemented, their causal mechanisms and their interaction with their contexts (Craig *et al.*, 2008; Medical Research Council, 2008). The guidance advocated process evaluation within trials (or other high-quality outcome evaluation designs) as a means of understanding these issues. However, it stopped short of providing recommendations on how to conduct process evaluation. Work funded by the MRC Population Health Science Research Network (PHSRN) has since served to fill this gap. This chapter, therefore, will summarize the more recent guidance on process evaluation of complex interventions and its key recommendations. Process evaluation is conceived as complementary to outcomes evaluation. We specifically discuss the role of process evaluation within trials of complex interventions, including feasibility and pilot trials and fully powered effectiveness trials. Though most authors are experienced primarily in public health research, the guidance is relevant to other domains such as health service and educational research.

Learning objectives

- Gain an understanding of the importance of process evaluation of complex interventions.
- Explore key considerations in planning, designing, conducting, analysing and reporting a process evaluation.

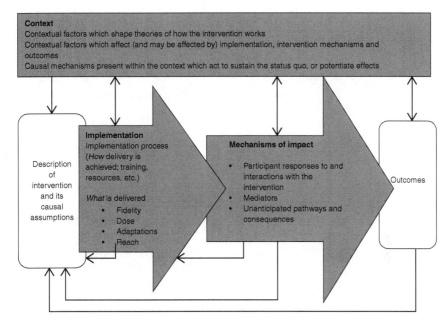

FIGURE 23.1 Key functions of process evaluation and relationships among them (shaded boxes represent components of process evaluation, informed by the intervention description, which inform interpretation of outcomes)

What key functions can process evaluations serve?

The UK MRC complex intervention guidance states that process evaluation 'can be used to assess fidelity and quality of *implementation*, clarify causal *mechanisms* and identify *contextual factors* associated with variation in outcomes' (Medical Research Council, 2008: 12, our emphasis). These functions, expanded upon below, form the basis of the MRC process evaluation framework, presented in Figure 23.1.

Implementation

Without a clear picture of what intervention components were implemented, it is impossible to conclude whether limited effects arise from flaws in the design of the intervention, or failure to implement it fully (Steckler and Linnan, 2002). Process evaluations should aim to capture whether the intervention was delivered as intended (fidelity) and the quantity (dose) of what was implemented. Complex interventions will often undergo adaptation when implemented across different contexts. Capturing adaptations, and their implications for intervention functioning, is vital. In addition, process evaluation should aim to understand *how* implementation is achieved (e.g. through training and support, management and communication structures). This is important, both to advance implementation science (i.e. understanding how to implement complex interventions) and provide policy-makers and practitioners with information on how the intervention might be replicated.

Mechanisms of impact

The 2008 MRC framework argues that understanding causal mechanisms is crucial in order to develop effective interventions and understand how findings might be transferred across settings and populations (Medical Research Council, 2008). Future interventions may not replicate the activities delivered within the original intervention, but may target similar mechanisms. Using evaluation to build theory through testing assumptions about how the intervention works, while also generating new theory, is a critical aim of process evaluation (Bonell *et al.*, 2012).

Context

The theme 'context' cuts across both previous themes, with process evaluation focused on how context shapes (and is shaped by) implementation, and how context influences whether or not mechanisms targeted by the intervention work. Evaluators may, for example, need to understand issues such as how implementers' readiness or ability to adopt new practices is influenced by pre-existing circumstances, skills, organizational norms, resources and attitudes. Evaluators will also need to understand how participant responses differ as a result of pre-existing contextual circumstances (e.g. whether the intervention works differently for groups of higher or lower socio-economic status).

Planning, designing, conducting and reporting a process evaluation

Different complex interventions pose different empirical uncertainties, suited to different methods. Hence, there is no one-size-fits-all process evaluation method. However, planning and conducting a process evaluation involve thinking carefully through a number of common issues. We now discuss key challenges faced by process evaluators and recommendations for overcoming them.

Planning a process evaluation

Working with programme developers and implementers

Process evaluation involves closely observing an intervention and understanding its workings. Good relationships with stakeholders involved in developing or delivering the intervention are necessary to enable this, but can be difficult to build, with evaluation often seen as threatening. It is also important that evaluators maintain sufficient independence to observe the work of these stakeholders critically. We recommend that:

- evaluators transparently report relationships with policy and practice stakeholders, and remain reflexive about how these affect the evaluation;

- evaluators consider occasional peer review by others external to the project who may help to identify where the researchers position has compromised the evaluation.

Evaluators also need to choose between a fairly passive role, feeding back findings at the end, or an active role of feeding back process findings as they emerge. We recommend that:

- systems for communicating information to stakeholders are agreed at the outset of the study, to avoid perceptions of undue interference, or that evaluators withheld important information;
- evaluators take an active role in shaping the intervention at the feasibility testing stage;
- where evaluating effectiveness, it will usually be appropriate to assume a more passive role, to avoid changing how the intervention is delivered and compromising a study's external validity.

Resources and staffing

Process evaluations involve prioritizing numerous potential research questions, combining quantitative and qualitative methods, and often draw upon theories across disciplinary boundaries. We recommend that:

- sufficient expertise and experience be included within the team to successfully decide and achieve the aims of the process evaluation;
- expertise includes quantitative, qualitative and mixed methods and relevant theory, drawing upon multiple disciplines (e.g. psychology and sociology) where appropriate;
- sufficient resources are costed for collection and analysis of large quantities of diverse types of data.

Relationships within evaluation teams

Process evaluation will typically form part of a study which includes outcomes and/or cost-effectiveness evaluation. These components should add value to one another, rather than act as parallel studies. We recommend that:

- attention is paid to assembling a team whose members respect and value one another's work;
- the overall study is supervised by a principal investigator who values integration (O'Cathain et al., 2008).

Some evaluators choose to separate process and outcome teams. In other cases the same people evaluate processes and outcomes. Defining the relationships between components of an evaluation at the planning stage is crucial. We recommend that:

- where allocated to separate teams, effective communications between teams be maintained to prevent duplication or conflict;
- where process and outcome evaluations are conducted by the same individuals, there is a need for openness about how knowledge of trial outcomes influences the analysis and interpretation of process data; and integration of process and outcome data be planned from the outset.

Designing and conducting a process evaluation

A lack of clarity about the aims of a process evaluation may lead to the collection of excessive data, or data which do not address the key questions. It is never possible to answer all potential questions. Over-intensive engagement with providers and participants may artificially change how the intervention is delivered and experienced, particularly alongside an evaluation of effectiveness. Process evaluation should thoroughly answer a small number of key questions, offering insights that advance intervention theory and practice.

Describing the intervention and its underlying 'theory'

A crucial starting point for process evaluation is a clear description of the intervention and its underlying 'theory' (i.e. the assumptions being made about how it will be implemented and how it will work in context). The assumptions underpinning complex interventions are often left unstated, but being clear about what these are will help to focus the evaluation and clarify potential contributions of the evaluation to the evidence base. This may include social science theories, and/or assumptions based on experience or 'common sense'. It is useful to develop a manual which describes the resources necessary to implement the intervention (and how they will be applied), intended intervention activities, hypothesized mechanisms and intended outcomes, and to represent key assumptions diagrammatically in a logic model (Kellogg Foundation, 2004). These activities may not form part of the process evaluation – a manual or logic model may have been developed prior to evaluation – but provide the basis for identifying key questions.

Deciding research questions

Research questions emerge from considering assumptions reflected by the intervention, the evidence base for those assumptions, and key policy and practice priorities. We recommend that:

- potential research questions are identified through systematically listing assumptions reflected within the intervention manual or logic model;
- agreement is sought on the most important questions through reviewing the literature, discussions within the research team and consultation with policy and practice stakeholders.

At some point, the study may be included in systematic reviews synthesizing evaluations of interventions with similar components or theories of change. Waters and colleagues (2011) argue that if reviews are to assist decision-makers, considering implementation and context is essential. We recommend that:

- process evaluations of similar interventions are identified, and consideration given to whether replicating aspects of these studies, and building on them to explore new issues is appropriate.

While a clear focus from the outset is vital, complex interventions are inherently unpredictable. Evaluators may identify additional questions which need to be addressed. For example, the context may change in unexpected ways which has implications for the intervention. The intervention may undergo unanticipated adaptations, whose implications for outcomes need to be understood. We recommend that:

- process evaluations be designed with sufficient flexibility to allow important emerging questions to be addressed.

Selecting methods

Process evaluations usually require a combination of quantitative and qualitative methods. For example, evaluators may need to quantify how much of certain components are implemented, while qualitatively capturing emerging adaptations. Qualitative investigation enables exploration of participant responses or pathways which are too complex to be captured quantitatively, and generation of theory regarding how an intervention works. Process evaluation should also use quantitative data to test pre-hypothesized causal pathways. Common process evaluation methods include self-report diaries/audits or questionnaires, observations (in person or via audio or video recordings), qualitative interviews and focus groups. All have different strengths and limitations. Diaries, audits and questionnaires may be cheap to administer on a large scale but are subject to reporting biases. Observations overcome self-reporting biases, but are resource intensive and may change how the intervention is delivered. We recommend that:

- decisions on research methods be guided by careful consideration of the strengths and limitations of each method in relation to the question posed;

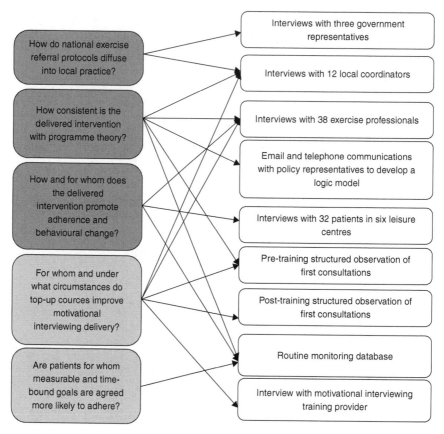

FIGURE 23.2   Research questions and methods used for the process evaluation of the National Exercise Referral Scheme in Wales (pre-specified questions are in dark grey, questions which emerged during the course of the study are in light grey)

- evaluators use an appropriate mix of quantitative and qualitative methods to address key process questions.

Some of the questions posed, and methods used to address them, within the evaluation of the National Exercise Referral Scheme in Wales (Moore *et al.*, 2013) are presented in Figure 23.2.

Sampling

A key consideration for process evaluation, particularly in large trials, is sampling. Interviewing every implementer, for example, may lead to overwhelming volumes of data. However, there are dangers in collecting data from only a few case studies and drawing conclusions from these regarding the intervention as a whole (Munro and Bloor, 2010). We recommend that:

- where feasible, evaluators consider collecting data on key process variables from all sites/participants;
- in-depth data are collected from samples purposively selected along dimensions expected to influence the functioning of the intervention.

Timing

Data, and the conclusions which can be drawn from them, will be situated in the time in which they are collected. For example, if collected during early stages of evaluation, data may capture teething problems, rectified soon after. Implementers' perceptions of the intervention, and their practices, may change as they receive feedback on what works. The organization may change to allow integration of the intervention. We recommend that:

- careful consideration is given to how data are situated in the time in which they are collected;
- data collection at multiple time points be considered to capture changes over time, while considering whether this can this be done without changing intervention delivery.

Analysis of process data, and integration of process and outcomes data

Quantitative analysis will likely include descriptive information on measures such as fidelity, dose and reach, while more detailed modelling will explore variations between participants or contexts in terms of implementation and reach. Qualitative process analysis may serve predictive or post hoc explanatory functions in relation to outcome evaluation. Where analysed prior to outcomes analysis, for example (Oakley et al., 2006), they may generate hypotheses regarding why positive or negative effects might be anticipated (overall or for certain subgroups). These hypotheses may then be tested quantitatively where suitable data have been collected or can be integrated into follow-up data collections. The integration of process and outcome findings in the process evaluation of the Southampton Initiative for Health (Baird et al., 2014) is presented in Figure 23.3. We recommend that:

- process evaluators work with those responsible for other aspects of the evaluation to ensure that plans are made for integration from the outset, and reflected in how the evaluation is designed;
- quantitative process data are integrated into outcomes data sets to examine whether effects differ by implementation or pre-specified contextual factors, and test hypothesized mechanisms of impact;
- where possible, initial analysis and reporting of qualitative process data take place prior to knowing intervention outcomes to avoid biased interpretation;

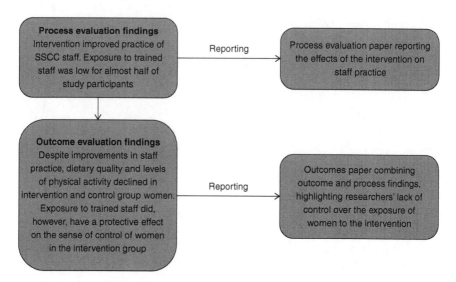

FIGURE 23.3 Integration of process and outcome findings in the Southampton Initiative for Health, a staff training intervention to improve the diets and physical activity levels of women attending Sure Start Children's Centres (SSCCs)

- qualitative analyses take advantage of the flexibility and depth of qualitative data to explore complex or unanticipated processes;
- quantitative and qualitative findings are coherently integrated.

Reporting findings of a process evaluation

What to report

Providing guidance on exactly what to report in a process evaluation is challenging because there is no one-size-fits-all method. Key considerations include clearly reporting relationships between quantitative and qualitative components, and the relationship of the process evaluation to the overall evaluation, including whether trial outcomes were known at the time process analyses took place. The theoretical assumptions underlying the intervention should be reported (ideally in a logic model), and evaluators should be explicit about how these informed the choice of questions addressed (Armstrong *et al.*, 2008). Separate ongoing work aims to extend CONSORT reporting guidelines (Montgomery *et al.*, 2013) to incorporate reporting of social and psychological interventions, including process evaluations.

Publishing in academic journals

Process evaluations usually generate more data than can be reported in a single journal article. A key challenge is dividing the process evaluation into pieces which stand alone, while not losing sight of the broader picture. It is common for process data not to be published in peer-reviewed journals, or for only parts to be published. We recommend that:

- all journal articles refer to other articles published from the study, or to a protocol paper or report, and make their relationship with the overall evaluation clear;
- articles emphasize contributions to advancing intervention theory, or methodological debates regarding how to evaluate complex interventions, to ensure a broader appeal to journal editors.

Reporting to wider audiences

While process evaluation aims to inform development of theory and a wider evidence base, it also aims to inform the actions of policy-makers and practitioners. We recommend that:

- findings are reported in lay formats to stakeholders involved in the delivery of the intervention or in decisions about its future implementation;
- findings are presented at conferences organized by service delivery organizations, which offers a means of promoting findings beyond academic circles, providing an opportunity to summarize the evaluation as a whole and highlight links between its components.

Conclusions

New MRC guidance for process evaluation provides assistance in planning, designing and conducting a process evaluation, and reporting its findings. It sets out a framework for linking the core functions of process evaluation. It argues for careful consideration of the relationships necessary to conduct a successful process evaluation, and a systematic approach to designing and conducting process evaluations, drawing on clear descriptions of intervention theory and identification of the empirical uncertainties within it.

Further reading

Moore, G., Audrey, S., Barker, M., Bond, L., Bonell, C., Cooper, C., Hardeman, W., Moore, L., O'Cathain, A., Tinati, T., Wight, D. and Baird, J. 2014. Process evaluation of complex public health interventions: the need for guidance. *Journal of Epidemiology and Community Health,* 68: 101–2.

24

INTERVENTION FIDELITY IN CLINICAL TRIALS

Henna Hasson

Introduction

Fidelity is often defined as the degree to which implementation of a particular program follows a program model. Thus, fidelity can act as a potential mediator of the relationship between interventions and their intended outcomes. Several studies have demonstrated that interventions implemented with high fidelity had better outcomes than interventions with lower fidelity (Blakely *et al.*, 1987; Dane and Schneider, 1998; Hansen *et al.*, 1991; Keith *et al.*, 2010; Rohrbach *et al.*, 1993). Some programs only had significant effects in the high-fidelity samples as compared with the entire intervention group (McGrew and Griss, 2005; Mihalic, 2004). From this it follows that measurement and control of fidelity is central in clinical trials. However, an intervention cannot always be implemented fully according to the program model since local conditions might require some adaptations to the predefined interventions. The present chapter presents the concept of fidelity and offers practical guidance in measurement of fidelity in clinical trials. The chapter also discusses the difficult balance between adhering to a clinical protocol and allowing some necessary local adaptations.

Learning objectives

- Have knowledge of the subcategories in fidelity and know how to address these in clinical trials.
- Be able to plan a study of fidelity for a clinical trial.
- Be able to reason about benefits of high fidelity and benefits of allowing local adaptations.

Background

In general, a process evaluation examines what the program is and how it is delivered to the target clients (Rossi *et al.*, 2004). Fidelity is a measure for the degree to which an intervention was implemented as was intended (Dusenbury *et al.*, 2003). Fidelity is often a part of a process evaluation. A measurement of fidelity implies a comparison of intervention's actual delivery to a standard of the intervention that describes the intended program and its intended delivery (Rossi *et al.*, 2004).

One of the primary benefits of fidelity analysis in clinical trials is the possibility to interpret results of the outcome evaluation. Thus, analysis of fidelity is important in order to understand what specific reasons caused an intervention to succeed or fail (Carroll *et al.*, 2007; Dobson and Cook, 1980; Fixsen *et al.*, 2005). This is especially relevant for complex interventions that consist of several active ingredients (Craig *et al.*, 2008). Otherwise, there is a risk of evaluating the effects of a program that have been described but not fully implemented.

Subcategories of fidelity

Two basic forms of violation to interventions fidelity, i.e. local adaptations, have been described. These involve modifications of intervention content and form of intervention delivery (Castro *et al.*, 2004). The content can be changed by omitting, modifying or adding intervention components. Changes concerning the delivery can deal with the manner or intensity with which the intervention components are delivered (Castro *et al.*, 2004). Fidelity can be defined in terms of five subcategories dealing with the potential areas of intervention modification, i.e. content and form of delivery. Subcategories of fidelity are content, frequency, duration, coverage and timeliness (Carroll *et al.*, 2007; Hasson 2010; von Thiele Schwarz *et al.*, 2013). These refer to whether the active ingredients of the intervention have been received by the participants as often and for as long as was planned. Timeliness refers to the degree of the intervention being conducted at the right time points. For instance, some methods might need to be delivered at certain time points during the day to have the most beneficial effects. Table 24.1 illustrates examples of process questions and potential data collection methods in relation to each subcategory of fidelity.

Factors affecting fidelity

Several conditions may require adaptations to an intervention model (Carroll *et al.*, 2007). The potential factors affecting intervention fidelity exist at individual, local and national levels (Tansella and Thornicroft, 2009). Factors such as financial incentives, effective monitoring and feedback systems are examples of potential factors at the national level affecting fidelity. These factors are especially important to consider when testing an intervention from one country in another country. For instance, the first evaluation of the evidence-based program for supported employment in

TABLE 24.1 Subcategories of fidelity, general process questions and potential data collection methods to measure each category

Subcategory of fidelity	General process questions	Potential data collection methods
Content	Was each of the intervention components implemented according to the intervention protocol?	Observations of work practices Staff/patient diaries or logbooks Interviews with relevant stakeholders
Frequency/duration (dosage, dose delivery)	Were the intervention components implemented as often and for as long as planned?	Observations of work practices Staff/patient diaries or logbooks Interviews with relevant stakeholders
Coverage (reach)	What proportion of the original target group participated in the intervention?	Recruitment protocols Interviews with relevant stakeholders Observations of work practices
Timeliness	Were the intervention components delivered at the right time?	Staff/patient diaries or logbooks Interviews with relevant stakeholders

the Swedish context showed that the national regulations for social benefits and work rehabilitation were the main factors affecting the success of the implementation (Hasson *et al.*, 2011). At the local level, availability of resources, leadership, champions, work culture, consistency of local policy and practice guidance and training affect fidelity. These are important to consider when conducting trials in several clinical settings or organizational units. Individual-level factors such as practitioners' preferences and knowledge regarding the intervention might also impact fidelity. Additional individual level factors for intervention adaptations include staff desire to increase a sense of ownership and create a better fit between a program and local needs (Blakely *et al.*, 1987), as well as a desire to improve program results (Fraser *et al.*, 2009). Others have suggested that poor staff training and uncommitted staff are reasons for low fidelity (Fraser *et al.*, 2009).

How and when should local adaptations be made?

Some authors argue that intervention implementation can be flexible as long as the essential elements of an intervention, i.e. the core intervention components, are implemented with high fidelity (Blakely *et al.*, 1987). According to the Replicating Effective Programs (REP) framework, the core elements of an intervention should be standardized, but the mechanism by which these are operationalized can be changed to allow flexibility in implementation (Kilbourne *et al.*, 2007). This suggests that articulating a priori the core elements and adaptation options of an intervention is necessary for its successful adaptation (Kilbourne *et al.*, 2007). This implies that the choices according to level of accepted fidelity in clinical trials should be made prior to the implementation of the intervention. Understanding the principles of intervention core components may also allow for flexibility in intervention content and delivery without sacrificing the potential benefits associated with each component (Fixsen *et al.*, 2005). With this approach, staff are not expected to follow process protocols exactly, but rather to work according to their own judgements of what fits with the client characteristics and context and the program theory (Mowbray *et al.*, 2003).

It has also been suggested that decisions about any program changes should be conducted together with practitioners who know the local conditions and administrators, experts or researchers who understand the underlying logics of the intervention (Fixsen *et al.*, 2005). In addition, it has been suggested that different hierarchical levels in an organization should be involved since the potential to make decisions and the reasons for them differ at different levels (von Thiele Schwarz *et al.*, 2013). Thus, staff, managers at different organizational levels and program experts could together develop their understanding about the program logic (program theory) and the underlying principles of intervention core components (Hasson and Topo, 2014).

Measurement of fidelity

Fidelity assessment should focus on the active ingredients of an intervention, i.e. the most crucial components of the intervention (Fixsen *et al.*, 2005). However, if such analysis has not been conducted it is suggested that evaluation of fidelity should be consulted for all intervention components. This is often the case for clinical trials that test a model for the first time, implying that all intervention components need to be carefully defined prior to the trial. In addition, evaluation of the delivery of each component during the trial should be compared to the description.

All of the subcategories of fidelity need to be measured in order to achieve a comprehensive picture of fidelity (Carroll *et al.*, 2007; Dusenbury *et al.*, 2003; Steckler and Linnan, 2002). However, many prior studies have solely focused on frequency or duration (Dusenbury *et al.*, 2003). Our recent study (see the description of the clinical case in Table 24.2) evaluated four fidelity subcategories (content, frequency, duration and coverage) and found that to be extensive and challenging, but also useful (Hasson *et al.*, 2012). Challenges concerned the flexibility that existed in the interpretation of the intervention components and delivery descriptions. It was challenging to describe content and delivery of the intervention components so that no lack of clarity existed. The study suggested that future trials could take into consideration the subcategories of fidelity when formulating descriptions of intervention components (Hasson *et al.*, 2012). This could help to specify the content, frequency and duration for each component prior to delivering

TABLE 24.2 Example of a fidelity assessment: case of a continuum of care program for frail older people in health and social care

Description of the intervention

The intervention consisted of developing a continuum of care model for frail older persons. The aim was to include all essential care providers, i.e. community health and social care, a university hospital and primary care. The intervention consisted of a systematization of collaboration between nurses with geriatric expertise situated at an emergency department, hospital ward staff and a multi-professional team with a case manager in community care services for older people. For more information about the intervention see Wilhelmson *et al.* (2011).

Evaluation of fidelity

Fidelity was evaluated during the entire trial period with observations of work practices, stakeholder interviews and document analysis according to a modified version of the Conceptual Framework for Implementation Fidelity (Carroll *et al.*, 2007; Hasson, 2010). All of the intervention core components, a total of 18 activities, were evaluated in accordance with the delivered content, frequency, duration and coverage.

Data analysis

Notes in the observation protocols were first discussed by two of the authors after each observation visit. Delivery of each intervention component was discussed, and the level of adherence was determined. The authors compared the interview and document data to the findings of the observed data of adherence. All non-adherences concerning the actual delivery of the intervention components were further investigated with specific interview questions in the next interview with the key stakeholders. The Conceptual Framework for Implementation Fidelity was used as a coding scheme for the analysis.

Results (in brief)

The level of the fidelity was high. A total of 16 of the 18 intervention components were always or most often delivered as these were described in the trial protocol. The non-adherences that were observed included components that were not delivered, were modified and were added to the original model. The dose delivered did not vary over time for the intervention core components, but variation was observed for the components that staff had added to the original model.

the intervention. This would reduce the need to interpret the content of intervention components. Another challenge was the fact that no standards exist for what is the optimal degree of adherence. High fidelity was defined as intervention components being delivered according to the protocol always or most often. This implies a need to define optimal levels of fidelity when planning clinical trials. There is also no agreement on whether or how to weight the fidelity of the different intervention components, i.e. whether high fidelity for core components compensates for low fidelity for less important components. This is an area of research that further studies could focus on in the field of fidelity.

Some authors have discussed whether it is enough to measure fidelity for the intervention group or whether fidelity should also be measured for control groups (Bond *et al.*, 2000). Measurement for the control group would naturally imply a need for more resources, but it could also offer an opportunity to analyze the real differences between the groups. Otherwise, there is a risk that intervention components are implemented also in the control groups. It is suggested that the risk of having intervention components implemented in the control condition should be evaluated prior to the clinical trial. This evaluation is then used to decide whether fidelity analyses are conducted only in the intervention condition or also in the control conditions. In our study of the care continuum model, we decided not to evaluate fidelity in the control condition. There was no possibility that the intervention components could have been delivered to controls due to organizational routines. There were strict care processes in the organizations and no real changes of contamination from the intervention group to control were considered realistic. Thus, after a careful evaluation, a decision was made that the research resources were not to be put into the evaluation of the control group.

Among the main strengths of our study are the use of multiple data collection methods and the longitudinal design. It is strongly recommended to collect fidelity data during the entire intervention period since fidelity may change over time. It is often also recommended to use a multi-method approach with observations, interviews and document analysis. Observations have been shown to be more efficient in evaluation of fidelity than using only interviews, since many practitioners do not reflect on the adaptations they conduct in practice (Hasson *et al.*, 2012). Components that are added to the original intervention model are challenging from the measurement point of view since staff often do not recover components they have added (Hasson *et al.*, 2012). The added components are often only captured in direct observations of work practices. Therefore, it is strongly recommended that observations, although a time-consuming and expensive data collection method, are used repeatedly during the trial to measure fidelity and especially added components. There are also some previously developed and validated instruments to evaluate the fidelity of well-established evidence-based interventions. For example, the Supported Employment Fidelity Scale (Becker *et al.*, 2008) could be used to inspire the development of fidelity measurement techniques.

There is a great need to combine process evaluation in the intervention outcome evaluation. More specifically, fidelity measurement should be connected to outcomes such as participants' health. That would allow analysis of intervention subgroups in terms of fidelity. The different types of non-adherence such as modified or added intervention components could in this way be analyzed in relation to patient outcomes. Some authors have suggested that local additions to an original model tend to enhance effectiveness (Blakely *et al.*, 1987). This is an interesting point since most prior studies showing that low fidelity was connected to worse intervention outcomes did not include the evaluation of added components. Future studies should investigate the possible positive (and/or negative) impact of added components on intervention outcomes.

There are different ways to publish the results of a fidelity measurement. Some scientific articles describe solely the measurement and results of a fidelity assessment. These articles are often published in journals interested in advancing the science of evaluation or implementation and often adopt an advanced methodology or an innovative evaluation model. Most of the results of a fidelity evaluation are published as part of an outcome evaluation in order to describe the success of the program implementation. This helps the reader to understand the validity of the outcome measurement.

Programs implemented as part of research projects usually receive considerable support to achieve high fidelity (Dusenbury *et al.*, 2003). Outside of the research context, implementation usually takes place in less ideal circumstances (Dane and Schneider, 1998). Some authors have argued that fidelity is often high when conducting clinical trials and that the real challenge is to implement the same methods in real-life settings with high fidelity. Thus, it is possible that the factors affecting fidelity in trials are not totally comparable to real-life situations. The step after a clinical trial would be to study the fidelity of the program in real-life settings. There is also a need to develop practical models to guide professionals in their choices concerning fidelity and local adaptations in practical settings.

Acknowledgements

The Vårdal Institute financed the development and evaluation of the intervention 'Continuum of care for frail elderly persons, from the emergency ward to living at home intervention'. In addition, the project received funding from the Vinnvård research program. The first author also received postdoctoral funding from ERA-AGE2, Future Leaders of Ageing Research in Europe (FLARE)/Swedish Council for Working Life and Social Research.

Further reading

Moore J, Bumbarger B, Cooper B. 2013. Examining adaptations of evidence-based programs in natural contexts. *J Primary Prevent.* 2013/06/01;34(3):147–161.

Stirman S, Miller C, Toder K, Calloway A. 2013. Development of a framework and coding system for modifications and adaptations of evidence-based interventions. *Implementation Science*; 8(1):65.

Zvoch K. How 2012. Does fidelity of implementation matter? Using multilevel models to detect relationships between participant outcomes and the delivery and receipt of treatment. *American Journal of Evaluation*.

25

QUALITATIVE PROCESS EVALUATION FOR COMPLEX INTERVENTIONS

*Salla Atkins, Willem Odendaal, Natalie Leon,
Elizabeth Lutge and Simon Lewin*

Introduction

Qualitative process evaluations focus on assessing how interventions are implemented through the systematic collection of data related to the intervention itself and its context. These studies are increasingly used to deepen our understanding of the findings of randomized controlled trials (Glenton *et al.*, 2011) of complex public health, health promotion and health systems interventions.

Whilst the findings of RCTs of complex health interventions provide information on whether an intervention is effective or not, these findings seldom explain *why* these effects have occurred. A process evaluation alongside such an outcome evaluation can address this lack of explanatory power.

Learning objectives

In this chapter, the researcher will:

- Gain an understanding of the importance of qualitative process evaluation.
- Understand key issues in conducting qualitative process evaluations.

Process evaluations are particularly suited to assessing participant views of intervention implementation, their acceptability and suitability (Reeves *et al.*, 2010), and can address questions related to:

- the mechanisms through which an intervention operates and moderates changes; identifying possible underlying reasons for the change in the outcomes assessed (Rawat *et al.*, 2013);

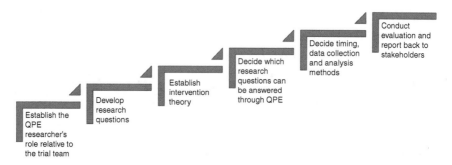

FIGURE 25.1   Steps in planning a qualitative process evaluation (QPE)

- the fidelity of the intervention (the extent to which an intervention was implemented as intended; see case study 1);
- contextual influences on the implementation of the intervention (factors that may have affected implementation and modified intervention effectiveness) as well as factors that could affect health systems decisions about the feasibility of future interventions, their transferability (to similar or different settings) and up-scalability and sustainability (Rapport *et al.*, 2013).

In short, qualitative process evaluations can answer, at least in part, whether the intervention will work here, and if it will work at scale (Pawson and Tilley, 2001).

This chapter is a resource for researchers aiming to design and implement a qualitative process evaluation alongside a randomized controlled trial. While these evaluations may use a mixed-methods approach, including both qualitative and quantitative data, we focus here on qualitative process evaluations. Figure 25.1 outlines the steps involved in designing a qualitative process evaluation alongside a trial.

Deciding on the researcher's role: independent versus participatory evaluations

The lead investigator in a qualitative process evaluation may be part of the trial team or an external evaluator (throughout this chapter, we refer to trial implementers as 'trialists' and persons conducting the evaluation as 'evaluators'). Being an external evaluator may be helpful in maintaining an independent viewpoint and producing fresh insights regarding the implementation of the intervention, but may be more challenging in terms of understanding the intervention and the trial and gaining the confidence of a trial team. In both cases, it is important for evaluators and trialists to work together throughout the evaluation (Rapport *et al.*, 2013), and to discuss and agree on roles and on the evaluation process before starting the study.

Stakeholder perspectives are important when developing research questions and methods. Involving stakeholders, including intervention designers, implementers and recipients, may help to focus the evaluation and clarify expectations (including scope), enhance usefulness and credibility and improve the uptake of evaluation results (Bryson *et al.*, 2011; Howell and Yemane, 2006). It is important to note, however, that a careful balance is needed in contacts with the trial team. If one recruits participants in the evaluation from both arms of the trial, one should ensure recruitment does not compromise blinding. This can be achieved through selecting participants on site or randomly, without knowledge of trial allocation and finding this out in the interview or focus group only.

Developing the question(s) for the qualitative process evaluation

Determining the question(s) that the evaluation will answer is critical to the choice of methods. Is the objective to explain the trial outcomes, to explore health systems factors affecting delivery of the intervention, or both? Consultation with stakeholders and understanding the intervention theory (i.e. the pathway through which the intervention is meant to produce change – which may be informed by a specific change theory) can help develop questions (Rossi *et al.*, 2004) which can be refined as the trial progresses.

Using theory to inform the evaluation

Using theory to inform qualitative evaluations alongside trials has several advantages. Firstly, theory can help to focus the research question and select a study design. Secondly, theory can facilitate data analysis and interpretation by providing a framework for examining, categorizing and making sense of data (Reeves *et al.*, 2008). It is also important to reflect on one's own preconceptions and theories about the intervention, in order to maintain reflexivity (reflecting critically on the researcher's influence on data analysis).

There are at least two types of theory that may be useful. Firstly, evaluators can draw on programme theory – the set of assumptions (often implicit) about the mechanisms of the intervention and its effects or outcomes (Rossi *et al.*, 2004).

Secondly, evaluators can utilize theories from disciplines such as sociology and psychology and apply these to the intervention. These may include behavioural theories (see Munro *et al.*, 2007) or health systems conceptual frameworks.

Choosing a study design

The choice of study design and methods should be guided by the research questions. Different research questions require different methods – for some, but not all, questions a qualitative approach is appropriate.

Study design decisions also include the timing of the evaluation. Ideally the evaluation should be designed and implemented alongside the trial (Oakley *et al.*, 2006). This implies a *longitudinal* design spanning the life of the trial from conception to completion (Bouffard *et al.*, 2003). This has several advantages: it helps to ensure that key issues relating to the implementation of the trial intervention and its reception among stakeholders are captured as they emerge. It may be easier to recruit evaluation participants while the trial is being implemented. This approach may also reduce the problems introduced by retrospective data collection including participants' recall (Hoddinott *et al.*, 2010), and allows for regular feedback to the trialists during implementation. However, one should avoid the danger of the evaluation becoming an intervention in itself as evaluation findings should not impact on trial outcomes. This includes making sure that, for example, treatment allocation is not revealed to trialists when interviewing trial participants.

Retrospective and *cross-sectional* (collecting data only at one point of the intervention) designs are sometimes used, and may be less costly to conduct. However, retrospective designs have to take into account how participants' recall of key events and issues impacts on data.

Collecting data

Qualitative evaluations may use a range of qualitative data collection methods, including interviews, focus group discussions, observation of practice and document review. Participant diaries, photographs and video can also be used. Each method has its advantages and disadvantages and the choice of data collection tools depends on the evaluation questions. A range of qualitative methods texts provide more information on selecting appropriate data collection methods (e.g. Patton, 2012).

The evaluation questions will also determine the range of participants included. This could encompass intervention designers and implementers, intervention recipients (including health service users and providers) and key stakeholders such as managers and policy-makers.

Case study 1 (Box 25.1) provides an example of the use of interviews within a qualitative process evaluation, while case study 2 (Box 25.2) describes the use of participant diaries as a data collection method.

BOX 25.1 CASE STUDY 1. ECONOMIC SUPPORT TO IMPROVE TUBERCULOSIS (TB) TREATMENT OUTCOMES IN SOUTH AFRICA: A QUALITATIVE PROCESS EVALUATION OF A PRAGMATIC CLUSTER RANDOMIZED CONTROLLED TRIAL (LUTGE *ET AL.*, 2013)

This trial was undertaken to evaluate whether a monthly voucher given to patients with active TB would improve their treatment outcomes. The qualitative process evaluation, consisting of in-depth interviews with patients, health care providers and health care managers, was designed to understand how participants perceived the intervention and how these perceptions affected the implementation and results of the trial. The interviews indicated that the nurses who administered the vouchers felt that the vouchers should be 'rationed', i.e. given to those whom they regarded as being most poor rather than being given to all people with active TB, as planned in the trial. This led to poor fidelity to the trial protocol (36.2 per cent of eligible patients did not receive a voucher at all) and contributed in part to its inconclusive findings.

Sampling is determined by the research questions, the methods chosen and the available funding and time (Flick, 2007). Often participants are selected purposively for their ability to be good informants in relation to the research questions and the phenomena that are being explored. The sampling strategy will also be driven by the trial. For example, sampling may need to include both intervention and control sites and individuals allocated to different interventions. It may also need to be designed to address questions emerging from the trial, such as why a particular participant subgroup did not adhere to an intervention. The sample size should be sufficient in number and diversity to provide a meaningful understanding of the issues under investigation. Sampling needs to be flexible, so that it can respond to emerging themes and data, and should include a range of participants and contexts, including those that may not be typical of the 'mainstream'.

CASE STUDY 2. USING DIARIES TO CAPTURE STAFF EXPERIENCES OF COMPLEX INTERVENTIONS (ODENDAAL *ET AL.*, 2008)

This process evaluation was undertaken alongside an RCT of a home-visit intervention to reduce the risks of unintentional childhood injuries in low-income neighbourhoods. Staff delivering the intervention were supplied with a diary sheet for each home visit. This diary sheet included a mix of structured and open-ended questions to record their views on how the visit went, recipients' responses to the intervention, and staff's views about the programme at that point. This method was useful in providing an ongoing assessment of staff perceptions. However, such intensive data collection can become a burden to programme staff.

Analysing the data

There are a number of different research traditions and analysis techniques for qualitative analysis and this can often be the most complex and time-consuming part of qualitative research (Pope *et al.*, 2000). The technique selected will depend on the aim of the evaluation, the research questions and theoretical orientation, and time and resources. A number of texts provide guidance on qualitative analysis methods (e.g. Pope and Mays, 2006). All of these approaches require an in-depth understanding of the data collected. The process may differ in terms of the level of analysis (manifest versus latent – Graneheim and Lundman, 2004), and the orientation towards inductive or deductive approaches (see e.g. Denzin and Lincoln, 2000).

In evaluations alongside trials, it may be more common to use the manifest, or descriptive approach, as the evaluation often focuses on specific, trial-related questions. However, the analysis can also be used to develop a conceptual model of how an intervention works or how recipients respond to it. A potentially useful method is framework analysis, which allows the combination of inductive and deductive methods (Ritchie and Spencer, 1994).

All analyses should be conducted rigorously and systematically (Pope *et al.*, 2000). Electronic software tools such as Nvivo or Atlas.ti can help to systematize analysis but are not a substitute for engagement with the data.

Case study 3 presents an example of qualitative content analysis.

CASE STUDY 3. PRESENTING YOUR ANALYSIS (ATKINS *ET AL.*, 2010)

This process evaluation explored patient experiences of a new tuberculosis treatment programme modelled on the community antiretroviral treatment programme in South Africa. Patients with different treatment outcomes – for example, those who had defaulted treatment and those that had been adherent – were included in interviews and focus groups. The resulting data were analysed using qualitative content analysis (Graneheim and Lundman, 2004). An example of the analysis process is shown in Table 25.1.

TABLE 25.1 The qualitative content analysis process

Meaning unit	Condensed meaning unit	Code	Subcategories	Main categories
(female, intervention): '... I think people need to take responsibility for their health because it is not the care-giver's fault to catch the bug in the air and you also as a patient did not choose to have TB therefore you need to love yourself and your health and be responsible as we are when we take our treatment at the clinic'	People need to take responsibility for their own health	Taking responsibility for yourself	Taking control over one's own life	Agency

(female intervention):	Things have	Change and	Taking	Agency
'My life has changed	changed	respon-	respon-	
for the better, I used	and patient	sibility	sibility for	
to be out there all	has to	over own	one's own	
the time but now	be more	health	health	
I know I have to	responsible			
look after my health				
everyday ...'				

Ensuring quality in qualitative process evaluations

As with any research, systematic, rigorous and transparent application of methods is key to ensuring quality. Good-quality qualitative research should provide a rich, 'thick description' (Creswell and Miller, 2000) and meaningful appraisal of the phenomena under investigation, and should be credible and trustworthy.

Some of the challenges to quality include the need for fast data collection and analysis. In addition, the quality of the evaluation is in part related to the extent to which it is able to create a credible explanation of how the trial was implemented and received. This requires ongoing interaction between the evaluator and the trialists.

Among of the ways to increase the trustworthiness of these evaluations is through the use of a theoretical framework (see above and case study 4). Another commonly used technique is triangulation (case study 4), which involves the use of multiple data sources or data collection methods as well as the employment of more than one researcher to analyse the data. Triangulation may be expensive and time consuming, but is considered useful.

CASE STUDY 4. IMPLEMENTING A PROVIDER-INITIATED TESTING AND COUNSELLING (PITC) INTERVENTION IN CAPE TOWN, SOUTH AFRICA: A PROCESS EVALUATION USING THE NORMALIZATION PROCESS MODEL (LEON *ET AL.*, 2013)

This qualitative process evaluation was implemented alongside a non-randomized clinical trial in an operational setting, aimed at increasing uptake of HIV testing among adult patients. The trial effect size was small, despite a high level of implementation support. Triangulation through multiple data sources provided insights on the reason for this. Staff focus groups, management interviews and observation of clinical practice provided a more comprehensive picture of implementation strength and challenges. In particular, through observation of clinical practice we discovered the difficulty faced by nurses in efficiently implementing the new intervention on the level of the clinical consultation. Thus triangulation of our findings through studying micro-level delivery in the consultation was essential for enriching understanding of implementation challenges.

Reporting and feedback

Conducting qualitative process evaluations alongside trials constitutes a form of mixed-methods research. Similarities and differences between the evaluation and trial findings need to be discussed and explained in the report. All parts of data collection, sampling and study design should be discussed transparently (Rapport *et al.*, 2013).

At the conclusion of the trial, findings should be presented to stakeholders, including trialists. This may serve as a useful feedback mechanism to contextualize and refine study findings. Appropriate formats for disseminating evaluation findings include reports to the intervention participants, policy briefs for policy-makers and peer-reviewed papers.

Final note

More qualitative process evaluations are needed alongside trials of complex health interventions to improve our understanding of trial effects and to inform practice and policy decisions on the further development of interventions (Lewin *et al.*, 2009; Glenton *et al.*, 2011). However, qualitative evaluations are often not able to address all the possible influences that may have impacted on trials and their findings (Munro and Bloor, 2010), or to identify all the possible facilitators and barriers to implementing the intervention on a larger scale in similar or different settings. As Pawson and Tilley (2001: 232) succinctly said: 'Never expect to know *"what works,"* just keep trying to find out'.

Summary

- Qualitative process evaluations can help us understand reasons for trial success or failure and provide knowledge on the feasibility, transferability, up-scalability and sustainability of trial interventions.
- Stakeholder involvement and continued interaction with trialists is important in determining the expectations, focus and reporting of the evaluation in relation to the trial.

- The underlying programme theory of the trial or theory of health systems functioning can help investigators focus the qualitative process evaluation.
- The choice of qualitative design depends on the research question(s).
- Methods for enhancing quality include applying systematic and transparent research design, data collection, analysis and quality assurance methods.

Further reading

Flick, U. 2007. *The Sage Qualitative Research Kit*. Thousand Oaks, CA: Sage.

Patton, M. Q. 2003. *Qualitative Evaluation and Research Methods*, 3rd edn. Thousand Oaks, CA: Sage.

Patton, M. Q. 2011. *Developmental Evaluation: Applying Complexity Concepts to Enhance Innovation and Use*. New York: Guilford Press.

Pope, C. and Mays, N. (eds). 2006. *Qualitative Research in Healthcare*. Oxford: Blackwell.

26

ECONOMIC EVALUATIONS OF COMPLEX INTERVENTIONS

Katherine Payne and Alexander J. Thompson

Introduction

The general impression from published economic evaluations is that the majority focus on quantifying the costs and benefits of 'simple' interventions. In practice, however, there are many examples of complex interventions. Indeed, by definition, all health care interventions are complex to some extent but some can be viewed as being more 'complex' than others. Such different levels of complexity need to be acknowledged when applying methods of economic evaluation to inform the allocation of scarce health care resources.

Learning objectives

- To understand the underlying concepts that inform the economic evaluation framework.
- To be able to describe the types of economic evaluation.
- To understand some key principles in the design and analysis methods for economic evaluations of complex interventions.
- To understand some key challenges for the design, conduct and use of studies to evaluate the incremental costs and benefits of complex interventions in practice.

Health care budgets and making choices: the role of economic evaluation

Economics is a social science that aims to understand the production, distribution and consumption of any good or service and to generate information on how to achieve the most efficient use of scarce resources. Health economics has emerged as a sub-discipline in economics and involves the application of economics to health and health care. The existence of fixed health care budgets and finite health care resources means there is an opportunity cost for every decision made to provide any intervention. The decision to allocate resources to a particular service excludes those resources from alternative possible uses within a health care system. Hence complex interventions, like simple interventions, need to be assessed to understand whether they offer added value, in terms of the relative costs and benefits, compared to established best practice. Each complex intervention introduces its own particular set of challenges for the design and conduct of a robust economic evaluation. Two general challenges must always be addressed: (i) how to identify, collect resource use data for the intervention, subsequent treatments and pathways of care compared to current practice, and (ii) how to identify and quantify the impact of the intervention and current practice on the relevant patient population, which may sometimes include family members and carers.

Methods of economic evaluation

Economic evaluation is one method available to health economists who want to generate evidence to inform decision-making and is defined as 'the comparative analysis of alternative courses of action in terms of both their costs and consequences' (Drummond et al., 2005: 9). The economic evaluation framework enables assessment of an intervention's incremental benefits and costs over existing treatment options, or, if appropriate, the alternative of doing nothing. Health economics uses this evaluative framework to generate evidence on how to best spend finite health care resources in order to guide decision-making. Other economic methods, such as budget impact analysis (Sullivan et al., 2014), cost of illness and costing studies (McGuire et al., 2002), are also seen in the literature. These types of studies may sometimes have a place in the evaluation of complex interventions, but their role is generally very limited because they only describe the current situation and what might happen if a certain intervention is implemented (a 'positive statement'). Burden of illness and costing studies do not provide evidence of the opportunity cost of the proposed complex intervention.

To make clear statements about what decision-makers *should* do (a 'normative' statement) economists require explicit normative principles, which also guide the technical application of methods of economic evaluation. Generally, applied methods of economic evaluation fall broadly into two categories: cost-effectiveness (or cost-utility) analysis and cost–benefit analysis. Thompson et al. (2014) provide an example of a published cost-effectiveness analysis of a pharmacogenetic test to predict a side effect (neutropaenia) associated with a drug (azathioprine) for treatment of autoimmune diseases. In this study, the effectiveness of the intervention was quantified using quality-adjusted life years. Whynes et al. (2003) illustrate how to value monetary benefits for use in a cost–benefit analysis of colorectal screening.

Cost-minimisation analysis has been used in the literature but is no longer considered useful for decision-making due to assumptions made in the analyses and limitations in the methods used to handle uncertainty (Briggs and O'Brien, 2001). Cost–consequences analysis is another potentially useful method, particularly in the context of complex interventions (Coast, 2004) but has been criticised because it places the onus on the decision-maker to decide which outcome is of primary interest (Brazier *et al.*, 2005; Claxton *et al.*, 2005).

Value judgements

In practice, all economic evaluations require the identification and quantification of the costs and benefits of competing uses of resources associated with a complex intervention and relevant comparators. Economists disagree, however, on the underlying value judgements, such as what constitutes a benefit and how practical these benefits are in terms of informing decision-making. The most notable collection of value judgements resides in the approaches called welfarism and extra-welfarism (Brouwer *et al.*, 2008).

Welfarism and cost–benefit analysis

Welfarism assumes that individuals are the best judge of their own welfare (or utility) and welfare is taken to be the satisfaction of an individual's preferences. Decision-makers should only enact policies which improve the welfare of some within society whilst harming no others (called a Pareto improvement). However, very few policy changes can meet this goal because typically for any potential policy there are costs and benefits which are distributed between the different individuals and groups in society. Instead, interventions which provide a *potential* Pareto improvement should be introduced (Ng, 1983). This is where the gainers of the policy can compensate the losers and still be better off.

To gauge the strength of preference for an intervention when market provision is absent, which is typical in the health care sector, contingent valuation methods (most commonly applied using willingness to pay – (WTP) – techniques) are used. Contingent valuation methods provide a measure of benefit on the same monetary scale as costs. Hence both the costs and benefits can be compared directly in a cost–benefit analysis (CBA).

Extra-welfarism and cost-effectiveness analysis

The extra-welfarist perspective has been argued to 'transcend traditional welfare' (Culyer, 1991) and provides the theoretical foundation for the use of cost-effectiveness analysis (CEA) (sometimes labelled 'cost-utility analysis'). The extra-welfarist perspective suggests it is legitimate for decision-makers, seeking to promote the social good, to use 'non–utility' information in their decision-making (Brouwer *et al.*, 2008). For policies associated with health care, it is argued that the appropriate measure of benefit is 'health' or health status. As the comparison of benefits and costs is on a different scale, the evaluative framework used is labelled cost-effectiveness analysis. Decision-makers seek interventions which provide the most benefit (measured in whatever natural unit chosen) for a given cost in what is then called cost-effectiveness analysis.

Alternative interpretations of benefit, such as capability, are also feasible in the context of the extra-welfarist perspective and are being used in economic evaluations of health interventions, in general, and complex health, social care and public health interventions, specifically (Coast *et al.*, 2008a, 2008b; NICE, 2013a).

Design and conduct of economic evaluations

Within the method of cost-effectiveness and cost-utility analysis, two main vehicles to produce evidence for decision-making exist: trial-based and model-based (Sculpher *et al.*, 2006). Trial-based evaluations (also called prospective economic evaluations) provide decision-makers with information given an analysis based on the resource use, cost and outcome data collected for an individual-level patient sample recruited to a randomised controlled trial. The collection of data necessary for the economic evaluation, such as resource use, effectiveness and health status, should be an integral component of the clinical trial protocol. Design and statistical issues similar to those necessary for a robust clinical trial, such as considerations of clustering, sample size calculations and appropriate methods of data analysis, must also be considered in the design of a prospective economic study along with specific challenges to the analysis of economic data (Elliott *et al.*, 2014b; Mihaylova *et al.*, 2011). Trial-based studies can be time and resource intensive, requiring considerable funding; the results are often not sufficiently timely for decision-making in practice and will clearly only generate results for the specified complex intervention and comparator. This may limit the generalisability of the trial findings to other settings.

The use of model-based evaluations is preferred by some decision-making bodies as the appropriate vehicle with which to inform decision-making. Model-based evaluations, as opposed to trial-based evaluations, can incorporate all the available evidence, the appropriate time horizon for the follow-up of the patient sample and all relevant comparators (Sculpher *et al.*, 2006). A model-based economic evaluation allows data from many different sources, such as data from the literature, trial-based effectiveness data, observational studies, micro-costing studies and expert opinion (Leal *et al.*, 2007; Philips *et al.*, 2006; Sullivan and Payne, 2011), to be compiled systematically. The advantage of model-type studies is that they are generally less time and resource intensive, and allow for extrapolation of data for the lifetime horizon and exploration of the sources and impact of uncertainty in the data. Uncertainty in a model-based study can arise for a number of reasons (Philips *et al.*, 2006). Therefore sensitivity analysis is a key component of any model-based economic evaluation. Probabilistic sensitivity analysis, which is used to explore the joint impact of uncertainty across all parameters simultaneously, is a recommended approach to conducting sensitivity analysis.

Both trial and model-based economic evaluations have important roles within different stages of the iterative process of evidence gathering. This iterative process fits alongside the MRC framework for evaluating complex interventions that suggest early modelling work to inform a larger definitive trial. Model-type studies are useful when assessing the costs and benefits of an intervention in the early life of the intervention and, by including value of information analysis (Claxton *et al.*, 2004), could be used to inform the value of further research. Value of information analysis involves quantifying the extent of uncertainty in the parameters used to populate the model-based economic evaluation and assign a cost to indicate the value for further research. This iterative approach to economic evaluation, as recommended by Sculpher *et al.* (1997), is then supplemented by further evaluations as and when new evidence becomes available.

Study perspective

Economic evaluation can take different perspectives. The objective of health care providers is often how to spend resources to achieve maximum benefit, which is synonymous with the concept in economics of technical efficiency: given a defined set of inputs, how can the outputs be maximised? This objective is consistent with assuming the viewpoint of a health care system policy-maker. Other viewpoints are, however, possible ranging from the societal view, in which the aim would be to maximise population well-being given government-level budget constraints, down to individual patients aiming to maximise their own well-being given their income. Each perspective will have different objectives and budget constraints. The perspective used in economic evaluation, specific to individual countries, is described by the International Society for Pharmacoeconomics and Outcomes Research (ISPOR) (ISPOR, 2014). For example, in jurisdictions such as The Netherlands the societal perspective is recommended (ISPOR, 2006). Such a perspective would have the aim of maximising population well-being, taking into account benefits and costs which fall outside of the health care system.

In the UK, the generally applied viewpoint by the National Institute for Health and Care Excellence (NICE) is that of the National Health and Social Services (NHS). In contrast, the Social Care Institute for Excellence (SCIE) suggests adopting a broad analytic perspective to include the impact of an intervention on all relevant stakeholders, including the people who use services and their families (SCIE, 2011).

Identifying and quantifying the costs

The costs included in an economic evaluation are measured by identifying and quantifying the resources consumed in the process of delivering a health intervention and the relevant alternative use of the budget (the comparator intervention or interventions). To be able to identify the relevant items of resource use it is necessary to be clear about the chosen study perspective (for example, health system or societal) and also the time horizon for the analysis (for example, duration of a clinical trial or patient lifetime). The process of identifying the different types of costs is described in many excellent textbooks (for example: Drummond *et al.*, 2005; Elliott and Payne, 2005). Identifying the items of resource use in the context of complex interventions is often challenging because the use of resources may be associated with (i) providing the complex intervention itself, which can involve multiple members of staff or interacting components, and (ii) subsequent care pathways, which may be numerous and diverse. Items of resource use for complex interventions can be identified by conducting systematic reviews of the existing literature or collecting patient-level health care resource use, using for example patient surveys, diaries or extracting data from medical records, for a specific intervention in a specific patient population. A useful resource is the Database of Instruments for Resource Use Measurement (DIRUM) which lists example data collection forms (DIRUM, 2014). The resource use data, once identified, are combined with published unit cost data to generate the total costs of the care pathways for the complex intervention and its comparator(s). The relevant care pathways should represent all the processes involved in providing the complex intervention and subsequent management strategies. A judgement needs to be made by the analyst, supported by other stakeholders involved in delivering care, as to which processes are linked to the complex intervention. Linking processes to the complex intervention is not a trivial task, and sensitivity analysis needs to be conducted to test the robustness of the results of the economic evaluation to the assumptions made.

Identifying and valuing benefits

Benefits should be readily identified and measured and focus on quantifying the impact on patients. In some cases, particularly for complex interventions, it may also be relevant to consider the benefits for family members and carers, which are termed 'spillover' effects (Basu and Meltzer, 2005). For example, a clinical genetics service for inherited cancers could generate benefits for the person presenting to the service for a diagnosis of hereditary breast cancer, but also for other female family members.

In the context of CEA, using health as the benefit to be valued implies there must be a reliable way of quantifying changes in health status, which can be described using generic or disease-specific measures (Bowling, 2005). The most commonly used measure of health status is the EQ-5D (Euroqol, 2014), which is now available in two versions with three (EQ-5D-3L) or five levels (EQ-5D-5L) (Herdman *et al.*, 2011). The main advantage of using the EQ-5D-3L is the availability of a published social tariff of preference scores (Dolan *et al.*, 1995). There is currently no equivalent social tariff for the EQ-5D-5L and so regression-based mapping from the

EQ-5D-3L is required (Van Hout *et al.*, 2012). Typically in health economics, preference scores for health states are measured on a scale ranging from zero (representing death) to one (representing perfect health), but scores less than zero are feasible if a health state is viewed as being as worse than being dead (Brazier *et al.*, 2007).

When valuing the benefits of a complex intervention in a trial-based analysis, it is necessary to collect EQ-5D data and then attach the appropriate preference scores (weights). Alternatively, in a model-based economic evaluation, it is necessary to assimilate published utility values from the literature to the respective health states included in the economic model. Catalogues of EQ-5D scores have been made available in the literature in order to help with this process (Sullivan *et al.*, 2011). The final outcome is then estimated by calculating the change in quality-adjusted life years for comparative technologies. Quality-adjusted life years (QALYs) are calculated using simple multiplication of the preference scores with the time spent in the health state measured using the EQ-5D.

The QALY approach, however, is not always viewed as ideal and there are numerous debates in the literature focusing on issues of theoretical validity, measurement methodology and the ethics of using them to inform health policy decisions (see Coast *et al.*, 2008a; Dolan, 2008). In the context of complex interventions it may not be appropriate to focus on change in health status alone, and other measures of benefit can be used. If the analyst wants to capture benefits beyond changes in health status, while maintaining the extra-welfarist view, then this is when measures such as the ICECAP-O (in older people) or ICECAP-A (in adults), with published social tariffs, can be used to capture benefits such as improvements in capability (ICECAP, 2014).

An alternative approach that moves beyond the extra-welfarist view is to calculate monetary benefit by constructing a contingent valuation market and use of willingness-to-pay (Smith, 2003). These methods, and their application, are described in the health economics literature but are not currently advocated, or being used, in health policy decisions. The paucity of examples of full CBA in health care (Smith and Sach, 2009, 2010) may be the result of ongoing methodological challenges as well as the recognition by decision-makers of the ethical challenges in applying contingent valuation methods to measure health benefit. However, the method is potentially useful in the context of complex interventions because it allows the benefit associated with improvements in non-health and process attributes in addition to gains in health to be quantified.

Using economic evaluation in decision-making

Economic evaluations have become an integral component of health technology, social care and public health assessments used by decision-making bodies to inform resource allocation decisions. CEA has become the primary method of economic evaluation used to inform decision-making. The output of a CEA is the incremental costs and incremental QALYs of at least two competing interventions, one of which is generally current practice. In instances when more QALYs are gained but at an increased cost, the incremental cost-effectiveness ratio (ICER) is calculated to show the incremental cost per additional QALY. Once an ICER has been calculated, this needs to be compared to a threshold to gauge whether the health technology represents a 'cost-effective' use of scarce public resources. Decision-making bodies can use the concept of an ICER threshold to guide whether an intervention is a cost-effective use of resources.

The alternative welfarist view, involving the calculation of a monetary metric for benefit in CBA, allows decision-makers to use a consistent framework to assess the allocation of scarce resources both within, and across, public sector budgets. In applied work, the use of WTP results in a monetary valuation of the perceived benefit attached to the technology and this is compared to the costs which are also measured using money as the metric. The cost–benefit principle implies decision-makers should only take those actions where the benefits exceed the costs. The use of cost–benefit analysis is the application of this process (Brouwer and Koopmanschap, 2000).

Care must be taken when generalizing the results of an economic evaluation to a different setting than that described in the study. A number of guidelines or methods to critically appraise the quality of published economic evaluations have been generated. Guidelines for methods of economic evaluation across the world are described by ISPOR (ISPOR, 2014). Specific guidelines for the authors of published manuscripts are also available (Husereau *et al.*, 2013). Other useful resources include the NHS Economic Evaluation Database Handbook (Centre for Reviews and Dissemination, 2007) and associated searchable database that provide critical appraisals of published economic evaluations.

Conducting economic evaluations of complex interventions

Table 26.1 summarises some example key issues for the conduct of economic evaluations of complex interventions. In practice, complex interventions have been produced to manage a range of conditions in many diverse patient populations. There are published examples of economic evaluations of complex interventions. Some illustrative examples are now described.

Byford *et al.* (2010) present a detailed analysis that collected data on the differences in the number, length of stay and cost of admissions for residential alternatives to standard psychiatric admissions. This observational cohort study is a good example of how to collect resource use and available outcome data from computerized patient activity records. Elliott *et al.* (2014a) show how it was necessary to conduct a prospective RCT, to characterize the cost and short-term benefits, followed by a substantive model-based economic evaluation, to identify long-term costs and benefits of a pharmacist-led information technology intervention for reducing rates of clinically important errors in medicines management in general practices. Thompson *et al.* (2014) conducted a prospective trial-based cost-effectiveness analysis of a pharmacogenetic test to predict a side effect (neutropaenia) associated with

TABLE 26.1 Example key issues for the conduct of economic evaluations of complex interventions

Design criterion	Issue for evaluating complex interventions
Study perspective	It may be necessary to take a broad societal perspective to capture the impact of the intervention on all relevant stakeholders, including the people who use services and their families. Ideally, the analysis should also present the health care perspective.
Define the relevant study population	The definition of the relevant study population can be complicated by the need to consider the number of eligible patient groups or organizational levels targeted by the intervention.
Define intervention and comparators	By definition, complex interventions involve a number of interacting components and a variety of behaviours by those providing the intervention. There may also be a number of different and potentially relevant comparator interventions. It is therefore vital to be able to provide a clear and transparent description of the intervention and comparators and provide a rationale for including these comparators in the analysis.
Vehicle for the economic evaluation	With a complex intervention it may be necessary to combine two vehicles for the economic evaluation and use a prospective study to collect resource use data, followed up with a robust model-based economic evaluation to capture the long-term costs and benefits.
Type of economic evaluation	In line with simple interventions, the most commonly used type of economic evaluation is likely to be cost-effectiveness analysis. However, in some instances it may be necessary to consider using cost–benefit analysis to reflect the impact of the complex intervention on outcomes other than health status.
Identify resource use	Clear patient pathways should be identified and quantified in the analysis. All relevant items of resource use should be included and it is necessary to be able to distinguish between the resources used to produce the intervention and the subsequent use of resources that can be directly linked to the complex intervention.
Link effectiveness with patient benefits	Careful consideration should be given to how to establish a causal link from the intervention, and relevant comparators, to the benefits to patients because of the complexity of the intervention.
Quantify benefits	Complex interventions will have different types of potentially relevant outcome. The evaluation needs to be able to capture these multiple benefits and, in some instances, a focus on valuing gain in health status alone may not be sufficient.

a drug (azathioprine) for treatment of autoimmune diseases. First impressions may suggest the pharmacogenetic test is a simple intervention; however, because the test requires clinical interpretation and subsequent change in prescribing behaviour it does meet the MRC definition of a complex intervention. This study illustrates the challenge of designing a trial to show the benefit of an intervention that requires change in clinician behaviour before patient benefits may be realised.

Summary

Decision-makers charged with allocating finite health care budgets require timely and robust clinical and economic evidence on complex interventions before recommendations for funding in clinical practice can be made. Complex interventions will incur costs in the short term that influence patients' care pathways, which will translate into an impact on resource use and patient outcomes downstream of the intervention.

This chapter has shown how to apply methods of economic evaluation in the broadest sense. Sometimes it will not be pragmatic or feasible because of the complexity of the intervention to identify costs and outcomes in a single study. Therefore, study designs may need to combine data collected prospectively together with a robust model-based economic evaluation. A key aim of the economic evaluative framework for complex interventions is to be clear about the number of pathways, and relevant use of health care resources, reflected in the analysis and results. By doing so, decision-makers have access to transparent and understandable evidence, allowing informed decisions to be made on the allocation of scarce resources for complex interventions.

Further reading

Brazier, J., Ratcliffe, J., Salomon, J. A. and Tsuchiya, A. 2007. *Measuring and Valuing Health Benefits for Economic Evaluation*. Oxford: Oxford University Press.

Briggs, A., Sculpher, M. and Claxton, K. 2006. *Decision Modelling for Health Economic Evaluation*. Oxford: Oxford University Press.

Brouwer, W. B., Culyer, A. J., van Exel, N. J., Job, A. and Rutten, F. 2008. Welfarism vs extra welfarism. *Journal of Health Economics*, 27: 325–38.

Drummond, M. F., Sculpher, M. J., Torrance, G. W., O'Brien, B. J. and Stoddart, G. L. 2005. *Methods for the Economic Evaluation of Health Care Programmes*. New York: Oxford University Press.

Elliott, R. A. and Payne, K. 2005. *Essentials of Economic Evaluation in Health Care*. London: The Pharmaceutical Press.

Glick, H. A., Doshi, J. A., Sonnad, S. S. and Polsky, D. 2007. *Economic Evaluation in Clinical Trials*. New York: Oxford University Press.

Gray, A. M., Clarke, P. M., Wolstenholme, J. and Wordsworth, S. 2011. *Applied Methods of Cost-Effectiveness Analysis in Healthcare*. New York: Oxford University Press.

McIntosh, E., Clarke, P. M., Frew, E. J. and Louviere, J. J. 2010. *Applied Methods of Cost–Benefit Analysis in Healthcare*. Oxford: Oxford University Press.

SECTION 4

Implementation of complex interventions

Introduction to Section 4

Theo van Achterberg

Once complex interventions are sufficiently supported by evidence for their beneficial effects on individuals, populations or the health care system, we face the question of how to implement them. A key element in the revised Medical Research Council (MRC) framework for the development and evaluation of complex interventions (Craig *et al.*, 2008) is its explicit emphasis on implementation. Whereas the MRC framework provides a brief discussion of why considering implementation is important, and some of the key issues in implementation processes, this section provides additional guidance for those facing implementation-related challenges.

Implementation refers to putting an innovation (complex intervention) in place; it is more active than dissemination, and includes effective strategies that use facilitators and overcome barriers to change in practice settings (see Davis and Taylor-Vaisey, 1997 for a discussion of terminology). In recent decades, the implementation of (complex) interventions, guidelines and innovations in general has received ever-growing attention. 'Implementation in health care settings' has become increasingly important, which is reflected in the rise of journals such as the *International Journal of Quality in Healthcare*, *Implementation Science* and *British Medical Journal Quality and Safety*. Apart from the MRC, the importance of investing in implementation – and therefore quality improvement – in health care has been stressed by key policy organizations such as the World Health Organization (WHO, 2010) and the European Science Foundation (ESF, 2011). In addition, these organizations stress the need for implementation *research*.

The fact that both health policy and health sciences increasingly stress the need to focus on implementation issues can be explained from ample examples of sub-optimal performance of health care systems and its workers (Grol and Wensing, 2013). These examples indicate that even when health care workers know about new insights on effective patient care, their practice does not change. Insufficient use of best evidence in clinical decisions threatens all key aspects of health care quality, namely: safety, effectiveness, efficiency, acceptability/patient centredness, timeliness and equitability/accessibility (IOM, 2002; WHO, 2006).

A book on complex interventions in health care would not be complete without a focus on implementation issues, as self-implementing complex interventions would qualify as an endangered species. Thus, this section offers six chapters for those seeking to get acquainted with the idea of implementation, issues to consider, pitfalls on the route to implementation and helpful insights and tools for those who seek to actively add to the implementation of complex interventions.

The stage is set by Ted Skolarus and Anne Sales, who introduce relevant terminology and provide a first insight into the complexity of implementation issues. In addition, their chapter discusses the level of implementation that could be desired or realistically expected. Skolarus and Sales propose a stepwise approach from *assessing practice gaps* to *designing implementation interventions* that can help lessen gaps in health care delivery.

Two chapters in this section add to understanding *why* implementation issues can be notoriously difficult. Carl May applies Normalization Process Theory to the implementation of complex interventions. Normalization Process Theory can help our understanding of the implementation and operationalization of complex interventions in everyday practice. *Capacity*, *Potential*, *Contributions* and *Capability* are introduced as key concepts of the theory, which is further explained through four guiding propositions.

Elizabeth Dogherty and Carole Estabrooks provide us with an operational overview of factors that may help or hinder the implementation of complex interventions. Their chapter describes evidence on these *facilitators* and *barriers* and ways to categorize these. Apart from describing commonly found factors, the chapter presents methods and tools to identify these factors in specific situations. The authors argue that knowledge of facilitators and barriers for implementation is the key to finding successful implementation strategies.

The final three chapters in this section present ways to help implementation and arrive at improved health care provision. The first of these chapters (Theo van Achterberg) proceeds from a scenario where barriers and facilitators for implementation are known and describes *how to build an implementation plan* from there. Here the range of potential change strategies to be considered is discussed, and the importance of linking strategies to barriers and facilitators is stressed. Furthermore, using theory and available evidence for implementation strategies is presented and illustrated as a way to optimize chances of successful implementation of complex interventions.

Brendan McCormack describes *action research* for the implementation of complex interventions. His chapter introduces action research methodology and its application in the implementation of complex interventions. Here, assessing relevant context, engaging stakeholders in all relevant steps and decisions, considering the 'fit' between interventions and the implementation context, and taking a collaborative and participatory approach to outcome evaluations are key messages. McCormack discusses different types of action research, and illustrates the value of action research for the implementation of beneficial interventions in health care settings.

Finally, Martin Pitt, Thomas Monks and Michael Allen present *systems modelling* as a valuable approach to improving health care. Systems modelling includes problem-structuring methods, conceptual modelling, mathematical programming and analytical techniques, and simulation techniques; all to be used for understanding system effects that can hinder or promote the implementation of complex interventions. From this perspective, insights from systems modelling can contribute to successful improvement in health care practice, which is illustrated by several case presentations in this chapter.

All chapters in this section ask the reader not just to jump into action. Clearly, the implementation of complex interventions should not be taken lightly. Though intuitive approaches might prove lucky, approaches using an analysis of the context and its facilitating and hindering factors, and linking these to well-considered implementation strategies are likely to be more successful.

An additional word of caution is given here, and relates to the very first step in the implementation process. At the very start of deciding to invest in implementation efforts, considering implementation readiness, the distance between practice and a potential innovation, and realistic expectations is crucially important.

Implementation readiness relates to the complex intervention at hand, which should have been built through the various elements proposed in the MRC framework (Craig *et al.*, 2008). Such interventions should include clear descriptions of their mechanisms, should be operationalized for use in practice and should be sufficiently tested for acceptability, feasibility and their desired effects. Though it is not always clear-cut when these criteria are sufficiently met, project initiators should always consider their own arguments. Promoting the implementation of interventions that are insufficiently developed or tested can – rightfully – frustrate the project at hand, and, regretfully, frustrate future implementation projects regardless of the level of implementation readiness.

A second aspect to be considered is the *distance between current practice and complex interventions* to be implemented. Often, innovative interventions are presented as totally new. In reality, they nearly always show overlap with current practice. The degree of overlap between 'new' complex interventions and current practice should always be carefully considered. If target users sense that they are asked to make a major change and then get the impression the proposed change is negligible, their motivation is probably at risk. Also, the project initiators may conclude that they have put a lot of effort into a change that is much smaller than they had foreseen.

Thirdly, *realistic expectations* are always important. So what level of implementation should we strive for? The answer is not an easy one, but an attempt at answering this question will be important in all cases. Here valid deviations from the proposed practice can occur, for instance in case of contra-indications or other preferences in patients. Also, health care workers and health care systems will always be imperfect. Acknowledging a likely level of mistakes is realistic, rather than defeatist. So setting a realistic target for implementation in practice can be tricky, but remains important.

Finally, the introduction of innovative practices in health care has grown into *implementation science*, an area of scientific endeavour with input from various disciplines and links to implementation issues in other areas, such as industry. This section provides a solid introduction into this area, and should help those who are relatively new to the area to make a flying start.

27

IMPLEMENTATION ISSUES

Towards a systematic and stepwise approach

Ted A. Skolarus and Anne E. Sales

Introduction

The study of implementation has received considerable attention in health care settings over the last few decades, spurred in part by the evidence-based practice (EBP) movement, but also drawing from a considerable literature that focuses on the use of research evidence in clinical practice (Brownson *et al.*, 2012; Estabrooks *et al.*, 2008; Squires *et al.*, 2011). Implementation is defined as 'the use of strategies to adopt and integrate evidence-based health interventions and change practice patterns within specific settings' (http://www.fic.nih.gov/News/Events/implementation-science/Pages/faqs.aspx). In this chapter, we address issues of terminology, the use of frameworks to guide intervention planning and design, discuss some examples of implementation efforts, and describe emerging systematic approaches to launching an effort to implement EBPs.

Learning objectives

- Recognize several important terms for understanding what implementation is, what is to be implemented, and how the process is accomplished.
- Identify differences between factors, constructs, domains and frameworks and how they relate to the context in which evidence-based health interventions are to be implemented.
- Understand some of the complexities of doing implementation and implementation research through review of two examples of implementation processes and their varying outcomes.
- Describe an emerging, stepwise approach to planning an implementation process and using linkages of barriers and facilitators to theory-based strategies for implementation intervention design.

Defining terms

Several terms are very important in understanding what implementation is, what is to be implemented, and how the process is accomplished. However, many different terms are used by different authors, sometimes from different disciplinary backgrounds, to describe similar processes. While there have been attempts to standardize definitions and terminology, as yet no standard terms have been agreed on. As a result, we feel it is important to provide the terms we will use in this chapter, with synonyms given when there are clear synonyms. We will use these terms as we describe the current state of the science in implementation research, and emerging systematic approaches to implementation.

Adoption: we use adoption to mean the implicit or explicit decision made by an individual or organization to change practice. As a result, adoption is internal to the individual or organization, while implementation can be internal, external or both. Adoption can occur at multiple points during an implementation process, and may require reinforcement; it may not be a single decision, but iterative instances of decision-making that result in a state in which the evidence-based health intervention is being practised on an ongoing, routine basis.

Dissemination: refers to a process of providing and spreading information, typically about an evidence-based health intervention. This is often an essential step prior to or concurrent with engaging in implementation processes; dissemination may occur prior to implementation efforts, or may be part of an implementation intervention, as a strategy for ensuring that all participants have the necessary information.

Evaluation: assessing whether the processes of both dissemination and implementation are effective. Evaluation is often geared to assessing the state or degree of adoption.

Evidence-based health intervention: synonymous to some extent with evidence-based practice or evidence-based clinical practice, but as noted earlier, may also include innovations related to service delivery or system approaches.

Innovation: following the definition of implementation above, 'innovation' refers to the evidence-based health intervention – which could also include a change in delivery systems or mechanisms – that is the focus of implementation efforts, or the 'thing' to be adopted.

Implementation intervention: we refer to implementation intervention as one or more implementation strategies and tools designed to assist in implementing a specific innovation (Sales and Helfrich, 2006; Sales *et al.*, 2006). In our discussion, we treat implementation interventions as planned approaches to implementation, the active ingredient that pushes an implementation effort forward. An implementation intervention can be regarded as complex when it includes multiple implementation strategies that can act on more than one organizational level (multilevel) or in different ways (multifaceted) (Craig *et al.*, 2008). In general, the design of implementation interventions should be geared toward overcoming known or anticipated barriers, and making use of known facilitating characteristics of the environment or context, the individuals who are the target of the implementation intervention and the characteristics of the innovation. Note that we are not referring here to 'clinical interventions' (or medical interventions) in this discussion. Clinical interventions are specific clinical practices used by providers to address patient, family or community needs. An evidence-based health intervention may be synonymous with a clinical intervention. In cases where intervention is used as a stand-alone term in this chapter, we intend to refer to an implementation intervention.

Tailoring: refers to a process of adapting a set of implementation interventions using specific strategies and tools to address environmental or contextual issues identified through a process of assessing barriers and facilitators to implementing a specific evidence based-health intervention.

The practice gap

The most common reason to engage in a process of implementation is the realization that there is a gap between the way people are practising and the best current, available evidence about how people should practice – and then, usually by logical extension, the outcomes that patients and other system users experience. Discerning this gap is not trivially easy. It requires identification and critical appraisal of the current evidence supporting the best practice(s), often through evidence synthesis (e.g. systematic review, meta-analysis). It also requires data to understand current practice patterns and, ideally, also the outcomes associated with those practice patterns (McGlynn *et al.*, 2003). Obtaining current data describing practices is often very difficult, as most health care systems struggle to even measure outcomes of care, much less the processes and practices that produce those outcomes. In addition, in the case of most evidence-based practices, outcomes are dependent not only on the practices used to deliver care and services, but also on factors outside the control of the individual provider, including patient health status, patient adherence to recommendations such as diet, exercise and medication, and contextual factors, or the environment surrounding care delivery.

The environment, or context, can include proximal factors such as available staffing or types of providers available for consultation, whether or not resources exist within the environment, and the culture or receptivity to new evidence or innovations in practice (Damschroder *et al.*, 2009; Greenhalgh *et al.*, 2005). The existence of tools such as guidelines or care pathways and the degree to which they draw on credible, current evidence is another important contextual factor. Other factors are less proximal, and may include overall policies within the health care sector or regulatory factors, such as national bodies regulating the supply of different types of medication, or scope of practice regulations defining what providers such as clinicians, therapists and nurses may or may not do. Defining, measuring and understanding the effects of these types of proximal and distal contextual factors is a major endeavour in implementation research.

The degree to which we measure and attempt to control for factors that affect uptake of evidence-based health interventions or practice may be related to our use of frameworks that have been developed to explain the factors that affect implementation efforts. There are a large number of such frameworks. In a recently published review, Tabak and colleagues identified 61 different frameworks (Tabak *et al.*, 2012). As they found, these often operate at different levels within the health care system, and focus on different levels of factors. Some frameworks attempt to cover multiple levels and provide extensive coverage of a number of different factors affecting implementation, while others are much simpler and include only a few factors. We note that 'factors' is a relatively vague term in implementation research. A factor may be simple, such as noting the age of the people who are the target of an implementation effort, or it may be complex, such as 'leadership', which almost certainly includes multiple factors grouped together. The sub-factors within a large, complex factor, and simple factors, can be referred to as 'constructs'. In addition, a number of factors and constructs can be grouped together to form a 'domain', which is usually a broad term that is considered an important building block in the framework.

One of the complicated aspects of current frameworks in implementation research is that each framework has its own list of domains, and groups factors and constructs differently, even if the factors or constructs mean the same thing across frameworks. In addition, different frameworks use different words to describe the same construct, or the same word to describe different constructs. This makes it very confusing to review across frameworks, and decide which framework to use to plan an implementation process. Despite this confusion, we offer some suggestions, based on relatively straightforward criteria, about frameworks to consider using.

Legitimate differences: why evidence-based health intervention uptake is unlikely to be 100 per cent

Think about your practice setting, and how you and your colleagues practice. Think about a specific clinical intervention or practice that you commonly use. Do you and your colleagues or teammates all do this practice exactly the same way? Is it even the case that you mostly do it the same way? The chances are that you don't. There are good reasons for this. In some cases, there may be different policies or procedures endorsed by the hospital or health care setting in which you work. There may not be policies or procedures that cover the specific practice or clinical intervention that you need to use. You and your colleagues may have been educated at different times and in different ways, resulting in different ways you practice specific clinical interventions.

There is a fairly large body of literature that describes the factors that influence health care professionals (e.g. physicians, nurses) in the way they practice (Cabana *et al.*, 1999; Eccles *et al.*, 2005, Grimshaw and Hutchinson, 1995; Grimshaw *et al.*, 2001, 2002, 2004; Oxman *et al.*, 1995). The evidence from these bodies of literature is that many different factors influence health care professionals, from personal factors to assessment and understanding of the evidence for and against a specific evidence-based health intervention to the context in which professionals work (Box 27.1.). Key differences among professional groups, and between professions, also create reasons for different uptake of evidence-based practices (Godin *et al.* 2008; Grimshaw *et al.* 2004). Despite these legitimate differences, which suggest that it is very unlikely that any implementation process will result in full or 100 per cent adoption of the desired evidence-based health intervention, the goal of implementation research is to study and assess how implementation efforts can more reliably result in desired change, and be designed to achieve desired practice more efficiently and effectively.

BOX 27.1 DIFFICULT CHANGE: EXAMPLES OF HAND HYGIENE IMPLEMENTATION INTERVENTIONS

Examples of implementation processes and their outcomes illustrate some of the complexities of doing implementation and implementation research. Two recent examples of cluster randomized trials of implementation interventions to improve health care workers' use of hand hygiene exemplify the difficulties of conducting complex interventions despite considerable planning and use of theory (Fuller *et al.*, 2012; Huis *et al.*, 2013a, 2013b).

In the first example, a group of scientists adapted a theory-based intervention to add on to a national campaign for improved hand hygiene in hospitals. The implementation intervention focused on use of feedback, given in three different ways. The intervention was based on goal-and-control theory. This was implemented using a cluster randomized controlled trial design to allow evaluation of the effectiveness of this approach. While the approach was marginally effective, the real-world barriers to fully implementing this carefully designed implementation intervention made it very difficult to assess effectiveness fully, and the realities of units entering and leaving the study made evaluation very difficult. While this team attempted to engage in a full process evaluation to monitor the progress of the intervention, they found themselves unable to get full process information.

In the second example, another group of scientists designed an implementation intervention using multiple levels of the organization and multiple intervention components to improve adherence to hand hygiene recommendations. The focus of the implementation intervention was on teams and team leaders, using social influence theory in a multifaceted intervention that included reminders, education and feedback. In this trial, also cluster randomized and controlled, the units involved in the study were selected more deliberately and the process of implementing the intervention, while complex, was more successful. In this case, the effectiveness of the implementation intervention was greater.

Both groups carefully planned their implementation interventions, based on good theoretical bases, and linked the expected barriers to the intervention design. However, the first group did not plan for barriers associated with implementing the intervention in the busy, chaotic world of intensive care and hospital wards, while the second group carefully planned their intervention to take account of the realities of organizational priorities, resources and barriers from the time pressures of delivering care. These two examples illustrate the importance of planning not only the intervention based on individual factors, but also the implementation of the intervention in the organizational contexts of busy hospital units.

Improving chances of success: toward a stepwise approach

Even though implementation research currently offers a vast smorgasbord without a lot of signposts to guide you to good choices, there are some emerging signs to follow to develop a stepwise approach to planning an implementation process. Figure 27.1 provides an overview and highlights the steps we describe.

Assessing the gaps in practice that are most important in your setting, and assessing the quality of the evidence to guide selecting one or more evidence-based health or health care delivery interventions (innovations) to address those gaps is an essential first step. While there are resources to help guide this step (US Department of Veterans Affairs, 2013), it remains highly localized and sensitive to topic and context. In fact, the interplay between observed gaps in practice, whether they remain substandard after further investigation, and the strength of the evidence base for the health or health care delivery intervention is critical to understand before moving forward with any implementation effort. Other resources within this handbook will assist in this initial, critical step.

Once a clear practice gap has been identified, and appropriate innovations in the form of evidence-based health interventions have been identified that will reduce the practice gap, the next step is to perform assessment of barriers and facilitators that will affect the effort to implement the evidence-based health intervention(s). This step is tightly linked with deciding which framework will guide the approach to assessing barriers and facilitators. In the next section, we make recommendations, based on the current state of the literature, about which frameworks will provide the most direct and easy to use guidance in this and subsequent steps.

Following assessment of barriers and facilitators, the next logical step is to design the implementation intervention, using the information about barriers and facilitators. Gradually, developers of frameworks are beginning to offer ways to link specific barriers identified to strategies based on theory that addresses methods of promoting behavior change (Cane *et al.*, 2012; French *et al.*, 2012; Michie *et al.*, 2005; Taylor *et al.*, 2013). While most of these are at the individual level, some are at organizational levels.

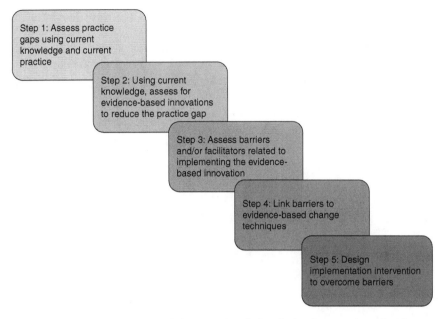

FIGURE 27.1   Steps to systematic intervention design for implementation of evidence-based practices

The final step, based on our current knowledge, is to test the implementation interventions designed using barriers and facilitators assessed in specific contexts and settings to see whether these theory-based interventions are successful in implementing evidence-based health interventions, and in promoting adoption of evidence-based innovations in health care settings that lessen the gaps in care. This final step is still being developed and tested, and represents one important cutting edge in implementation research.

Specific recommendations based on current literature

The Theoretical Domains Framework (TDF) (Francis *et al.*, 2012; French *et al.*, 2012) provides clear linkages from assessment of barriers and facilitators to designing implementation interventions through theory-based strategies. While most of the barrier assessment using the TDF to date has used qualitative methods for assessment, primarily interviews and focus groups with key representatives of provider groups whose behavior is the subject of change, a survey instrument to allow researchers and implementers to survey participants rather than conduct interviews has recently been published. Use of this survey instrument is still very new, but it offers an approach that may make barrier assessment easier (Huijg *et al.*, 2014).

Once barriers have been assessed and linked to key constructs within the TDF, a mapping of identified barriers to implementation strategies that has been developed and published (Michie *et al.*, 2008) may be useful. Using this map, some research groups have taken the further step of designing implementation interventions to overcome barriers, and launch implementation efforts using theoretically based interventions (French *et al.*, 2012; Taylor *et al.*, 2013). While it is still too early to know the results of these efforts, carefully planning and designing implementation interventions offers considerable advantage over idiosyncratically designed and developed implementation interventions without much basis in theory (Colquhoun *et al.*, 2013; Ivers *et al.*, 2014).

Summary

This introductory chapter defines several important terms related to implementation and offers a systematic and stepwise approach to planning an implementation process and addressing implementation issues. Through identifying gaps in practice, assessing barriers and linking them to key constructs within frameworks, and designing subsequent theory-based implementation interventions we can effectively lessen gaps in health and health care delivery. Below we list suggested reading for those interested in theory-based implementation.

Further reading

French, S. D., Green, S. E., O'Connor, D. A., McKenzie, J. E., Francis, J. J., Michie, S., Buchbinder, R., Schattner, P., Spike, N. and Grimshaw, J. M. 2012. Developing theory-informed behaviour change interventions to implement evidence into practice: a systematic approach using the Theoretical Domains Framework. *Implementation Science,* 7: 38.

Godin, G., Bélanger-Gravel, A., Eccles, M. and Grimshaw, J. 2008. Healthcare professionals' intentions and behaviours: a systematic review of studies based on social cognitive theories. *Implementation Science*, 3: 36.

Michie, S., Johnston, M., Abraham, C., Lawton, R., Parker, D. and Walker, A. 2005. Making psychological theory useful for implementing evidence based practice: a consensus approach. *Quality and Safety in Health Care,* 14: 26–33.

28

WHY DO BARRIERS AND FACILITATORS MATTER?

Elizabeth J. Dogherty and Carole A. Estabrooks

Introduction

Translating research into clinical practice remains a challenge and suggests the existence of a number of barriers to practice change. Researchers have examined the barriers and facilitators to research use encountered by health care professionals generally reaching consensus, specifically in nursing, as to what the barriers are. A number of tools and strategies exist for identifying barriers and facilitators to evidence implementation. However, recognition of barriers and facilitators, while a necessary first step, is not sufficient to ensure evidence uptake. To advance the field, research must focus on the development of implementation interventions that target barriers and facilitators to increase the use of evidence in practice.

This chapter outlines the importance of identifying barriers and facilitators to evidence implementation and we offer examples of those most commonly reported in the literature. In the second section, we review instruments that can be used to assess barriers and facilitators and measures that examine the context within which research is to be implemented. Finally, we offer suggestions for future areas of research and emphasize the relevance of researchers conducting a thorough process evaluation alongside studies of effectiveness of implementation interventions that aim to enhance evidence uptake.

Learning objectives

*   Develop an understanding of common barriers and facilitators to the implementation of evidence.
*   Identify methods and tools to analyse organizational context and instruments to assess specific barriers and facilitators that may influence implementation.

Why do barriers and facilitators to evidence implementation matter?

Practice settings are stubbornly resistant to successful and sustained achievements in implementing evidence-based practice changes. Interventions targeting such changes demonstrate variable effectiveness (Grimshaw *et al.*, 2004) and there remains a lack of evidence about which strategies are effective at getting evidence into practice, under what conditions and contextual influences (Kitson *et al.*, 2008). One explanation for the variable impact of different change strategies is that the barriers to implementation vary across settings and at different points in time (Cheater *et al.*, 2005).

Barriers are factors that inhibit the implementation of practice change (Cheater *et al.*, 2005) and facilitators are factors that make implementation easier. In the literature, barriers are more often referred to than facilitators. Additionally, the same factor can sometimes be considered both a barrier and a facilitator (Légaré and Zhang, 2013). Légaré and Zhang conducted a search in PubMed up to 7 August 2012 using the terms 'barriers' and 'barriers AND implementation' that resulted in 57,665 and 4,359 hits, respectively (Légaré and Zhang, 2013). We reran the same search up to 22 February 2014 and produced 68,823 and 5,670 hits, respectively, evidence of increasing and accelerating interest in the field.

One strategy recommended for addressing the research to practice gap is, a priori, to identify barriers to practice change and develop strategies to address these barriers (Nilsson Kajermo *et al.*, 2010). Systematically exploring the barriers and facilitators to implementation of evidence-based practices and using this information to develop implementation interventions should enable these interventions to be more effective. Tailored implementation strategies will assist in overcoming or minimizing barriers to practice change and will potentiate the effect of existing facilitators of change.

What are some of the more commonly reported barriers and facilitators to evidence implementation?

Barriers and facilitators to implementing evidence-based interventions and practice changes exist at multiple levels – individual professional, group or team, patient-care unit, organization, and the larger structural (e.g. financial incentives) and social context of care provision. The Cochrane Effective Practice and Organisation of Care (EPOC) Group is a review group of the Cochrane Collaboration focusing on interventions designed to improve health care delivery, practice and organization of services (Cochrane Effective Practice and Organisation of Care Group, 2012). The EPOC Group classifies barriers to change according to nine categories (Cochrane Effective Practice and Organisation of Care Review Group, 2002):

(a)   Information management
(b)   Clinical uncertainty

(c) Sense of competence
(d) Perceptions of liability
(e) Patient expectations
(f) Standards of practice
(g) Financial disincentives
(h) Administrative constraints
(i) Others

Barriers and facilitators to implementation may exist at multiple levels and there may be interaction between levels.

Physicians encounter various barriers at several of these levels that may influence their ability to engage in practice change (Grimshaw *et al.*, 2002): clinician knowledge, attitudes and skills (individual level), local standards of care not aligned with best practice (peer group or social contextual level), financial disincentives (structural level), inappropriate skill mix and/or inadequate facilities or equipment (organizational level). Cabana and colleagues conducted a systematic review of barriers to physician adherence to practice guidelines (Cabana *et al.*, 1999), one form of evidence use. The authors included 76 articles that reported 293 potential barriers. Barriers included lack of awareness (n = 46 articles); external barriers (n = 34); lack of agreement with a particular guideline, recommendation, or guidelines generally (n = 33); familiarity with recommendations (n = 31) or self-efficacy (n = 19; belief in one's ability to perform the guideline recommendations); inability to overcome inertia of previous practice (n = 14); and lack of outcome expectancy (n = 8; expectation that performing the recommendations will have a certain result). External barriers were either guideline related (e.g. not easy to use), patient related (e.g. disconnect between patient preferences and guideline recommendations) or environmental (e.g. lack of time or support) (Cabana *et al.*, 1999).

Other barriers to physicians' use of evidence-based practices include concerns about the applicability of clinical trial data to specific patients, financial concerns, resource constraints and information overload (Grimshaw *et al.*, 2002). Facilitators to implementing knowledge in practice (shared decision-making in particular) as perceived by professionals, primarily physicians, are provider motivation and positive impact on the clinical process and patient outcomes (Légaré *et al.*, 2008). Barriers to guideline adherence in some cases may actually facilitate adherence in other cases. For example, patient pressure on a physician may be a barrier to adherence to guideline recommendations in specific situations but if the patient pressure is a request that is in line with the evidence, this promotes physician adherence (Cabana *et al.*, 1999).

Specific barriers and facilitators to research use are well documented in the nursing literature, with considerable consensus as to what constitute the main barriers (Hutchinson and Johnston, 2006; Micevski *et al.*, 2004; Nilsson Kajermo *et al.*, 1998, 2010; Parahoo and McCaughan, 2001;). Key barriers that nurses identified are insufficient time to read research or implement new ideas, lack of evidence and resources to access research, limited confidence in critiquing research and understanding statistical analyses, and a perceived lack of authority to implement practice change. Facilitators include participatory management, culture building, higher academic education, positive attitudes and beliefs about evidence-based practice (EBP), colleague and professional association support, mentorship and inter-organizational collaboration and networking (Brown *et al.*, 2008; Koehn and Lehman, 2008; Ploeg *et al.*, 2007; Smith and Donze, 2010). Again, these barriers and facilitators are situated at the organizational level the interdisciplinary team level, and individual nurse level (Smith and Donze, 2010). Rycroft-Malone and colleagues argued as early as 2004 that research in this area had been exhausted (Rycroft-Malone *et al.*, 2004).

In 2010, Nilsson Kajermo and colleagues reported the findings of an exhaustive longitudinal review of the 'BARRIERS' research that had been conducted in nursing using the Funk *et al.* BARRIERS scale (Nilsson Kajermo *et al.*, 2010). Following their analysis of over 60 studies, they concluded that not only had no new information been reported since the early studies, but that this general style of assessing barriers was inappropriate, calling for more site-specific and process-oriented assessments. Recognition of the barriers and facilitators is a necessary first step but of course, not a sufficient step to ensure evidence implementation. To advance the field, research needs to focus on the development and evaluation of knowledge translation interventions that target barriers and enhance facilitators.

Although some of the barriers nurses encounter are the same as those affecting physicians (e.g. lack of awareness, inadequate resources), there are variations in cultural and professional norms between the two professions. One example relates to autonomy and ability to influence change in practice (Hodnett *et al.*, 1996; Kitson, 1995). Physicians do not perceive feeling a lack of authority to change practices as a barrier to implementation; however, it is a significant barrier for nurses (Hutchinson and Johnston, 2006; Nilsson Kajermo *et al.*, 2010). Similarly, nurses identified other staff not being supportive or physicians not cooperating with the implementation as barriers (Nilsson Kajermo *et al.*, 2010). Although we have only focused on physicians and nurses in this chapter, there are likely differences in the barriers and facilitators to evidence implementation that other professional groups encounter. Researchers should keep this in mind in the design and delivery of implementation interventions to change practice. Another area often overlooked that requires consideration is the explicit ways that clinicians conceptualize evidence. In addition to evidence-based guidelines, clinicians rely on collectively reinforced, internalized, tacit guidelines also as referred to as 'mindlines' (Gabbay and Le May, 2004). 'Mindlines' could be either barriers or facilitators so this is an important area to explore.

Some instruments and methods for identifying barriers and facilitators and analysing context

Interest in evaluating organizational features, context, culture and climate in the fields of implementation science and quality improvement is high, and a number of measures and tools with which to assess barriers and facilitators and analyse context are emerging.

Evidence-Based Practice Attitude Scale

Aarons and colleagues presented a tool in 2004 that measures mental health and social service provider attitudes towards EBP, called the *Evidence-Based Practice Attitude Scale* (EBPAS; Aarons, 2004). EBPAS uses a five-point Likert scale and scores relate to provider characteristics, organizational characteristics and leadership (Aarons *et al.*, 2012). The scale contains four domains of attitudes towards EBP: appeal of an EBP, requirements to adopt an EBP, openness to innovation and perceived divergence between current work processes and those required by an EBP. An overall Cronbach's alpha of 0.77, with subscale alphas ranging from 0.90 to 0.59, has been reported (Aarons, 2004).

The BARRIERS Scale

In 1991, Funk *et al.* published the *Barriers to Research Utilization Scale* (Funk *et al.*, 1991). The 28 items are rated on a four-point scale depending on the degree to which the item is perceived to be a barrier. Respondents can also add and score other possible barriers, rank the three greatest barriers and list factors they perceive as facilitators (Nilsson Kajermo *et al.*, 2010). Items are categorized in four dimensions: characteristics of the adopter, characteristics of the organization, characteristics of the innovation and characteristics of the communication. Cronbach's alpha values for the four subscales were 0.80, 0.80, 0.72, and 0.65, respectively (Funk *et al.*, 1991). Preliminary estimates of test–retest reliability of the scales resulted in Pearson correlations ranging from 0.68 to 0.83. The scale has been used extensively in nursing to identify barriers to research utilization, but there is no evidence of its use for tailoring implementation interventions to overcome identified barriers (Nilsson Kajermo *et al.*, 2010).

The Context Assessment Index

The *Context Assessment Index* (CAI) is a 37-item, five-factor model that helps clinicians assess and make sense of the context in which they work and the effect that context has on the use of evidence in practice (McCormack *et al.*, 2009a). The CAI contains a four-point Likert response format and five constructs: collaborative practice, evidence-informed practice, respect for persons, practice boundaries and evaluation. The final score represents the level of readiness of the context to implement evidence into practice. The Cronbach's alpha for the complete questionnaire was 0.93. McCormack and colleagues report test–retest reliability and that all five factors reached adequate levels of internal consistency in scoring (range 0.78–0.91;

McCormack *et al.*, 2009a). The CAI demonstrates evidence of acceptable validity and reliability, and feedback obtained from focus group participants indicates that the CAI has practical utility.

Organizational Readiness to Change Assessment

The *Organizational Readiness to Change Assessment* (ORCA) is a tool for gauging overall site readiness and identifying particular barriers (Helfrich *et al.*, 2009). The instrument contains 77 items within a number of subscales and three primary scales: strength and extent of evidence for the clinical practice changes, quality of the organizational context, and capacity for internal facilitation. ORCA uses a five-point Likert scale and takes approximately 15 minutes to complete (see Box 28.1 for a clinical example; Helfrich *et al.*, 2009). Generally, the authors reported adequate reliability and validity estimates. Cronbach's alphas for reliability were 0.74, 0.85 and 0.95 for the evidence, context and facilitation scales, respectively. The authors observed low reliability for three evidence subscales. Additional validation is required.

BOX 28.1 USE OF THE ORGANIZATIONAL READINESS TO CHANGE ASSESSMENT (ORCA) TOOL IN A RANDOMIZED TRIAL

Researchers in the United States are conducting a cluster randomized clinical trial to test the effectiveness of an evidence-based quality improvement plus facilitation intervention to improve the monitoring and management of the metabolic effects of antipsychotics (Owen *et al.*, 2013). As part of the pre-implementation phase of their study (the six-month period prior to initial site visits), investigators administered the ORCA instrument to all provider participants to measure the effect of organizational readiness-to-change on implementation. The tool will be administered again at the conclusion of the sustainability, or final, phase of the study (Owen *et al.*, 2013).

The Alberta Context Tool

In 2009, Estabrooks and colleagues reported on the *Alberta Context Tool* (ACT), an eight-dimension measure of organizational context for health care settings (Estabrooks *et al.*, 2009). The tool was designed to be brief enough to be completed in busy health care settings and assess concepts of organizational context that are potentially modifiable. The eight contextual dimensions are culture, leadership, evaluation, social capital, informal interactions, structural and electronic resources, and organizational slack. The tool contains 56 items, a five-point Likert-scale and takes 8–10 minutes to complete. Cronbach's alpha for the 13 factors ranged from 0.54

to 0.91 with four factors performing below the accepted cut-off of 0.70 (Estabrooks *et al.*, 2009). Bivariate associations between what the ACT was developed to predict (instrumental research utilization levels) and the 13 factors were statistically significant at the 5 per cent level for 12 out of 13 factors. Construct validity was also demonstrated. Subsequent reports of its use and adaptation, as well as its validity and reliability, have appeared (Estabrooks *et al.*, 2011; Hoben *et al.*, 2014).

These tools represent promising directions in instrument development; however, it may not be practical or feasible to administer tools, especially lengthy ones, in the interest of time and to large numbers of individuals. Additionally, tools provide a general assessment and responses are usually aggregated to the group or setting level to make them usable. Other methods, specifically process-oriented methods, offer richer and more context and innovation specificity. For example, the barriers to implementing a hand hygiene routine may differ significantly from those pertaining to an innovation that reduces injury falls. Stetler *et al.* used a strategic change model and examined key contextual elements that may need attention for the institutionalization of EBP (Stetler *et al.*, 2009). They identified that the most critical element was key people leading change, which impacted on operationalization of other key elements of the model. Other methods include focus groups, interviews, non-participant observation, case studies, brainstorming, and informal discussion (see Box 28.2 for a clinical example; National Institute of Clinical Studies, 2006).

BOX 28.2 EXAMPLE OF THE USE OF INTERVIEWS, OBSERVATION AND FOCUS GROUPS TO IDENTIFY BARRIERS AND ENABLERS (FACILITATORS)

Squires *et al.* are developing a theory-based knowledge translation intervention to improve physician hand hygiene compliance (Squires *et al.*, 2013a). Phase 1 of their study focuses specifically on identifying barriers and enablers to hand hygiene compliance. This will involve key informant interviews with physicians using a structured interview guide, non-participant observation of hand hygiene audit sessions, and focus groups with hand hygiene experts. The researchers will use the data collected in Phase 1 to inform Phase 2: development of a knowledge translation intervention that incorporates behaviour change strategies to overcome barriers and enhance enablers to hand hygiene compliance (Squires *et al.*, 2013a).

Another approach is the use of intervention mapping (IM; Bartholomew *et al.*, 1998; French *et al.*, 2012). IM begins with a needs assessment including analysis of behavioural and environmental causes of the problem(s); a preliminary description of what is known about predictors or determinants of the behavioural and environmental causes; and community resources. The needs assessment can be used to identify barriers and facilitators that could be mapped in the development of an implementation intervention to enhance research utilization. Conceptual frameworks regarding barriers to knowledge use in health care have also been developed (see Box 28.3; Cabana *et al.*, 1999; Moulding *et al.*, 1999).

BOX 28.3 A CONCEPTUAL FRAMEWORK FOR EFFECTIVE MANAGEMENT OF CHANGE IN CLINICAL PRACTICE

Moulding and colleagues developed a framework for guideline dissemination and implementation based on diffusion of innovation theory, the trans-theoretical model of behaviour change, health education theory, social influence theory, social ecology and evidence from literature reviews on the effectiveness of various behaviour change strategies (Moulding *et al.*, 1999). The framework emphasizes the importance of conducting a pre-implementation assessment of barriers to change as experienced by clinicians. The authors also provide suggested strategies to assess barriers to change (e.g. use of local opinion leaders, small group discussions).

Summary

Implementation interventions to enhance evidence uptake target different organizational levels and a variety of health care professionals. These levels and actors are not mutually exclusive; researchers are often working across levels in many settings (e.g. hospitals, nursing homes, home care). Although there are commonly reported barriers and facilitators to implementing EBP reported in the literature, there is no substitute for a thorough assessment in relation to the local practice environment or context. In this way, interventions can be tailored prospectively to improve care and patient outcomes. (Cheater *et al.*, 2005). Barriers are referred to more often than facilitators in the literature in reference to enhancing EBP; however, it is important to remember that the same factor can sometimes be considered both a barrier and a facilitator. There is still limited evidence regarding the most effective strategies to use for identifying barriers and facilitators of practice change but there are best practices emerging: for example, use of suitable tools with setting relevance and demonstrated validity evidence; careful pre-assessment of barriers and facilitators using interview or focus group methods and careful process evaluation before, during and post implementation (see Box 28.4). Knowledge about which barriers are most important or which knowledge translation interventions are effective for overcoming different barriers is nascent but developing.

BOX 28.4 USE OF THE ALBERTA CONTEXT TOOL IN A PROCESS EVALUATION

The Facilitating Implementation of Research Evidence (FIRE) study is investigating the effectiveness of facilitation (as a knowledge translation intervention) on the implementation of research findings into practice (Seers *et al.*, 2012). Researchers are using the tool to assess the context in which care is delivered within nursing homes, as well as any factors that may account for implementation activity and outcomes. The survey will be administered at baseline and then 12 and 24 months post-intervention.

29

HOW TO ARRIVE AT AN IMPLEMENTATION PLAN

Theo van Achterberg

Introduction

As was addressed in the previous chapters in this section, the implementation of complex interventions is not self-evident. Even when all previous phases of the MRC framework for the development and evaluation of complex interventions (Craig et al., 2008) were followed systematically, many factors may still hinder the actual uptake of complex interventions in health care practice. Choosing implementation strategies in relation to these facilitating or hindering factors is crucial and can make the difference between implementation success and failure. But how to go about this, and where to begin?

Learning objectives

Be aware of the range of change strategies to be considered.

- Be aware of the need to link barriers and facilitators for implementation to relevant concepts.
- Find and consider theories that can inform the selection of implementation strategies.
- Consider the effectiveness of common strategies.
- Be critically aware of the need to tailor strategies to barriers and facilitators.

Considering options for implementation

Figure 29.1 provides a first overview of options, organized from involuntary to voluntary strategies, using extrinsic motivation through environmental changes and intrinsic motivation through addressing individual professionals as a main distinction

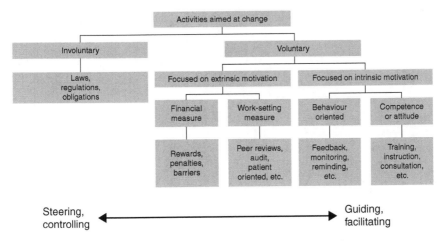

FIGURE 29.1   An overview of optional implementation strategies*
*Derived from van Woerkom (1990)

to be made within the group of voluntary strategies. Though this figure helps to consider options, it does not necessarily lead the way for those who need to decide on strategies in a particular case. Also, the figure triggers an ethical reflection on how *voluntary or involuntary* the implementation of evidence-based interventions should be. A clear proposition from the evidence-based practice literature is that patients should benefit from optimal use of evidence in practice. Yet overall, the implementation literature indicates that projects in Western health care choose voluntary approaches to change health care professionals' actions (e.g. Holleman *et al.*, 2006), and dominantly focus on the least steering strategies (training, consultations etc). On the positive side, these voluntary strategies respect the professionalism and autonomy of health care providers. Such strategies encourage evidence-*informed* decision-making, which can be valuable for patients who are the exception to the rule and who may not benefit from interventions that suit most. Also, these voluntary strategies recognize how specific situations can ask for deviations from guidelines (e.g. not performing hand hygiene when re-animation is needed). On the negative side, however, voluntary implementation approaches count on professionalism which may not always be there, and may implicitly tell professionals it is still 'okay' not to implement evidence. Thus, involuntary strategies may protect patients more effectively, especially where interventions are very likely to suit all patients and situations (such as in infection prevention measures in the operating room).

This chapter will start from a situation where the first essential steps in each implementation process are taken: an implementation issue is known, clear implementation goals are described, and hindering or facilitating factors have been explored (Grol *et al.*, 2013). At this stage choices are crucial. But again, where to go from here? Where to look for matching implementation approaches and how to optimize chances of successful change in practice? This chapter will discuss considering concepts, theories and evidence as the keys to preparing for success.

TABLE 29.1 Relevant factors and related concepts for pain management in emergency care

Factor related to pain management in emergency care	Barrier or facilitator	Potentially relevant concepts*
Lack of knowledge on pain management	Barrier	Knowledge
Staff see pain as 'part of the deal' and minor priority	Barrier	Attitude
Emergency department physician promotes pain management	Facilitator	Leadership Social influence
No shared perspective on pain management	Barrier	Social norms Attitude
Not one guideline for all emergency care	Barrier	Facilitation
Protocol use not evaluated	Barrier	Feedback leadership
Inadequate multidisciplinary communication on pain	Barrier	Skills Teamwork Organization

* More information may be needed to choose the most relevant concept.

From facilitating and hindering factors to concepts

Any scientist investigating factors that may hinder or facilitate implementation is likely to end up with various factors that were observed, named in interviews or identified from the literature. Often, such factors are phrased in everyday language, thus reflecting issues reported by those involved in implementation of complex interventions in patient care. A first and critical step is to think about these factors from a conceptual point of view. What are these factors which health care workers, patients or managers report? What is the conceptual equivalent of the factors they name?

Considering concepts is crucial in developing an implementation plan, as it will point us towards potential answers.

Table 29.1 provides some examples of factors named by health care workers with a view to why adequate pain management may or may not be accomplished in emergency care settings (Berben *et al.*, 2012). Respondents in the qualitative study by Berben *et al.* were physicians, nurses, paramedics and managers who were asked to reflect on what hindered or facilitated adequate pain management in emergency care. Only a fraction of all factors named are reflected in the left-hand column of Table 29.1; in the right-hand column an attempt to relate these factors to concepts is shown. Here the main purpose is to think of what reported factors relate to; for example, do respondents' comments relate to facilities, attitudes or skills of health care workers?

Matching factors as reported in everyday language to concepts is not necessarily an easy task. For some of the respondents' factors in Table 29.1 the analytical exercise is easy, yet with other factors more information and going back to the target group might still be needed to choose between potentially relevant concepts (e.g. *why* does multidisciplinary communication not happen? Is it a matter of skills, organization or team dynamics?). Also, definitions of concepts should be checked to see whether the concepts actually include the factors in operational terms.

Though a bit of a puzzle and perhaps not as tempting as jumping into action, the analytical step of considering concepts related to factors hindering or facilitating implementation is important. It provides an important link between implementation problems and implementation approaches. Without it, providing solid arguments for an implementation approach will be difficult as conceptual links are needed for the selection of strategies.

Considering useful theories and theory proposed strategies

'There is nothing so practical as good theory.' This famous quote from the German psychologist Kurt Lewin certainly applies to the development of implementation plans, to which consideration of relevant theories is a key. Here, keeping an open mind should be tried as choosing a theory one knows best or prefers for other reasons could be a pitfall. Ideally, theories should be sought based on the concepts linked to implementation barriers and facilitators in practice. Such theories could be based in any scientific discipline. As health care is mostly delivered through human behaviour, behaviour change theories from (social) psychology will often be important. Yet, depending on relevant factors and concepts, theories from other disciplines such as economics, occupational health or management sciences might be very relevant.

Knowing all potentially relevant theories is next to impossible. However, several authors have provided handy overviews. Table 29.2 illustrates how concepts behind hindering and facilitating factors can be linked to theories and provides examples of strategies for change proposed by these theories. The table is freely inspired by the book *Planning Health Promotion Programs* (Bartholomew *et al.*, 2011), which was originally written to design health promotion interventions but which can be applied to implementation issues as well (see Abraham *et al.*, Chapter 11 for more details of intervention mapping). The book provides an overview of theories relevant to behaviour change, including theories relevant to changing environments in which behaviours should be performed. A valuable asset of the book is that it helps those who set out to develop approaches for change to find relevant theory and change strategies proposed in these theories.

A second useful reference for linking concepts to theory-proposed strategies is provided by Michie *et al.* (2008), who worked on consensus for a theoretical frame of reference for implementation research. Michie and colleagues identified 12 domains to explain behaviour change: (1) knowledge, (2) skills, (3) role and identity, (4) beliefs about capabilities, (5) beliefs about consequences, (6) motivation and goals, (7) memory, attention and decision processes, (8) environmental context and resources, (9) social influences, (10) emotion regulation, (11) behavioural regulation

TABLE 29.2 Concepts linked to examples of relevant theories and theory-proposed strategies*

Concept	Theory addressing the concept	Theory-proposed change strategies
Knowledge	Social Cognitive Theory	Active learning
	Theories of Information Processing	Advanced text organizers
Attitude	Health Belief Model	Shifting perspective
	Persuasion Communication Matrix	Anticipated regret
Self-efficacy	Social Cognitive Theory Attribution &	Modelling
	Relapse Prevention Theories	Planning coping responses
Social norms	Social Cognitive Theory	Role modelling
	Theory of Quality Management	Leadership
Funding	Economic Theories	Financial incentives
Organization	Theories on Organizational Culture	Priority setting

* Adapted from Bartolomew *et al.* (2011).

TABLE 29.3 Fragment of the Classification of Behaviour Change Techniques*

Concept	Theory-proposed change strategy (examples)
Knowledge	Provide general information
	Active learning
Awareness	Risk communication
	Self-monitoring of behaviour
	Delayed feedback of behaviour
Social influence	Provide social comparison
	Use of social support
Self-efficacy	Guided practice
	Role modelling
Facilitation of behaviour	Provide materials
	Provide continuous professional support

* Abraham and Michie (2008); de Bruin *et al.* (2009).

and (12) nature of the behaviour. In relation to this work, Abraham and Michie (2008) and De Bruin and colleagues (2009) published a Taxonomy of Behavior Change Techniques. This classification is based on behaviour change theories and provides a handy overview of theory-proposed change strategies one could use in a context with given implementation barriers or facilitators. A fragment of this classification is provided in Table 29.3.

Evidence for implementation strategies

Apart from theory, scientific studies and overviews of such studies can inform the implementation of complex interventions in health care. For this, the website of the Effective Practice and Organisation of Care Group (EPOC) is a key source (http://www.epoc.cochrane.org). EPOC is a review group of the Cochrane Collaboration and aims to create insight into evidence for interventions designed to improve the delivery, practice and organization of health care services. The EPOC website can be used to access overviews of studies on specific types of improvement strategies (e.g. education, feedback, financial interventions) as well as specific types of practice (e.g. discharge planning, patient referral, patient education, etc.).

In recent years, the number of publications on implementation research has dramatically increased, also in relation to the success of the journal *Implementation Science* (http://www.implementationscience.com), which now is an additional source of evidence in this area. The downside of this is that is has become increasingly difficult to give an overview of all evidence in this area.

One of the last and most comprehensive systematic reviews on the effects of health care improvement strategies dates back to 2004 and was performed by Grimshaw and colleagues. Their results from a decade ago indicated modest effect sizes of implementation strategies in health care settings, of around 10 per cent more performance of the desired practice. Today, providing an overview of all studies reporting on the effects of implementation strategies used in health care is next to impossible. Yet reviews on the effect of common strategies such as feedback (Jamvedt *et al.*, 2006), continuing education (Forsetlund *et al.*, 2009) and providing educational materials (Farmer *et al.*, 2008) indicate modest effect sizes are still common. This is also underlined from a review of systematic reviews on the effects of implementation strategies (Boaz *et al.*, 2011). With all these reviews one should keep in mind, however, that modest or absent effects of implementation strategies can probably also be explained by a lack of matching theories and strategies to barriers and facilitators of change. Grimshaw *et al.* (2004) indicated a lack of reporting on the rationale for implementation strategies in the studies included in their review. Though this seems gradually to have improved in more recent papers on the effects of implementation strategies in health care settings, a lack of reporting on the rationale behind choices is still common. This implies that modest effects of education can probably also be explained from the use of ill-chosen strategies, for example the use of education in situations where education did not match with knowledge issues as barriers or facilitators of change (see Dogherty and Estabrooks, Chapter 28). An implication of this is that evidence from studies should always be seen in relation to clarity on theory-informed mechanisms behind choices.

From strategies to implementation plan: a practice example

Once strategies for the implementation of complex interventions have been chosen, an operational implementation plan needs to be developed. At this stage, thinking about practical content and organization is most important. An example of how strategies can be translated into a practical implementation plan is shown in Table 29.4. The content of this box is derived from the work of Huis *et al.*

TABLE 29.4 Implementation plan in a project on improving hospital nurses' hand hygiene*

Implementation strategies	Activities and materials
Education	Distribution of written materials addressing • importance of hand hygiene • Misconceptions about alcohol-based hand disinfection • theory and practical indications for hand hygiene Website providing • similar content education (above) • knowledge quiz • reward for nursing ward with most website visitors Educational sessions with • infection prevention education • launch of hospital campaign • hand hygiene demonstrations
Reminders	Distribution of posters emphasizing • hand hygiene importance • particular importance of using hand alcohol Messages and interviews in newsletters/hospital magazine
Feedback	Feedback reports on hand hygiene rates to ward managers Comparison of ward performance and hospital performance
Products and facilities	Screening for adequate products and facilities; adjustments when necessary
Setting norms and targets within team	Three interactive team sessions that include goal setting in hand hygiene performance at group level • analysis of barriers and facilitators to determine how they could best adapt their behaviour in order to reach their goal • nurses talking to each other in the case of undesirable hand hygiene behaviour
Gaining commitment and initiative of ward management	Ward manager designates hand hygiene as a priority • ward manager actively supports team members and informal leaders • ward manager discusses hand hygiene compliance rates with team members
Modelling by informal leaders in wards	Informal leaders demonstrate good hand hygiene behaviour • informal leaders model use social skills in addressing behaviour of colleagues • informal leaders instruct and stimulate their colleagues in providing good hand hygiene behaviour

* Based on Huis *et al.* (2011).

(2011), who set out to improve hand hygiene among hospital nurses. In their research project, they studied whether setting norms, gaining management commitment and providing role models added to the effects of standard approaches for promoting hand hygiene including education, feedback, reminders and the provision of adequate products and facilities. The reported results of the study (Huis *et al.*, 2013b) indicated that norm setting, gaining management commitment and providing role models indeed added to the effect size and resulted in more hand hygiene adherence than standard campaigns alone. In addition to what is presented in Table 29.4, a well-developed implementation plan should always contain further practicalities (e.g. number of meetings, duration of meetings, numbers of prints to be made, website maintenance, etc.), descriptions of roles and responsibilities and a financial paragraph. Without such practicalities, any plan might fail at an early stage.

Summary

Several steps should be taken to arrive at a potentially successful implementation plan. Knowing about factors that hinder or facilitate the uptake of evidence-based complex interventions provides an essential departure point. After this, a first step is to think about the concepts these often practical factors represent, as this will allow linking them to relevant theories. From there, helpful theory-proposed strategies can be identified after which evidence for these strategies can be collated. Once a well-considered choice for one or more implementation strategies has been made, practical activities and materials can be developed.

A common pitfall is to start at the end of this series of steps and to jump to practical plans and activities. Though one may make lucky intuitive choices, the chances of choosing ill-matched approaches and a lack of change in practice are substantial with such immediate-action approaches. The steps offered and explained in this chapter should help in arriving at more well-considered and successful implementation plans. An integrated illustration of all successive steps is provided in Table 29.5.

TABLE 29.5 Taking successive steps towards a well-considered implementation plan, illustrated for three (out of many) factors influencing hand hygiene in hospital nurses

Desired practice	Hand hygiene in line with WHO guidelines for health care workers		
Factors (reported by hospital physicians and nurses)	Doubts on evidence for guideline recommendations	Forgetting	Management not interested, nobody controls it
Consider concepts & theories	Knowledge	Intention cue to action	Leadership social influence
Considering useful theories & theory-proposed implementation strategies	*Information Processing Theory* *Social Cognitive Theory* Education (active learning & information provision)	*Theory of planned behaviour* Reminders	*Leadership Theory* *Social Learning Theory* Norm & target setting
Evidence for implementation strategies	*General literature:* Mixed effects of education as strategy. *Hand hygiene literature:* education not sufficient to change behaviour but important as element of combined strategies	*General literature:* effective strategy; probably more effective than education or feedback. *Hand hygiene literature:* reminders usually an element of effective strategies	*General literature:* leadership and social influence effective in changing behaviours, not often used in health care improvement. *Hand hygiene literature:* few studies, but early evidence for effects

Activities & materials for improving hand hygiene (hh)

∨

Distribution of written materials addressing
- hh importance
- misconceptions about alcohol-based hh
- theory and practical indications for hh

Website providing
- similar content (above)
- knowledge quiz
- reward for ward with most website visitors

Educational sessions with
- infection prevention
- launch hospital campaign
- hh demonstrations

∨

Distribution of posters emphasizing
- hh importance
- particular importance of using hand alcohol
- messages and interviews in newsletters/hospital magazine

∨

Three interactive team sessions that include
- goal setting for hh performance at group level
- analysis of barriers and facilitators to determine how they could best adapt behaviour in order to reach goals
- how nurses talk to each other in the case of undesirable hh

Further reading

Bartholomew, L., Parcel, G., Kok, G., Gottlieb, N. and Fernández, M. 2011. *Planning Health Promotion Programs: An Intervention Mapping Approach*, 3rd edn. San Francisco, CA: Jossey-Bass.

Cochrane Effective Practice and Organisation of Care Group (EPOC). http://epoc.cochrane.org.

Grol, R., Wensing, M., Eccles, M. and Davis, D. (eds). 2013 *Improving Patient Care: The Implementation of Change in Healthcare*, 2nd edn. Chichester: John Wiley.

30

APPLYING NORMALIZATION PROCESS THEORY TO THE IMPLEMENTATION OF COMPLEX INTERVENTIONS

Carl May

Introduction

Implementing new ways of conceptualizing, enacting or organizing health care is a complex business. In this chapter I set out a theoretical model that can help us to understand implementation as a *process*, and which we can use to plan (Murray *et al.*, 2010) and evaluate (May *et al.*, 2009) implementation processes. There are innumerable theories of implementation, ranging from high-level organizational theories through to psychological theories of individual behaviour change (Tabak *et al.*, 2012), but Normalization Process Theory (May, 2013; May and Finch, 2009) – the subject of this chapter – is useful because it focuses on action rather than attitudes, and is organized around factors that have been empirically demonstrated to matter in implementation processes, and that are policy relevant (McEvoy *et al.*, 2014). Normalization Process Theory (NPT) has mainly been used in qualitative studies of implementation, but a quantitative instrument – the Technology Adoption Readiness Scale (Finch *et al.*, 2012) – to measure important NPT constructs is available and others are in development (Finch *et al.*, 2013).

Learning objectives

- To assert the value of applying explanatory models of implementation processes.
- To describe the scope and application of Normalization Process Theory.
- To show how Normalization Process Theory can be applied to understand implementation dynamics of different complex health care interventions.

The starting point for this chapter is that understanding the dynamics of practice change demands theoretical models that can be applied to problems of design and evaluation of complex interventions in health care, but – despite the plethora of available theories – published studies in this area are often descriptive and atheoretical. They tell us what happened, without helping us to understand why. Description is fine as far as it goes, but theory provides explanations for observed processes, and a point of departure for forecasting the parameters of future action and its outcomes. Theory is important, but theory-informed work has a paradox at its heart. Because to apply theory is always to seek to explain (and sometimes to predict), the kinds of theories that we apply need to be able to handle complexity, but at the same time massively simplify it. So theories are never – in themselves – complete pictures of the world. Recent research on the structure of theories suggests that we can find in them two kinds of assumptions or propositions: generic assumptions which describe and explain the core processes at work relating to some phenomenon, and which are highly transportable between contexts (Lieberson and Lynn, 2002); and a contingent periphery of assumptions that describe and explain processes that are unique (and are thus not transportable) between contexts. This division seems to hold for all kinds of theories: from economics to astrophysics (Machta et al., 2013), and it suggests that theories that offer generic, and generative, assumptions are more likely to be successful as explanations. This chapter is organized around a set of core generative propositions, and I am going to focus on complex health care interventions. This is an area where NPT has been widely used to develop and evaluate implementation processes.

Applying NPT to understanding the implementation of complex interventions

To understand the dynamics of implementing complex health care interventions is to attempt to understand how they are operationalized in practice, how practice is shaped by different human and technical factors, and how these shaping effects lead to particular outcomes. NPT helps us do this by first explaining important aspects of the capabilities inherent in a complex intervention. (The constructs of the theory are summarized in Figure 30.1.) NPT began with the development of a set of propositions that explain routine incorporation of a complex intervention in everyday practice (May, 2006), and these are set out below. Spangaro et al. (2011) were amongst the first researchers to use NPT when they evaluated the implementation of a complex intervention – a screening tool – to identify women who were at risk of violence from their partners in Australia. Results from their study are set alongside NPT propositions about intervention capabilities so that we can see what these context-independent statements mean in practice.

- Interactional workability: *A complex intervention is disposed to normalization if it confers an interactional advantage in flexibly accomplishing congruence of action between participants and their disposal of tasks* (May, 2006). Spangaro et al. (2011) showed how the screening tool became embedded in practice because its carefully

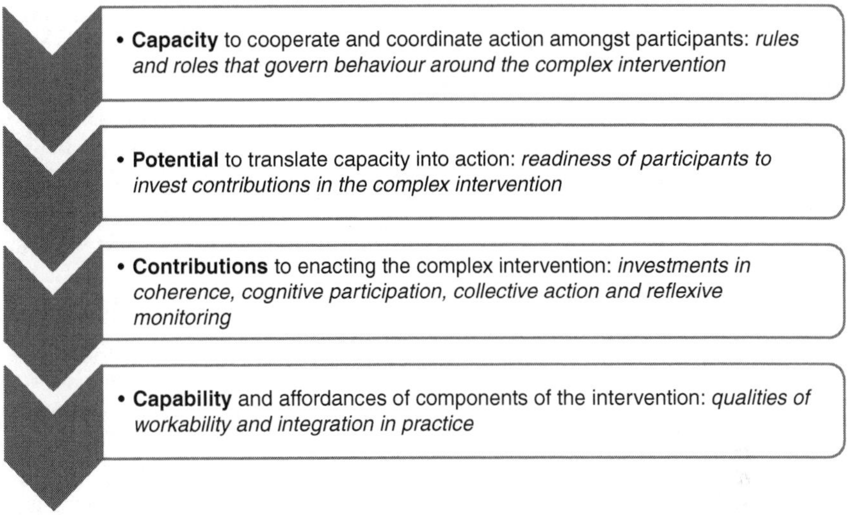

FIGURE 30.1 Core concepts of Normalization Process Theory

scripted and direct questions were easily performed and thus *interactionally workable* in the encounter between women and community health workers.

- Relational integration: *A complex intervention is disposed to normalization if it equals or improves accountability and confidence within networks of participants* (May, 2006). In Spangaro *et al.*'s study, the creation of robust referral pathways for women meant that community health workers shared accountability for outcomes, improving collective commitment.

- Skill-set workability: *A complex intervention is disposed to normalization if it is calibrated to an agreed skill-set at a recognizable location in the division of labour in which it is to be operationalized* (May, 2006). In Spangaro *et al.*'s study the intervention fitted well with existing role definitions, and was built into expectations of practice performance.

- Contextual integration: *A complex intervention is disposed to normalization if it confers an advantage on an organization in flexibly executing and realizing its work* (May, 2006). Spangaro *et al.* show how the intervention was linked to both a clear plan for resource allocation and operational execution, and that performance and delivery were consistently monitored.

Where this conceptualization of practice has been applied, we can see very quickly that complex interventions fail when their proponents do not pay equal attention to *workability* (how it is used, and how people learn to use it) and *integration* (confidence in its use and the resources available to execute it). NPT starts by considering how a complex intervention and its users are mutually engaged. We can encapsulate the four constructs that relate to *capability* in a single proposition that will contribute to a general theory of implementation (May, 2013):

(1) *The capability of users to enact a complex intervention depends on its potential for workability and integration in their everyday practice.*

Paying attention to workability and integration is important, because it speaks directly to the problem of practice that is often left untouched by intervention designers. The complexity of complex interventions does not, however, only reside in the properties or capabilities of the intervention to be implemented – whether this is a new way of thinking, enacting or organizing health care, or – more likely – a combination of all three. For example, the effective delivery of new models of care for people with depression does not simply depend on the capabilities of the model itself, but on the ways that its users operationalize the model and accomplish it in practice. This is revealed by important studies in primary care (Gunn *et al.*, 2010; Hermens *et al.*, 2014) that point to the role of participants' investments in the implementation process itself.

To think about participants' investments in an implementation process focuses our attention on their *contributions* to it. These contributions are the things that they do as they work with each other, and interact with the contexts in which they work, to realize the capabilities of the complex intervention. The work that people do with the different elements of a complex intervention is central (May and Finch, 2009). Once again, we can link underpinning mechanisms of *contribution* (coherence, participation, action and monitoring) to a proposition that informs a general theory of implementation.

(2) *Participants' contributions to enacting a complex intervention depend on them investing in meaning, commitment, effort and understanding.*

In relation to *contribution*, we can define four social mechanisms. Each of these is associated with a kind of work through which individuals and groups contribute to implementation processes. We can unpack this, too, in relation to actual practice. Here, studies using NPT have consistently shown that focusing on action helps to explain outcomes in clinical trials. For example, Kennedy *et al.* (2013) undertook a process evaluation of the WISE trial – a trial of supported self-management for long-term conditions in primary care.

- Coherence: *Normalization of a complex intervention is dependent on work that defines and organizes its component practices as a coherent cognitive and behavioural ensemble.* The production and reproduction of coherence in a practice requires that participants collectively invest meaning in it. Kennedy *et al.* (2013) showed how primary care nurses' stated commitments to supported self-care were restricted to routinized practices of monitoring necessary to obtain fee-for-service under the UK's Quality Outcomes Framework in primary care.
- Cognitive participation: *Normalization of a complex intervention is dependent on work that enrols participants and legitimizes their participation.* The production and reproduction of participation requires that participants collectively invest

commitment in it. In the WISE trial, Kennedy *et al.* showed how participating nurses found it difficult to enrol themselves and others into interactions that sought to promote self-care, and that they found it difficult to legitimize the actual practice of this work however much they were attitudinally inclined to be sympathetic to it.

- Collective action: *Normalization of a complex intervention is dependent on work that defines and operationalizes the enacting of its component practices.* The production and reproduction of action requires that participants collectively invest effort in it. In the WISE trial, the work of promoting self-care disrupted nurses' routine interactions with patients, and did not fit well with the financial incentives that structure British primary care services for long-term conditions.

- Reflexive monitoring: *Normalization of a complex intervention is dependent on work that defines and organizes the everyday evaluation of its effects.* The production and reproduction of evaluation requires that actors collectively invest in appraisal. In the WISE trial, negative outcomes of the trial itself could be explained by the complex intervention requiring nurses to invest in commitment and effort to do something that almost every aspect of their participation revealed was not rewarded by their employers or supported by other elements of their work.

So far, we have seen that participants in the implementation of complex interventions invest in contributions that mobilize the capabilities of intervention components. Plainly these contributions do not arise in a vacuum. They draw on social and cognitive resources. The first set of resources that are relevant here are structural resources of the kind characterized by Damschroder *et al.* (2009) as outer and inner settings. These include the culture, norms and values of the institutional or organizational settings in which the complex intervention is implemented and enacted, and the material and informational resources available to their users. Importantly, these properties of an organizational and institutional setting are those that shape the rules that govern participants' behaviours towards each other, and towards the work that they do. In other words, they structure participants' *capacity* to engage with a complex intervention. The second body of resources includes cognitive resources of the kind characterized by Bandura at a higher level of psychological theory (2001) and which are explored by Weiner (2009) under the more practical ambit of 'readiness'. These resources make it possible to mobilize participants' *potential* to engage with a complex intervention. When we look at capacity and potential, we find that they play a fundamental role in informing implementation processes, and that they form two further propositions towards a general theory of implementation of complex interventions.

(3) *Implementing a complex intervention depends on participants' capacity to cooperate and coordinate their actions.*

(4) *Translating capacity into action depends on participants' potential to enact the complex intervention.*

These propositions characterize important processes. With Andy Sibley and Katherine Hunt, I have shown how the implementation of clinical practice guidelines in hospital settings depends on nurses' capacity to operationalize changing clinical norms and professional roles, especially in relation to medical staff; and to coordinate changing informational resources. Translating capacity into practice required that structural and cognitive resources were mobilized in such a way as to build inter- and intra-professional collaborations and commitments to both the task set (the requirements of 'doing' the guideline in practice) and to its underlying body of evidence. Here, we can return to the four constructs of NPT as a general theory of implementation, and show how the data collected in a systematic review of qualitative studies of nursing guideline implementation (May *et al.*, 2014) contribute to a grounded analysis of factors that promote or inhibit these processes.

In Proposition (1), above, I stated that *the capability of users to enact a complex intervention depends on its potential for workability and integration in their everyday practice.* In our systematic review of qualitative studies of nursing practice guideline implementation (May *et al.*, 2014), we ought to have been able to comment on this in detail. After all, we were reviewing studies of guideline implementation, an area where there is much research and where problems of guideline design and delivery are well understood. In fact, none of the studies that made it into our review described the guideline in sufficient detail for us to explore their inherent qualities.

In Proposition (2) of the proposed general theory, I stated that *participants' contributions to enacting a complex intervention depend on them investing in meaning, commitment, effort and understanding.* Here we found that guidelines are likely to become embedded in practice when they have high levels of *coherence*. Their users can make sense of their purpose, and differentiate them clearly from other kinds of practice. They are also likely to become embedded in routine practice when they are associated with a group of staff who form a community of practice around them and enrol others into it. In these circumstances, a guideline implementation process is likely to be characterized by high levels of *cognitive participation*. As we would expect, the review found that when guidelines were not easily operationalized in practice – if they interfered with other interactions with patients, undermined confidence in professional knowledge and practice, or were poorly supported by their host health care provider organizations – then *collective action* to implement them was subverted and implementation processes were likely to fail. A final, but evidently important factor revealed by our review was that *reflexive monitoring* matters. Guidelines seemed more likely to be embedded when they were associated with improvements in professional knowledge of its users, and when that knowledge could be meaningfully integrated into individual nurses' workflow.

Two further propositions were also supported by our systematic review of guideline implementation studies. In Proposition (3) I asserted that *implementing a complex intervention depends on participants' capacity to cooperate and coordinate their actions*, and in Proposition (4) that *translating capacity into action depends on participants' potential to enact the complex intervention.* Here, we found that guidelines are not likely to be embedded in everyday practice if they disrupt the professional and organizational behaviour norms that underpin agreements about the scope of professional practice – that is, if they changed ideas about what nursing work should be. But they appeared to be likely to be embedded in everyday practice if they led to new collaborative commitments between nurses, and improved relations with local medical staff.

Conclusion

In their systematic review of studies using NPT, McEvoy *et al.* (2014) point to the strengths of an approach to evaluation theory that focuses on action (the things that people do) rather than attitudes (what they feel about what they do). Understanding the implementation of complex interventions involves understanding a set of social and technical processes in which these multiple components are operationalized – perhaps in different ways, and at different times, by different participants. In this chapter I have set out a very simple theoretical model that can be used to explore the process of implementing and operationalizing a complex health care intervention. Using research models like that offered by Normalization Process Theory offers evaluators the opportunity to move beyond description of processes and outcomes, and to *explain* them.

31

ACTION RESEARCH FOR THE IMPLEMENTATION OF COMPLEX INTERVENTIONS

Brendan McCormack

Introduction

Action research (AR) is a systematic approach to the development of new knowledge whilst at the same time bringing about social change. As a research methodology it is unique in having this dual focus and indeed dual purpose. For this reason alone, action research is an important methodology to consider in the context of the implementation of complex interventions. In this chapter, AR will be considered from the perspective of implementation of complex interventions only. The challenge of 'context' will be discussed. An overview of action research in the context of implementing complex interventions will be provided. Key considerations in doing action research and being an action researcher in the context of implementing complex interventions will be explored. An example of action research being used to implement a complex intervention will be provided, as well as an overview of the processes used, the outcomes achieved and the new knowledge generated that is relevant to future implementation efforts.

Learning objectives

- Identify how action research as a methodology can be used for the implementation of complex interventions.
- Understand the methodological principles underpinning action research.
- Present a practical example of action research used in the implementation of a complex intervention.

Context and complex interventions

Methodologies used in the implementation of complex interventions need to be able to handle the dimensions of complexity that exist in every practice settings where the implementation occurs. Much of this complexity arises due to the context within which evidence is to be implemented, and Bate (2014: 3) suggests that 'nothing exists, and therefore can be understood, in isolation from its context'. This is particularly important from the perspective of implementing a complex intervention, as the evidence increasingly identifies (cf. Jacobs *et al.*, 2014; May, 2013; McCormack *et al.*, 2013) that despite the quality of the evidence being implemented, it is the context in which it is being implemented that will determine how the evidence is used (or not).

McCormack *et al.* (2002) highlighted the variability of contexts in which health care takes place and the breadth of factors that subsequently influence practice settings. The context of health care can be seen, on one level, as infinite as it takes place in a variety of settings, communities and cultures that are all influenced by a variety of socio-cultural, political, economic and historical (for example) factors. In a recent overview of perspectives on context, Robert and Fulop (2014) suggest that before beginning any implementation effort there is a need to take important contextual factors into account, that part of the implementation process should include trying to make the context more receptive and that understanding these (local) contextual factors should be used to tailor implementation programmes. In their concept analysis of context, McCormack *et al.* (2002: 96) used the term to refer to the environment or setting in which people receive health care services, or in the context of implementing complex interventions, 'the environment or setting in which the proposed change is to be implemented'. With this explicit focus on the significance of practice context, the 'Promoting Action on Research Implementation in Health Services' (PARIHS) framework (Kitson *et al.*, 1998, 2008; Rycroft-Malone *et al.*, 2004) was one of the first to pay particular attention to the ways in which context affected the uptake of evidence in practice. The PARIHS framework proposes that successful implementation occurs when the evidence to be implemented is strong, when the context is receptive to change and when the evidence to be implemented is actively facilitated, i.e. contextual strengths and weaknesses are addressed through the implementation process. Rycroft-Malone *et al.* (2004) argue that in order to effectively balance the relationship between evidence, context and facilitation in implementation efforts, participatory methods are needed that focus on the co-production of implementation strategies.

Action research and complex interventions

Action research responds to the challenges of context when implementing complex interventions, by:

- Systematically determining the action that needs to be taken based on an assessment of the context within which the action is to be operationalized.
- Reflexively engaging with stakeholders to ensure that all dimensions of the context are considered.

- Collaboratively engaging stakeholders in the design of the implementation strategies, thus maximizing the credibility of the intervention and the potential of implementation success.
- Providing a comprehensive 'map' of all the potential strategies for implementing the intervention and ensuring that the chosen implementation strategies 'fit' the context within which they are to be used.
- Mediating the different behaviours of stakeholders by building in strategies for working with these behaviours in advance of implementation commencing.
- Reflexively engaging with stakeholders during each stage of implementation to minimize the impact of potential barriers to success.
- Adopting a collaborative, inclusive and participatory approach to evaluation that links outcomes with processes used and that minimizes the impact of stakeholder bias.

The origins of AR extend back to the 1940s when Kurt Lewin, a German social psychologist, developed group participatory processes for addressing problems in organizations. Lewin discovered that social change was more effective when team members collaborated on reaching solutions to problems of effectiveness in organizations (Lewin, 1946). Lewin coined the phrase 'action research' to capture the cycles of problem identification, planning for action, taking action, reflection on action, learning from action and re-planning for action, etc.

He observed that meaningful change arose from group collective action that was systematically planned through multiple cycles of problem identification, planning, action, reflection and learning (Figure 31.1). Thus Lewin defined action research as 'a comparative research on the conditions and effects of various forms of social action and research leading to social action'. By comparative research, Lewin was referring to the reflexive nature of the processes involved and the need to compare the outcomes for action to the social context in which they are located. However, whilst Lewin's approach was innovative and respectful of the contribution that all persons make to the changing of social conditions (be it work or society in general), his approach was largely considered to be a 'technical' approach where the researcher/change agent is the initiator of the idea/innovation for the action research and persuades others to try it out for themselves. They decide on the research questions and gather and analyse the data and feed them back to the 'subjects' and the organization to take forward the action. Since Lewin's work, there have been many developments in advancing the theory and practice of action research. These are summarized in Table 31.1 and are applied to the practice of complex intervention implementations.

Whilst each of these modes of action research provides contrasting perspectives on how action research can be used in the implementation of complex interventions, there are a number of principles that are common to all approaches to action research:

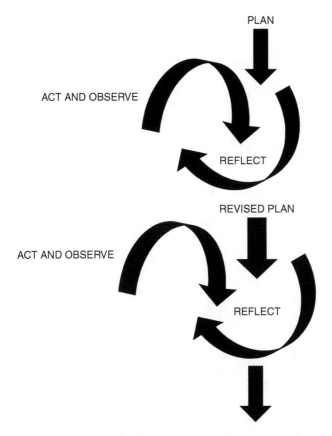

PLAN

ACT AND OBSERVE

REFLECT

REVISED PLAN

ACT AND OBSERVE

REFLECT

FIGURE 31.1 Graphical representation of action research cycles (Adapted from Kemmis and McTaggart, 2005)

- Collaboration of all key stakeholders is critical to success (where a key stakeholder is any person, group or organization that has an interest in the research).
- Developing shared understanding among all participants enables meaningful action to be implemented.
- Change is facilitated when the creativity of stakeholders is maximized in the implementation process.
- Change is realized by the adoption of a systematic approach to problem identification, planning for action, taking action, reflection on action, learning from action and re-planning for action.
- The potential for sustainability is realized when practitioners are helped to research their own practice.
- Evaluation of process and outcome is an integrated part of the methodology adopted and is a continuous process.

TABLE 31.1 Modes of action research

Types of action research	Focus in complex intervention implementation
Practical action research – The word 'practical' is derived from Habermas' (1981) theory of knowledge, where practical knowledge is about interpreting the nature of reality. An example of practical action research is that of Reason and Rowan (1981).	If you are working in the practical mode when implementing a complex intervention, although you as the researcher might be working in a traditional researcher–researched relationship with project participants, you would be trying to help these participants to become co-researchers with you, with the intention of developing a shared understanding about practice and what needs to be changed. For example, in the implementation of postoperative pain management guidelines, even though the guideline being implemented is based on the best available evidence, that is not taken for granted. A key stage in the implementation process using practical action research would be an interpretative stage with a focus on gaining a shared understanding of 'best practice' from the perspectives of all key stakeholders. So whilst the empirical evidence suggests what needs to be implemented, this interpretative stage helps practitioners to make sense of this evidence from their perspectives.
Emancipatory action research – Informed by Critical Theory (Fay, 1987; Freire, 1987; Habermas, 1981) with its focus on democratizing, enabling empowerment, emancipation and power with, rather than power over, for the purpose of overcoming obstacles to change. Examples of emancipatory action research include Elliott (2011), Kemmis *et al.* (2014) and Somekh (2005).	In the implementation of a complex intervention, if you are working in the emancipatory mode, you would be in similar roles to the practical mode but the intent is very different, i.e. as well as seeking new understanding of practice and innovation, you are also concerned with creating the conditions for empowerment, emancipation, social justice and transformation of self, others, cultures, workplaces and organizations. For example, in the implementation of postoperative pain management guidelines, developing a shared understanding of the evidence to be implemented (as in practical action research) is a first stage. The second stage would be that of identifying the most appropriate methods for implementation. Key to this stage is understanding practice context. Through understanding the context within which the evidence is to be implemented, processes are designed to enable, (i) the practice context to be changed; and (ii) the participants to become empowered to make changes and sustain the change long-term. The focus is on changing the culture of the practice setting within which the practice of (for example) pain management occurs.

Transformational action research – also informed by Critical Theory, transformational action research promotes action through creative imagination and artistic expression, and derived from an eclectic understanding of knowledge – whilst empirical knowledge is important, transformational action research aims to access embodied and artistic knowledge, as well as emotional and spiritual intelligence. These varying forms of knowledge and intelligence are seen as critical to enable 'human flourishing', which is the ultimate purpose of transformational action research. Examples of transformational action research include McCormack and Titchen (2006) and Titchen and Armstrong (2007).

If you are working in the transformational mode when implementing a complex intervention, then you are concerned with the intent of emancipatory action research but you operationalize it through critical and creative strategies. Being critical (through reflection) and creative (encouraging and adopting alternative views, stances and ways of being) enables individuals, groups and organizations to be transformed. For example, in the implementation of postoperative pain management guidelines, the implementation process would not start with identifying 'the best evidence', but instead processes (such as action learning) would be put in place to help staff reflect on their existing practices, to explore their own embodied knowledge about pain management derived from their practice experience and to draw on image and metaphor to shape new ways of thinking and being. This creative engagement would then be linked with the empirical evidence (best practice guidelines, for example) in order to develop a shared understanding of how practice needs to change and how to change it.

Action research has many advantages for implementing complex interventions because of its focus on collaboration, inclusion and participation – thus having the potential for enduring impact and sustainability of implementation programmes. However, like all research and development, action research has some limitations. These include challenges in ensuring objectivity in outcome evaluation as the nature of the methodology directs towards multiple perspectives on outcome definition, delineation and evaluation. The use of standardized measurement tools in an implementation programme can help with overcoming this limitation. Managing ethical processes is a second limitation and challenge in action research. Whilst no research can completely predict ethical challenges in a research study, because of the participatory nature of action research, predetermining ethical challenges is more complex. Therefore researchers need to ensure that an ethical framework is in place for managing the decision-making and relational processes in a project. Finally, a significant limitation can be the handling of a large quantity of data. In action research projects there is a tendency to view 'everything as data'. This can be overwhelming in implementation work and so researchers need to be judicious about what data to collect and what processes and outcomes these will inform.

Developing an implementation strategy: improving pain management with older people

Background

This study drew upon an 'Emancipatory Action Research' approach that aimed to explore and address the factors in the practice context that inhibited effective pain management practices with older people (Brown and McCormack, 2011). Adequate pain management can be seen as complex health care interventions, as standards and protocols on pain management include series of interlinked interventions and several decision points for health care staff. Despite extensive advances in the availability of evidence-informed standards and protocols for postoperative pain management, evidence continues to indicate that frequently the management of acute and chronic pain is inadequate (Doctor Foster, 2004; Donnell et al., 2003). Inadequate relief of acute pain increases the incidence and severity of postoperative complications and adverse outcomes, consequently increasing the cost of health care (Donnell et al., 2003; Kehlet and Dahl, 2003). Older people offer distinct challenges, because pain not only lowers the individual's quality of life but also predisposes them to a number of medical conditions, including depression, sleep disturbances, anxiety and occasionally aggressive behaviour, as well as increasing their vulnerability and eroding individual autonomy (AGS, 2002; Feldt et al., 1998).

Context

The study was undertaken over a two-year period, in an abdominal surgical unit that consisted of two wards. Engagement of the lead nurse, ward sister/charge nurse

(2) and deputy ward managers (2) on each ward was essential to the success of the project. These leaders, along with 85 per cent of nursing staff (n = 48), agreed to participate: 11 senior registered nurses, 32 junior registered nurses and 5 health care support workers.

Designing the strategies for implementation

The design of the implementation strategy was informed by the PARIHS framework (Kitson *et al.*, 1998) which argues that three key elements – evidence, context and facilitation – should be considered when implementing evidence into practice. Using PARIHS as a theoretical framework, a 12-month ethnographic study was conducted to explore the practice context of the abdominal surgical unit and gain an understanding of the factors that hindered effective pain management with older people (Brown and McCormack, 2006). The findings from this research showed:

- limited/absent pain assessment;
- inflexible analgesic prescriptions;
- limited use of non-pharmacological strategies;
- dominance of family and physician opinion on use of analgesics rather than protocols;
- fear of addiction;
- patients not being believed;
- patients having decisions made 'for' rather than 'with' them. (Brown and McCormack, 2006)

Using these findings, reflective groups were set up with all staff. Over a period of three months, clinical staff participated in reflective groups (six reflective sessions were held and each lasted one and a half hours) and discussed the findings from the ethnographic study. The researchers and participating staff co-constructed three 'action cycles' that were representative of the ethnographic data and that had the potential to improve pain management practices:

- Action cycle one: Pain assessment and practice.
- Action cycle two: Organization of care.
- Action cycle three: Knowledge and insight to deal with problematic pain.

Delivery of the implementation intervention

Adopting the principles of cooperative inquiry (Reason and Bradbury-Huang, 2013), all consenting nursing staff had the opportunity over a two-year period to work in: structured facilitated reflective sessions (n = 18); ad hoc-facilitated reflective sessions (n = 26); and consolidation workshops (n = 3), to explore their experiences and reflect together. The lead nurse and ward sister/charge nurse also had one-to-one reflective coaching (n = 27) with the facilitator. All group work was negotiated in line with the nursing roster, resulting in any member of the nursing team who was on duty and had consented being able to participate. To assist individuals/teams to work with the fluidity of the project, to understand the process and set the scene for all group work, ground rules and a facilitation framework were formulated, verified and adhered to throughout the project.

Data collection and analysis

The lead researcher maintained field notes of each reflective session and workshops. A reflexive approach was adopted, whereby the lead researcher used the field notes to engage in reflective dialogue with participants to ensure shared interpretations of the need for change and develop agreed actions. Data obtained throughout the lifetime of the project were constantly reflected upon, fed back to participants and examined to identify possible themes arising. Additionally, findings were fed back to the wider team through discussions, workshops and interim reports. In addition, data were collected to specifically inform the evaluation of outcomes arising from the implementation processes used, including:

1   Two episodes of non-participant observation of nursing practice (46 hours in total) midway and at the end of the project.
2   Pre- and postoperative semi-structured interviews with six older patients.
3   Completion of the revised Nursing Work Index (NWI-R) Questionnaire (McCormack et al., 2009b) by 83 per cent of registered nursing staff to provide further insight into the culture and nurse decision-making in the unit.
4   Focus groups with participating nursing staff. The data were used to provide a focus for discussion on the issues raised; and to examine nursing staff's values and beliefs and promote problem solving.

Practice changes

Through these action cycles a number of changes to the context of practice were achieved, including:

- A pain management algorithm was designed and implemented by the nursing staff and embedded into everyday practice. This was used to guide pain assessment and management practices.
- A reflective approach to engagement between nursing and the multidisciplinary team (MDT) was implemented through the use of action learning and reflective strategies. Communication between nursing staff, patients and the multidisciplinary team was seen to improve and tools such as the pain management algorithm also helped with this.
- The leadership skills of lead nurses improved over the project period through the one-to-one coaching sessions they engaged in with the researchers.

- Interruptions to nurses during activities such as pain assessment and medication administration were reduced by reorganizing the way in which nursing teams worked and by introducing a 'care coordinator' who had an overview of all activities on the unit.

Box 31.1 provides an overview of how changes such as these were achieved.

BOX 31.1 OVERVIEW OF CHANGES IN PAIN MANAGEMENT WITH OLDER PEOPLE

Following a reflective session, one ward manager led on an action initiative to introduce an early morning medicine round. The nursing team reasoned that this change in practice would permit patients to receive analgesia prior to 'getting up and about' and allow nurses more freedom to attend the medical ward rounds to enhance MDT communication and reduce interruptions to patient care. Some nursing staff expressed concerns about giving analgesia to patients who were fasting prior to surgery, while others were reluctant to change from traditional practices. In response to these concerns, further reflection led to the nursing team completing an audit of medication adverse effects and the efficacy of the change being instigated. The results showed no increase in adverse effects and 92 per cent of nursing staff considered that MDT communication had improved. Consequently, this change was permanently adopted. One nurse commented: 'The change to working patterns in the morning has had a positive effect as it permits us to spend more time with patients; because older people have analgesia on board, they can now do more for themselves'.

This change in the morning routine signified a major shift in the culture and mindset of the nursing staff working within the ward. The success with which they carried out this change encouraged nursing staff to engage with enthusiasm in the reflective process, enhanced nurse morale and encouraged them to be innovative. Additionally, reflection assisted nursing staff to draw upon empirical evidence and their experience to develop a pain assessment algorithm (Brown and McCormack, 2011: 17).

New knowledge generated

As well as guiding a systematic collaborative approach to the implementation of complex interventions, the adoption of action research as a methodology for implementation efforts enables the generation of new knowledge that contributes to the transferability of 'the specific [practice change] to the general [key considerations for future action]'.

Reflective critical engagement with the findings revealed that context is a dynamic, complex and somewhat anarchic phenomenon, with many issues blending together to create a complex collection of factors that enable or inhibit effective nursing practice. 'Ward culture' impacted not only on pain management practices, but also influenced all aspects of ward life and patient care. Three key themes (psychological safety, leadership, oppression) and four sub-themes (power, horizontal violence, distorted perceptions, autonomy) were found to influence the way in which not only pain management with older people, but all nursing practice could be effective or not. Within the theme of 'context', effective leadership and the creation of a psychologically safe environment were key elements in the enhancement of all aspects of nursing practice. Therefore, it is probable that the theme of pain management practices with older people could be substituted with other areas of speciality nursing practice (for example, tissue viability) to achieve enhanced patient outcomes. It would be imperative therefore that in future implementation efforts these dominant themes of psychological safety, leadership and oppression are considered in implementation plans.

Conclusions

Contemporary health care policy and strategy emphasizes the need for care systems to be responsive to individual patient needs and to be adaptive in the way that care is delivered. Nursing work exists in a context where there is a constant tussle between conflicting priorities and where everyday practice is challenging, often stressful, sometimes chaotic and largely unpredictable. Interventions to improve practices are implemented in these contexts and so it is imperative that the implementation processes used are adaptive to, respectful of and concerned for the dynamic relationships that exist. Action research provides a systematic and theory informed approach to doing this and ensures that determined outcomes are context-specific. Key steps in the process include:

- A systematic analysis of the context using mixed-methods prior to designing the implementation process.
- Stakeholder analysis (through questionnaires, interviews or focus groups) to ensure that key issues in the context are considered.
- Planning strategies for implementation intervention that are collaborative and inclusive of all stakeholders who need to be involved in the implementation and ensuring that these processes are collaborative.
- Agreeing the implementation steps and stages with all key stakeholders and building in (reflective) strategies for dealing with the different behaviours of stakeholders in advance of implementation commencing.
- Adopting an approach to facilitation that is consistent with the context and the evidence to be implemented and that as far as possible is guided by theory (e.g. the PARIHS framework).
- Using systematic data collection to evaluate the effectiveness of the implementation intervention strategies used and minimize the impact of potential barriers to success.

- Designing an evaluation method that links outcomes with processes used and that minimizes the impact of stakeholder bias.

Further reading

McCormack, B., Manley, K. and Titchen, A. (eds). 2014. *Practice Development in Nursing and Healthcare*. Oxford: Wiley-Blackwell.

Reason, P. and Bradbury-Huang, H. 2013. *The Sage Handbook of Action Research: Participative Inquiry and Practice*, 2nd edn. London: Sage.

Somekh, B. 2005. *Action Research: A Methodology for Change and Development*. Maidenhead: Open University Press/McGraw-Hill Education.

32

SYSTEMS MODELLING FOR IMPROVING HEALTH CARE

Martin Pitt, Thomas Monks and Michael Allen

Introduction

Systems modelling studies in the health services date back to 1965 (Fetter and Thompson, 1965); however the vast majority of research and development in this field has occurred in the last 20–30 years. This has been driven largely by the increasing pressure to ensure efficient and effective use of resources within health services against a background of rising demands and limited budgets, coupled with the increasing availability and accessibility of computer technology which has enabled its rapid evolution. There is hence a growing interest in the use of techniques such as modelling and simulation to identify potential service improvements and provide an evidence base for proposed changes in delivery.

Systems modelling (also referred to as operational research – OR) encompasses a wide range of techniques. A distinction is commonly drawn between so-called 'hard' methods characterized by mathematical approaches, clear metrics and quantitative outputs, and 'soft' methods which typically incorporate qualitative aspects and extensive interaction with stakeholders. An example of a soft approach is the Problem Structuring Methods (PSM) which aims through dialogue to develop a structured characterization of an area of concern. Importantly, different tools are appropriate for distinct contexts and differing levels of analysis (e.g. strategic, operational and tactical). Different methods can often complement one another and be used in combination. In this chapter we aim to introduce some of the key concepts in health care systems modelling and offer a flavour of how these both can be, and have been, applied to improve health care delivery, focusing specifically on the use of systems modelling in the implementation of complex interventions.

Learning objectives

- To understand the wide range of systems modelling techniques applicable to health care.
- To appreciate how distinct approaches can be applied to different health care issues to support decision-making.
- To understand the contribution that systems modelling can make to the implementation of complex interventions in health care.
- To recognize both the potentials and limitations of health care modelling techniques and the barriers and facilitators key to their successful application.

An overview of modelling

There have been several attempts to classify systems modelling methods as deployed within health care (Jun and Clarkson, 2008; Brailsford *et al.*, 2009). Table 32.1 outlines a range of the most commonly used methods giving typical areas of application in health care and some core references. In addition, it should be noted that there are a series of integrated improvement frameworks (incorporating modelling) which have been applied in health care and such as Lean Thinking, the Theory of Constraints, and Six Sigma (Young *et al.*, 2004), a discussion of which goes beyond the scope of this chapter but many of which are described by Sermeus in Chapter 12.

Table 32.1 illustrates the broad basis of systems modelling *research* across a range of modern health care settings. Evidence for the effective application of these methods, however, is less clear and, in contrast to other industries, take-up of systems modelling in health care *practice* is probably best described as patchy (Brailsford *et al.*, 2009). Moreover, evaluation of the effectiveness of such interventions is currently very weak (Virtue *et al.*, 2013). There is much still to be done, therefore, to establish an extensive evidence base for the effective use of systems modelling in health care. The reasons for these shortcomings, which are many and complex, are discussed below.

Despite these limitations, however, an increasing number of publications in recent decades (Brailsford *et al.*, 2009; Katsaliaki and Mustafee, 2011) demonstrate that systems modelling methods can, and have been, successful applied across a wide range of health care areas. Frequently the contribution of modelling may be to help define a problem, provide focus or provide a map/conceptual framework to facilitate understanding and dialogue amongst stakeholders. Soft OR methods such as PSM, for example, are commonly used in this context. In other instances, quantitative output metrics from models allow users to assess the relative benefits and costs for a range of service design options. Discrete event simulation, for instance, is often used to model alternative service design options and provide 'what if' analyses to show the likely impact of any planned changes.

It should be stressed here that in order to achieve effective change in an organization, these methods (modelling, simulation, etc.) are often applied in tandem with other disciplines such as health economics, statistics, management science, etc.

TABLE 32.1 List of methods used in systems modelling

Problem-structuring methods and conceptual modelling

Example technique	Summary description	Typical areas of application in health	References
Soft Systems Methodology (SSM)	A process to construct descriptive models of human activity systems in order to improve a team's understanding of the aims of a system and to ask questions of it.	• Performance improvement • Outpatient service modelling • Determining study objectives	Checkland and Poulter (2006), Rosenhead (1996), Rosenhead and Mingers (2001)
Strategic Options & Decision Analysis (SODA)	A process involving cognitive mapping and workshops to facilitate teams reaching a consensus and committing to strategic action.	• Health care/tele-health systems design	Rosenhead and Mingers (2001)
Strategic Choice Approach	A process to help teams compare strategic options, deal with uncertainty and commit to actions.	• Strategic employment relations	Rosenhead and Mingers (2001)

Mathematical approaches and optimization

Example technique	Summary description	Typical areas of application in health	References
Mathematical Programming	Problems are formulated as equations in order to maximize or minimize a function by systematically choosing input values from a constrained set.	• Resource allocation • Measuring performance/efficiency	Denton et al. (2007)
Data Envelopment Analysis	A technique to measure the relative efficiency of different decision-making units (e.g. hospitals) subject to a common set of inputs.	• Measuring performance/efficiency • Assessing quality and patient satisfaction	Charnes et al. (1978)

Meta-heuristics	Computational approaches to provide nearly optimal solutions to intractable mathematical programming problems.	• Scheduling • Staffing	Gupta and Denton (2008)
Vehicle Routing	Techniques to minimize vehicle travel distance and time to a discrete number of locations.	• Dispatch and routing of emergency vehicles	Ingolfsson et al. (2008)
Queuing Theory	Equations to estimate waiting time, space requirements and throughput in queuing systems.	• Waiting time/utilization analysis • System/pathway design • Appointment systems	Ernst et al. (2004), Gupta and Denton (2008),
Scheduling	Techniques to optimize schedules, e.g. clinical operations in order to minimize waiting times or maximize throughput.	• Theatre list management • Outpatient appointments	Gupta and Denton (2008)
Location Analysis/Facility Location	Decision support for geographic location and number of facilities needed to minimize customer travel distance or maximize use of a facility.	• Ambulance location analysis • Hospital/clinic placement	Daskin (2008), Smith et al. (2009)

(cont.)

TABLE 32.1 (cont.)

Simulation

Example technique	Summary description	Typical areas of application in health	References
Discrete Event Simulation	A stochastic discrete time step simulation for modelling the dynamics of complex queuing systems.	• Redesign of clinical pathways • Visualizing existing pathways • Waiting list and scheduling issues • Modelling impact on bed usage	Law (2006), Gunal and Pidd (2010)
System Dynamics	Deterministic continuous time simulation focused on feedback and delay in macro-level systems	• Predicting impact of local system changes on wider health & social care systems • Identifying areas for policy focus • High-level systems thinking	Dangerfield (1999), Sterman (2000)
Agent–Based Simulation	Study of emergent dynamics of a whole system by simulating the interactions of individual autonomous agents (e.g. patients).	• Modelling disease spread • Modelling uptake of interventions/ technology	Axelrod (1997)
Monte Carlo Simulation	A broad range of computational techniques to estimate the unknown distribution of a quantity of interest	• Disease screening modelling • Demand estimation • Disease transmission • Disease screening modelling	Berg (2004)

Furthermore, the successful application of systems models in health care generally requires the engagement and collaboration of relevant health service staff to be successful (Harper and Pitt, 2004). Typically, for instance, skills in change management, as well as resource and team planning need to be integrated with effective modelling to bring about sustained and meaningful improvements in service delivery. See Sermeus, Chapter 12 for details.

Case study examples

Perhaps the most direct way to understand the contribution modelling can make to improving health care delivery is to review some relevant examples of application. The three case studies below outline the potential for different approaches to addressing diverse aspects of health care. A more comprehensive listing of case studies in health care modelling can be viewed on the MASHnet (Modelling and Simulation in Healthcare Network) website (MASHnet, 2014).

OUTLINE CASE STUDY 1:

Redesigning emergency stroke pathways to maximize thrombolysis rates

Discrete event simulation is used to model patient pathways across a range of 'what-if' scenarios. The study hospital needed to improve its rate of thrombolysis for stroke patients, which involved engaging many stakeholders and implementing change across several organisations. Resultant changes demonstrated dramatic improvements in service delivery. (Monks *et al.*, 2012)

Context

Thrombolysis with the clot busting drug *alteplase* is currently the only licensed treatment worldwide for acute ischaemic stroke. The benefit is critically dependent on time from stroke onset to treatment, with an exponential decay in the odds of a favourable outcome from one 90-minute interval to the next up to 4.5 hours. It is therefore crucial to minimize in-hospital treatment delays both to increase the potential for thrombolysis and reduce the time from onset to treatment.

Method

Computer simulation (Figure 32.1) and quantitative analysis were used to evaluate proposed changes prior to any implementation. A key benefit of this model was a visualization of patient pathways, which provided a basis for communication and helped bridge barriers between different departments within hospitals. It allowed clinicians from the emergency department, the acute stroke

---

unit and the regional ambulance trust to work together and identify optimal changes to the stroke pathway ahead of any changes to the real process.

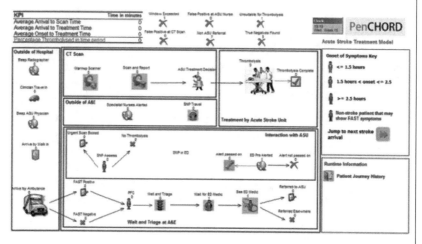

FIGURE 32.1   Screen-shot of computer simulation of the emergency in-hospital stroke pathway

Outputs

The pathway was modelled as it operated at the start of the study. A number of potential changes to the pathway were then evaluated using the model and compared against each other. The quantified benefit in terms of number and speed of treatments was output (Figure 32.2), and published research was used to convert these figures to additional patients with no disability post-stroke.

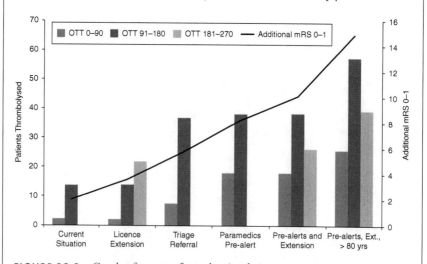

FIGURE 32.2   Graph of outputs from the simulation

Impact

The study recommended two changes that carried little to no cost for the hospital. Both of these were implemented in 2012. Paramedics now ring a dedicated acute stroke phone number to alert clinicians to the imminent arrival of potential stroke patients. This allows emergency resources to be in place as the patient arrives at the emergency department. Modelling also illustrated that for a robust pathway a second change was needed within the emergency department triage system. Triage nurses now share information with the stroke unit to facilitate patient management.

The figures showed that since study commencement, door to treatment times fell from 100 to 50 minutes on average and treatment rates increased from 4 per cent to 16 per cent. In real terms this equates to 100 strokes receiving treatment per year compared with 25 at study commencement (Figure 32.2). Discrete event simulation thus helped to overcome barriers in the implementation of timely treatment.

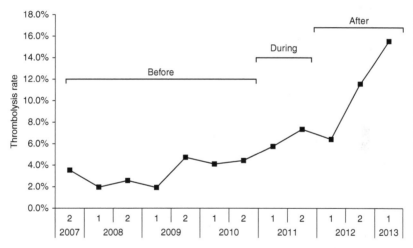

FIGURE 32.3 Thrombolysis rate by half-yearly intervals for period before, during and after intervention

OUTLINE CASE STUDY 2:

Emergency and on-demand care: modelling a large complex system

This illustrates how system dynamics can be used to generate a model of the complex relationships between acute and community care and provide important decision support to policy makers. This proved key to ongoing strategic initiatives. (Brailsford et al., 2004)

Context

The project concerned the pressure on emergency medical services and consequent increasing number of hospital admissions at the local hospital. This was having a detrimental effect on, amongst other things, the waiting times for treatment for those attending, difficulty in managing hospital wards at greater than expected capacity, and frequent cancellations of routine admissions for surgery. The project posed four main research questions: (1) identifying the current configuration of the system; (2) more precisely defining the present level of demand; (3) showing how the system could be developed; and (4) to what extent community preferences were driving use of the hospital emergency department. Before any modelling was undertaken, a conceptual map was drawn up of the system, which was elaborated in a series of interviews with health service staff and patient representatives. The final process map was used as the basis for the system model.

Method

Based on an initial conceptual map, the project created a System Dynamics (SD) model (Figure 32.4) which represented the essential elements of the region's emergency medical services as they existed at the time (2002).This choice centred on the need to model large numbers of patients, the importance of studying feedback effects and the fact that precise estimates of Key Performance Indicators (KPIs) were less important than overall trends.

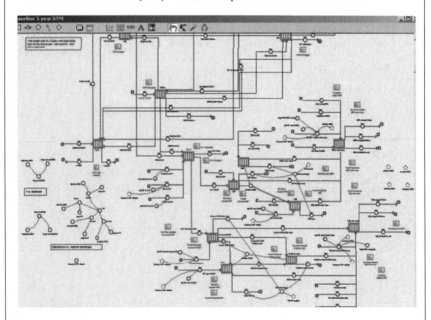

FIGURE 32.4   Part of the systems dynamics model used to look at the NHS Direct component of care

Outputs

Projections from the model suggested that if emergency admissions continued to rise at the rates experienced, average bed occupancy levels would be
unmanageably high within 2–3 years. The most promising intervention was
found to be the diversion of selected elderly patients to specialist investigation
centres.

Impact

The model was used to investigate patient flows and bottlenecks and as a tool
for provoking and facilitating discussion. The policy steering group used the
model to test and evaluate different scenarios of care. However, the primary
use of the model was for promoting greater understanding of the dynamics of
the system rather than in generating numerical outputs.

The essentially generic framework adopted and the model's use of routinely
collected data entails that this approach can readily be adapted elsewhere.

OUTLINE CASE STUDY 3:

Simulation and queuing theory to schedule community mental health assessment

This shows how discrete event simulation based on queuing theory was used
to analyse the impact of queue sharing for mental health appointments across
multiple organizations. Changes were implemented via an initial pilot phase
which showed significant reductions in patient waiting times.

Context

Devon Partnership Trust in the UK planned to implement a centralized 'choose
and book' telephone booking system for mental health assessment. This
would book patients into available diary slots for the appropriate local team.
As this system was new, the Trust requested help in forecasting the number of
appointment slots to schedule into the diary to provide good waiting times
for patients, but without allocating excessive spare capacity in the system. A
simulation-based approach also allowed for the examination of sharing work
between teams, especially to avoid breaching waiting time targets.

Method

A simulation model was developed in which patients arrive at random and in
proportion to the demand for each regional team (Figure 32.5). Patients may

be seen by any team as identified in a 'pooling matrix' – this may be used to limit patients being seen only by their local team or by being seen by neighbouring teams (or a hypothetical model may be tested when any patient may be seen by any team – to understand the maximum beneficial effect of queue sharing). The simulation model contains a virtual diary of appointment slots available for each team; patients are then allocated to these diary slots.

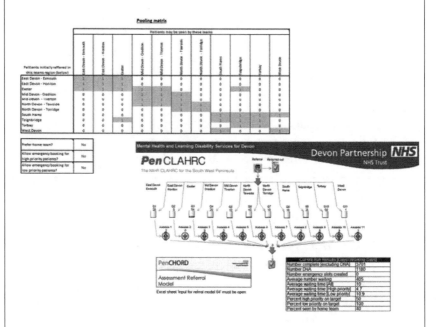

FIGURE 32.5   Screen-shot showing simulation model and pooling matrix used to configure queue-sharing options

Outputs

Scenarios were tested with varying capacity within each team and also with varying strategies of sharing of work. Figure 32.6 shows one example of queue sharing between teams and demonstrates how most of the potential benefits of queue sharing can be obtained with local sharing between neighbouring teams.

Impact

In this example, simulations helped the implementation of a choose-and-book system for community mental health assessment. The choose-and-book system has been implemented with local queue sharing – appointment slots within the target time and within the local area are available to be booked by the patient.

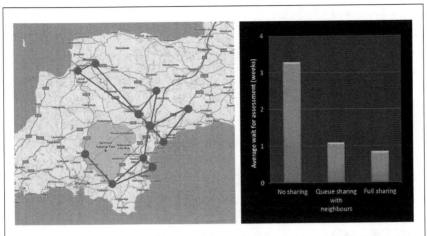

FIGURE 32.6 Sharing configuration chosen by Trust and resultant waiting time reduction predicted by simulation model (also shows effects of full sharing between centres – i.e. any patient can be seen anywhere)

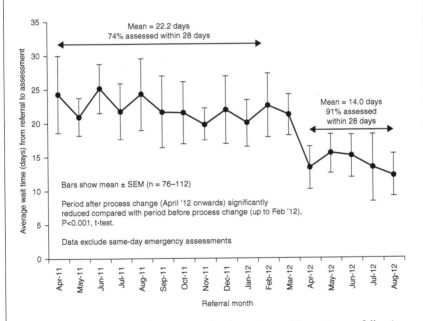

FIGURE 32.7 Graph showing reduction in waiting times following implementation of queue sharing

Figure 32.7 shows a significant reduction in waiting times achieved during the roll-out of the first area (with sharing between two teams as necessary).

Key issues and challenges

Undoubtedly the major limitation to the effective application of systems modelling in health care is the yawning gap between those who research and advocate these methods and health care staff (both managerial and clinical) at the coalface of service delivery. We are still a long way, for instance, from a world in which a health service improvement manager would fire up a computer simulation to analyse hospital operations as readily as a spreadsheet. However, it is worth remembering that only a few decades ago spreadsheets too were outside the comfort zone of most health service managers.

Though potentially valuable in the implementation of complex interventions, many factors influence the current lack of uptake of systems modelling in health. Some of these are cultural. The underlying ethos of most health care is (and should remain) a caring system built around human values. Many health service staff lack the technical background predisposed to the uptake of analytical and mathematical tools to support decision-making. Another key aspect is the complex, diverse and highly interactive dynamics of health service organization. Within this it is often difficult to devise generic and standardized approaches which can be applied across institutions and for different periods of time. It is also very difficult to devise viable methods to evaluate the contribution that modelling can make and hence develop a necessary evidence base for its use. In addition, problems are often experienced in marshalling the necessary data to drive usable models of health care. All these factors are prominent especially in the context of complex interventions.

Notwithstanding these challenges, systems modelling is arguably playing an increasing role in health care. The case studies above, for instance, illustrate some of the headway being made in the field and show how such approaches can contribute to impactful change to complex health care systems. There are also clearly identifiable areas for advancement. These include more concerted efforts to build greater understanding, capacity and capability among health service staff, increasing the user-friendliness of models, and developing better methods for data sharing and collection. In complex areas specifically, we need to integrate and align systems modelling better to other key methods of intervention to ensure that a concerted approach to effective change can be accomplished.

One emerging trend is the development of behavioural operational research in health as a means to encompass the human, social and behavioural factors into models (Brailsford et al., 2012). Another interesting area which is currently receiving attention is the involvement of patients and public in modelling and simulation (Pearson et al., 2013).

Conclusion

Despite the plethora of research papers bearing on systems modelling in health care, the application of these methods for the implementation of complex interventions is at best patchy and much still needs to be achieved. In addition, few studies clearly and systematically evaluate the benefits of adopting such solutions for the implementation of complex interventions and, without this evidence base, scepticism will remain as to their effectiveness. Many of the key challenges in the field have been discussed but, despite the obvious limitations, it seems clear there is enormous potential for systems modelling to contribute to many key areas of health care improvement, particularly in complex interventions. Perhaps the central lesson from our experience to date is that the major barriers and enablers to more extensive adoption of such techniques in health are focused around the human and social aspects of change rather than technical issues.

Further reading

Daskin, M. S. 2010. *Service Science*. Hoboken, NJ: John Wiley.

Ozcan, Y. A. 2009. *Quantitative Methods in Health Care Management: Techniques and Applications*. San Francisco, CA: Jossey-Bass.

Pidd, M. 2009. *Tools for Thinking: Modelling in Management Science, 3rd edn*. Chichester: John Wiley.

Sanderson, C. and Green, R. 2006. *Analytical Models for Decision Making*. Maidenhead and New York: Open University Press/McGraw Hill.

33

A FEW FINAL THOUGHTS

Ingalill Rahm Hallberg and David A. Richards

Introduction

In this concluding chapter, as editors we wanted to indulge ourselves by reflecting on some of the major themes underpinning this book. Our contributors have ranged far and wide through the whole process of developing, testing, evaluating, implementing and reporting complex interventions in health care. One might imagine that in covering such a broad subject matter there is a danger of the book lacking coherence. However, we find this not to be the case. Throughout the book, our contributors return again and again to some crucial messages. In this chapter we hope to summarize what those messages are and add a few of our own.

Methodological plurality

Despite the brevity of the available guidance on complex interventions research methods, even a cursory glance will lead to the obvious conclusion that one cannot investigate most health care interventions without using a mix of methods. Whether it be modelling intervention pathways, assessing feasibility, evaluating a natural experiment, understanding the relationship between intervention processes and outcomes, or undertaking quality improvement strategies to implement effective interventions, it will be necessary to use very different methodologies from different world-views. The extent to which these different methods can be seen as 'mixed' or 'multiple' depends on the context of inquiry.

The chapter by Borglin and that by Moore and colleagues highlight this most clearly. Both of these chapters emphasize how different methods must link together, but each method is chosen because it can best answer specific questions being posed. As in all research, mixed-methods research is driven by carefully articulated questions. The key challenge is in integration. Multiple methods only become mixed methods when different strands of data are explicitly integrated. This can happen at many different stages but currently it appears that most research reports integrate different data streams towards the end of the project, sometimes only in the discussion. Moore and colleagues recommend a much more integrated and explicit approach to process evaluation using mixed methods. The use of process evaluation as an exemplar is a masterstroke, since it has the potential not only to move the field forward methodologically, but also addresses a key 'intervention unpacking' aim of complex interventions research – the critical look into the black box of our evaluations. What works, for whom and when are just some of the questions a mixed-methods study can address.

This is not to say that single-research methods are no longer appropriate. We reiterate that all research must be driven by carefully written and specific questions. At certain times in the process of developing an intervention some very focused work will need to be done and suitable single methods chosen accordingly. It is during the feasibility and evaluation stages that *integrated* mixed methods really come into their own.

Further methodological development

We believe that methodological developments in mixed methods will gather pace over the next few years, helping to guide researchers in undertaking sophisticated evaluations of ever more complex interventions. However, methodological development is unlikely to be confined to mixed-methods approaches alone. Research methodology is developing all the time, along with an improved understanding of complexity and a change of attitudes and values. The MRC guidance (2008) was just such an example of this development.

We have included many examples of new methodological developments in this book. For example, systematic reviews of various kinds are presented in Section 1. The development of different kinds of systematic reviews, in particular mixed-methods reviews, is a recent development that helps us to open up the existing repository of research before embarking on the next step. However, other areas still need to be moved forward. There are still important questions to be asked so that we can translate the current knowledge base derived from systematic reviews into interventions to provide better outcomes. As well as clinical observations, systematic reviews need to address complex interventions in depth, understand the problem under study from the consumers' perspective, and untangle the context and the process in which the intervention is supposed to be applied. Indeed, Köpke and Meyer introduce this in their chapter, but at the same time indicate just how much thought and development still needs to occur before these challenges are adequately addressed

At this point, knowledge still needs to be translated into a model for the intervention to be tested. The chapter by Sermeus in Section 1 addresses this challenge and he correctly points out that successful research is not only about the intervention. Undertaking research in a productive manner is also about the context and the process of implementing the intervention to be tested. We clearly need even more knowledge concerning the task of translating review evidence into an intervention study. In particular we need publications critically describing this process and thereby serving as role models and providing new knowledge about developing the intervention to be tested.

Another area where more knowledge and shared experiences are needed is in the further development of 'traditional' designs such as those described in Section 3. A further challenge is in integrating them with process evaluations assessing fidelity or helping to understand the mechanisms promoting, hindering or explaining outcomes. Despite the exciting new work of Moore and colleagues (Moore et al., 2014), we still lack good examples of how this integration can be done. In particular we need methodological publications addressing the challenges that occur when integrating traditional research designs with new methods to understand the intervention black box. In particular we need more critical descriptions of studies in terms of how internal reliability and validity, and subsequently external validity, may have been threatened or kept under control, the presence of confounders, spill-over or other aspects that may bias the results and how these risks have been addressed by researchers publishing their results.

Unfortunately sometimes researchers like to think that there is only one way forward. In this book we have tried to point out the diversity of approaches already available but we have also tried to indicate that 'everything under the sun is not yet discovered'. Method developments are ongoing and should progress further. For example, despite impressions to the contrary, the manner in which we should undertake a traditional randomized controlled study is still not cast in stone. If we make the mistake of discarding the RCT as a suitable design because on the face of it it appears to be an inappropriate approach, we will miss the opportunity to develop the RCT to be more suitable for complex situations under study. Methods selection is simply a matter of determining and applying the design and methods best suited to provide a sound and trustworthy response to the main question, not a matter of choosing the method with which we ourselves are more comfortable.

The diversity of research programmes

There are many ways to build a research programme and we have previously made it clear that researching complex interventions will often require an integrated series of studies under an overarching programmatic framework. However, the principal aim of every research programme may not necessarily be that of intervening successfully to obtain a better outcome compared to that which would occur should we let nature run its course.

There is also the possibility that we could develop a programme on a specific method, design or analytical problem rather than solving or alleviating a specific health care issue. This book details some very good examples of research methods development and these are needed to improve the conduct of research itself. In the short term they may not contribute to knowledge that is fit for implementation into clinical practice, but in the long term methodological research programmes will most certainly contribute to the improvement of research quality and thus also contribute ultimately to a more solid knowledge foundation for practice.

Clearly, such work could be a research programme in its own right or, alternatively, be embedded in a clinical research programme that generates data to help solve methodological conundrums. All this needs expertise and experts. As pointed out by some of the authors of this book, setting up a complex intervention research programme requires collaboration across scientific and clinical disciplines and needs a variety of experts. The competences needed change from time to time depending on the questions in focus. This in turn requires an open mind in relation to other disciplines and scientific approaches. It also requires an open mind in relation to designs, methods, procedures or the like.

Another choice to be made is where one might contribute in a programme of research in order to produce knowledge for practice. As highlighted in Chapter 2, not all research contributes knowledge that is ready to be implemented in health care, and research undertaken within a research programme may not result in knowledge immediately ready for implementation. We must recognize that in order to progress, we as researchers may have to deviate at times from the main route of obtaining knowledge for practice. This deviation may be driven by a problem, process or context that needs to be more fully understood before a theoretical framework for intervention can be developed and tested. It could be that the hypotheses on how we might achieve improved benefit for the patient, family or society are still not solid enough to be tested. These digressions do not mean that as researchers we should lose sight of what we would like to obtain when we come to the end of the journey, but they might certainly be necessary divergences. Working in a research programme allows for these side trips, in fact they are expected. This back-and-forth process is explicitly referenced in the MRC guidance for developing and evaluating complex intervention (Medical Research Council, 2008) and we most certainly endorse the authors' view.

Patient and public involvement

At the beginning of our book, we devoted a chapter to the theory and practice of involving patients and the public in research. We want to reiterate here the importance of this concept. Health care, and health care research, is just too important an activity to be left in the hands of professionals and clinicians. It is all of our business. We use the term 'all' advisedly, since each of us is a member of the public and every one of us will at some time in our lives be a patient. As patients, most of us expect to be full participants in our own interactions with health care professionals, and we should demand no less of ourselves as researchers. There is no part of a research programme that cannot benefit from patient and public involvement (PPI). Topic selection, project management, questionnaire development, data collection and project dissemination can all be vastly improved through PPI.

When involving patients and the public in research, we urge researchers to carefully consider the ability of people to influence decision-making and the value placed on different forms of social capital such as knowledge (for example, how medical knowledge is often given greater status than lay experiences of illness in decision-making). We should be open to the fact that patients and family members may introduce surprises, in the sense that they may not experience a situation in the same way that we (as outsiders) do. They may not agree with professionals on what is best for them.

This situation calls for caution when we as researchers want to implement normative theories and models in practice, believing that this is best for patients and their families. Our views may not coincide with what the patients or families think is in their best interests. Normative theory stipulates what is right or wrong, desirable or not wanted in society or in the case of health care, how to view and behave in relation to patients and families. This theory outlines what should be the ideal situation and not what actually exists. There is, in particular in nursing science, an endeavour to develop such normative theories. However, these theories need to be questioned empirically in order not to take assumptions for granted as being suitable for every patient or family.

Thinking critically in this way will allow researchers to provide the best possible environment for people to be truly, and not tokenistically, involved in research. We encourage researchers to be guided by modern theories of participation, empowerment and engagement such as those referred to in Chapter 4.

Ethical considerations

Ethical considerations have been only briefly addressed in this book and that may seem a shortcoming. The main reason we have not engaged with ethical agendas in depth is the great variation in Europe and elsewhere in the world of laws, regulations, processes and organizations that provide permission to carry out research. This may seem surprising taking into account the Declaration of Helsinki (http://www.wma.net/en/30publications/10policies/b3/) that most countries in the world have agreed to follow. The declaration is a statement of ethical principles for medical research involving human subjects and human material and data. It was developed to protect the individual from harm and is regularly updated, the latest update being in 2013. Some, but not all, countries have expanded their laws on research ethics to include not only medical research but also all research involving human beings irrespective of academic discipline.

The declaration covers general principles for research including risks, burdens and benefits, vulnerable groups and individuals such as children and people unable to voice their opinion. It encompasses scientific requirements and research protocols, which may be even more important in interventions of the kind addressed in this book, given that adaptations or deviations from what is traditionally expected often occur. The declaration also includes material on how to determine that a new intervention is better than that already in place, the use of the placebo and how to proceed if there is no proven intervention in place. It also covers post-trial provisions.

The element of the declaration most often considered when discussing research ethics is that concerning privacy and confidentiality. A major challenge in much research is obtaining informed consent. This is commonly given by participants in a written format, preceded by printed information about items such as the research aims, methods, the expected behaviours of the research participant, and potential risks and benefits. It is by no means permissible to put any pressure on the individual to consent. Whilst extremely laudable in principle, individuals being asked to consent may have significant difficulties in understanding all the information provided. Sometimes the participant information and consent forms consist of several pages including complex information. In these situations one might actually question whether the person has truly provided informed consent. Simplification of information giving, whilst not compromising informed consent, is one important element of future attempts to increase recruitment into clinical research.

In order to make sure that research methods chosen and implemented are both ethically sound and not altered during the course of a study, the declaration includes statements about registering the research protocol in publicly accessible databases prior to starting the study. It also includes strictures on the responsibilities of researchers to follow reporting guidance when publishing findings. In particular, the obligation to present all our results, irrespective of the outcome, is emphasized in the declaration, a subject that brings us neatly to our next section on research reporting.

Research reporting

We now turn to the important issue of research reporting, and a companion concern – reducing 'research waste'. Although there are other reasons why resources being put into research efforts might be wasted, for example by asking the wrong questions, inadequate research design, over-fussy research regulation requirements, or inattention to existing research evidence, producing an intervention that is inadequately described and that no one can replicate with any degree of fidelity is a major contributor to wasteful research. It retards the implementation of evidence, delays improvement in routine practice and leads to weaker interventions being implemented in clinical environments.

The two most comprehensive attempts to address this are the CReDECI (Möhler et al., 2012) and TIDieR (Hoffmann et al., 2014) guidelines. The CReDECI guideline suggests criteria by which researchers can fully report the phases they have undergone in the development, feasibility and piloting, and evaluation of complex interventions. If researchers were to adopt the suggested CReDECI criteria, readers of research would be able to critically appraise the process by which a complex intervention has arrived at its evidence-based destination. We might all be able to determine not only the rigour of the methods, but also the thought and effort given to identifying theory, previous evidence, and addressing clinical, procedural and methodological uncertainties during that journey. CReDECI sets out to address many of the issues and reservations in the MRC guidance (2008) about poor and premature evaluations of complex interventions.

In contrast, the TIDieR guideline focuses exclusively on descriptions of interventions in trials. As such, TIDieR and CReDECI are complementary pieces of advice. TIDieR outlines 12 descriptive criteria that will provide the reader (and hence clinicians, patients and policy-makers) with clear information about the what, who, where, how and when of complex intervention delivery in clinical research. It also requires research reports to contain information about intervention theories or goals, tailoring and modifications of interventions, and finally, requires authors to report both the planned and actual adherence and fidelity to the intervention. We absolutely endorse this idea and we hope that in future journal editors will pay as much regard to reporting intervention content as they do to CONSORT and other guidelines for reporting research methods in their editorial policies and instructions to authors.

The research career

If we were to take a helicopter perspective on developing knowledge for practice, we could not avoid touching briefly upon one's development as a researcher. The research we choose to involve ourselves in is closely connected to our careers as researchers and professionals. Building a research career in academia or in health care practice is a road with many choices to be made.

Traditionally, university-based careers are built on scientific publications in high-impact journals together with grants from prestigious funding bodies. Such careers pay less attention to the impact research findings may have in practice. The pressure on publishing may well influence the research waste problem mentioned previously. Having said this, implementation and dissemination are at last being increasingly emphasized in some institutional and national research quality assessments and research council or academy personal funding awards. However, in general there is no system in place that takes such issues into account when adding up individual researchers' merits. A researcher who is more focused on high-impact journals may be more highly regarded and be awarded the big grant or be appointed to more senior positions than one whose work looks towards clinical practice development.

In any research career, it is helpful to keep in mind what counts as a contribution in the meritocratic system at most universities. Despite recent attempts to include 'impact' in some national research assessments such as that in the UK, research that has the power to inform practice may not be considered as valuable in the academic system as research conducted further upstream in the knowledge translation pipeline. Thus, for individuals building and carrying out a research programme, one choice to be made is in which arena one would like to contribute to the most. Making an informed choice protects us as researchers from disappointment and helps us to make decisions that are true to the journey we as researchers prefer. This book has its focus on research aiming at providing knowledge for practice and we are heartened by recent developments emphasizing research impact, but we acknowledge that much work still needs to be done before academic careers can be assessed fairly on one's endeavours to change clinical practice.

Implementation

We cannot let the book be completed without a final few words about implementation. Putting the findings of research into practice is the ultimate goal of any researcher engaged in intervention development, complex or otherwise. As Theo van Achterberg puts it in his introduction to Section 4, the fact that policy-makers increasingly stress the need to focus on implementation is explained by the far too numerous examples of health care systems and clinicians failing to delivering optimal performance, not least integrating evidence-based findings into their routine practice. Even when health care workers know about new interventions and techniques, their practice does not change, threatening care quality, safety, effectiveness, efficiency, acceptability/patient centredness, timeliness and equitability/accessibility.

For the research community, whilst we may not actively engage in the routine implementation of evidence-based complex interventions ourselves, it is absolutely our duty to ensure that the knowledge we generate is fit for this purpose. It is our obligation to make our results available to others in a format that is understandable and it is our responsibility to guarantee that such information is accurate, free from as many biases as possible and clearly described. We should consider the 'implementability' of our complex interventions from the moment we begin the process of design, testing and evaluation.

And maybe we should also actually tarry a while after we have produced our evidence. Dissemination is more than writing academic journal articles. Dissemination can include speaking to policy-makers and politicians. It can include writing educational training manuals for our new intervention. It can include helping patient groups to lobby for change. Whilst we accept that some researchers, particularly those with methodological specialities such as health economics or medical statistics, may find themselves somewhat remote from the clinical coalface, many other researchers are clinicians at heart. We strongly encourage the applied health services community to look beyond the next high-impact journal and consider what they might do to ensure that interventions get implemented routinely and with high fidelity. Improving the lives of patients and people is, after all, the fundamental goal of all health services research. We hope that this book will make that goal easier to achieve.

REFERENCES

Aarons, G. A. 2004. Mental health provider attitudes toward adoption of evidence-based practice: the Evidence-Based Practice Attitude Scale (EBPAS). *Mental Health Services Research,* 6: 61–74.

Aarons, G. A., Cafri, G., Lugo, L. and Sawitzky, A. 2012. Expanding the domains of attitudes towards evidence-based practice: the Evidence Based Practice Attitude Scale-50. *Administration and Policy in Mental Health and Mental Health Services Research,* 39: 331–40.

Abaid, L. N., Grimes, D. A. and Schulz, K. F. 2007. Reducing publication bias of prospective clinical trials through trial registration. *Contraception,* 76: 339–41.

Abbott, J. H., Robertson, M. C., McKenzie, J. E., Baxter, G. D., Theis, J. C., Campbell, A. J. and the MOA trial team. 2009. Exercise therapy, manual therapy, or both, for osteoarthritis of the hip or knee: a factorial randomised controlled trial protocol. *Trials,* 10: 11.

Abraham, C. and Michie, S. 2008. A taxonomy of behavior change techniques used in interventions. *Health Psychology,* 27: 379–87.

Abraham, C., Sheeran, P. and Johnston, M. 1998. From health beliefs to self-regulation: theoretical advances in the psychology of action control. *Psychology and Health,* 13: 569–91.

Adams, G., Gulliford, M. C., Ukoumunne, O. C., Eldridge, S., Chinn, S. and Campbell, M. J. 2004. Patterns of intra-cluster correlation from primary care research to inform study design and analysis. *Journal of Clinical Epidemiology,* 57: 785–94.

Altman, D. G. 1980. Statistics and ethics in medical research. III: How large a sample? *British Medical Journal,* 281: 1336–8.

Altman, D. G. and Bland, J. M. 2003. Interaction revisited: the difference between two estimates. *British Medical Journal,* 326: 219.

Altman, D. G. and Gardner, M. J. 2000. Regression and correlation. In: D. G. Altman, D. Machin, T. N. Bryant and M. J. Gardner (eds), *Statistics with Confidence.* Bristol: British Medical Journal Books, pp. 73–92.

American Geriatrics Society (AGS). 2002. Panel on persistent pain in older persons: the management of persistent pain in older persons. *Journal of the American Geriatrics Society,* 50, Suppl.: S205–24.

Anderson, L.M., Petticrew, M., Rehfuess, E., Armstrong, R., Ueffing, E., Baker, P., Francis, D. and Tugwell, P. 2011. Using logic models to capture complexity in systematic reviews. *Research Synthesis Methods,* 2: 33e42.

Anderson, L. M., Petticrew, M., Chandler, J., Grimshaw, J., Tugwell, P., O'Neill, J., Welch, V., Squires, J., Churchill, R. and Shemilt, I. 2013. Introducing a series of methodological articles on considering complexity in systematic reviews of interventions. *Journal of Clinical Epidemiology,* 66: 1205–8.

Antman, E. M., Lau, J., Kupelnick, B., Mosteller, F. and Chalmers, T. C. 1992. A comparison of results of meta-analyses of randomized control trials and recommendations of clinical experts. Treatments for myocardial infarction. *JAMA: Journal of the American Medical Association,* 268: 240–8.

Antonovsky, A. 1993. The structure and properties of the sense of coherence scale. *Social Science & Medicine,* 36: 725–33.

Arain, M., Campbell, M. J., Cooper, C. L. and Lancaster, G. A. 2010. What is a pilot or feasibility study? A review of current practice and editorial policy. *BMC Medical Research Methodology,* 10: 67. http://www.biomedcentral.com/1471–2288/10/67.

Armitage, P., Berry, G. and Matthews, J. N. S. 2002. *Statistical Methods in Medical Research.* Oxford: Blackwell Science.

Armstrong, R., Waters, E., Moore, L., Riggs, E., Cuervo, L. G. and Lumbiganon, P. 2008. Improving the reporting of public health intervention research: advancing TREND and CONSORT. *Journal of Public Health,* 30: 103–9.

Arnstein, S. R. 1969. Ladder of citizen participation. *Journal of the American Institute of Planners,* 35: 216–24.

Atkins, S., Biles D., Lewin., S. A., Ringsberg, K. C. and Thorson, A. 2010. Patients' experiences of an intervention to support tuberculosis treatment adherence in South Africa. *Journal of Health Services Research and Policy,* 15: 163–70.

Axelrod, R. 1997. *The Complexity of Co-operation: Agent Based Models of Competition and Collaboration.* Princeton: Princetown Univeristy Press.

Backman, C. L., Harris, S. R., Chisholm, J.-A. M. and Monette, A. D. 1987. Single-subject research in rehabilitation: a review of studies using AB, withdrawal, multiple baseline, and alternating treatments designs. *Archives of Physical Medicine and Rehabilitation,* 78: 1145–53.

Baird, J., Jarman, M., Lawrence, W., Black, C., Davies, J., Tinati, T., Begum, R., Mortimore, A., Robinson, S., Margetts, B., Cooper, C., Barker, M. and Inskip, H. 2014. The effect of a behaviour change intervention on the diets and physical activity levels of women attending Sure Start Children's Centres: results from a complex public health intervention. *British Medical Journal Open,* 4: e005290.

Bandura, A. 2001. Social cognitive theory: an agentic perspective. *Annual Review of Psychology,* 52: 1–26.

Barlow, D. H. and Hersen, M. 1984. *Single Case Experimental Designs: Strategies for Studying Behavior Change.* New York: Pergamon Press.

Barth, J., Munder, T., Gerger, H., Nüesch, E., Trelle, S., Znoj, H., Jüni, P. and Cuijpers, P. 2013. Comparative efficacy of seven psychotherapeutic interventions for patients with depression: a network meta-analysis. *PLoS Medicine,* 10: e1001454.

Bartholomew, L. K., Parcel, G. S. and Kok, G. 1998. Intervention mapping: a process for developing theory- and evidence-based health education programs. *Health Education & Behavior,* 25: 545–63.

Bartholomew, L., Parcel, G., Kok, G., Gottlieb, N. and Fernández, M. 2011. *Planning Health Promotion Programs: An Intervention Mapping Approach,* 3rd edn. San Francisco, CA: Jossey-Bass.

Basu, A. and Meltzer, D. 2005. Implications of spillover effects within the family for medical cost-effectiveness analysis. *Journal of Health Economics,* 24: 751–73.

Bate, P. 2014. Context is everything. In: Health Foundation, *Perspectives on Context: A Selection of Essays Considering the Role of Context in Successful Quality Improvement.* London: Health Foundation, pp. 1–30.

Becker, Swanson, S., Bond, G. R. and Merrens, M. R. 2008. *Evidence-Based Supported Employment Fidelity Review Manual.* Lebanon, NH: Dartmouth Psychiatric Research Center.

Belaid, H., Cossette, S. and Heppell, S. 2011. Effet d'une intervention infirmière de soutien favorisant l'autodétermination sur la pratique des auto-soins chez des patients atteints d'insuffisance cardiaque. *Canadian Journal of Cardiology,* 27: S348.

Berben, S., Meijs, T., van Grunsven, P., Schoonhoven, L. and van Achterberg, T. 2012. Facilitators and barriers in pain management for trauma patients in the chain of emergency care. *Injury,* 43: 1397–402.

Berg, B. 2004. *Markov Chain Monte Carlo Simulations and Their Statistical Analysis.* Hackensack, NJ: World Scientific.

Berg, R. C. and Denison, E. 2013. Interventions to reduce the prevalence of female genital mutilation/cutting in African countries. *Campbell Systematic Reviews,* 9. doi: 10.4073/csr.2012.9.

Bernhardt, J., Dewey, H., Thrift, A., Collier, J. and Donnan, G. 2008. A very early rehabilitation trial for stroke (AVERT). Phase II: Safety and feasibility. *Stroke,* 39: 390–6.

Berry, S. A., Doll, M. C., McKinley, K. E., Casale, A. S. and Bothe, Jr., A. 2009. ProvenCare: quality improvement model for designing highly reliable care in cardiac surgery. *Quality & Safety in Health Care,* 18: 360–8.

Biglan, A., Ary, D. and Wagenaar, A. C. 2000. The value of interrupted time-series experiments for community intervention research. *Prevention Science,* 1: 31–49.

Biomarkers Definitions Working Group. 2001. Biomarkers and surrogate endpoints: preferred definitions and conceptual framework. *Clinical Pharmacology and Therapeutics,* 69: 89–95.

Blakely, C. H., Mayer, J. P., Gottschalk, R. G., Schmitt, N., Davidson, W. S., Roitman, D. B. and Emshoff, J. G. 1987. The fidelity-adaptation debate: implications for the implementation of public sector social programs. *American Journal of Community Psychology,* 15: 253–68.

Bleijlevens, M., Hendriks, M., van Haastregt, J., van Rossum, E., Kempen, G., Diederiks, J., Crebolder, H. and van Eijk, J. 2008. Process factors explaining the ineffectiveness of a multidisciplinary fall prevention programme: a process evaluation. *BMC Public Health,* 8: 332.

Boaz, A., Baeza, J. and Fraser, A. (European Implementation Score Collaborative Group – EIS). 2011. Effective implementation of research into practice: an overview of systematic reviews of the health literature. *BMC Research Notes,* 4: 212.

Bolin, K., Lindgren, B., Lindström, M. and Nystedt, P. 2003. Investments in social capital, implications of social interactions for the production of health. *Social Science & Medicine,* 46: 2379–90.

Bond, G. R., Evans, L., Salyers, M. P., Williams, J. and Kim, H. W. 2000. Measurement of fidelity in psychiatric rehabilitation. *Mental Health Services Research,* 2: 75–87.

Bonell, C., Fletcher, A., Morton, M., Lorenc, T. and Moore, L. 2012. Realist randomised controlled trials: a new approach to evaluating complex public health interventions. *Social Science & Medicine,* 75: 2299–306.

Booch, G., Rumbaugh, J. and Jacobson, I. 2005. *The Unified Modeling Language User Guide,* 2nd edn. Upper Saddle River, NJ: Pearson Education.

Boote, J., Telford, R. and Cooper, C. 2002. Consumer involvement in health research: a review and research agenda. *Health Policy,* 61: 213–36.

Booth, A. 2011. Searching for studies. In: J. Noyes, A. Booth, K. Hannes, A. Harden, J. Harris, S. Lewin and C. Lockwood (eds), *Supplementary Guidance for Inclusion of Qualitative Research in Cochrane Systematic Reviews of Interventions Version 1* (updated August 2011), chapter 3. http://cqrmg.cochrane.org/supplemental-handbook-guidance.

Borglin, G. 2012. Mixed methods: an introduction. In: M. Henricsson (ed.), *Scientific Theory & Method: From Idea to Examination within Nursing Science.* Lund: Student Litteratur, pp. 269–87.

Bouffard, J. A., Taxman, F. S. and Silverman, R. 2003. Improving process evaluations of correctional programs by using a comprehensive evaluation methodology. *Evaluation and Program Planning,* 26: 149–61.

Bower, P., Gilbody, S., Richards, D., Fletcher, J. and Sutton, A. 2006. Collaborative care for depression in primary care: making sense of a complex intervention – systematic review and meta-regression. *British Journal of Psychiatry,* 189: 484–93.

Bower, P., Kontopantelis, E., Sutton, A., Kendrick, T., Richards, D. A., Gilbody, S., Knowles, S., Cuijpers, P., Andersson, G., Christensen, H., Meyer, B., Huibers, M., Smit, F., Van Straten, A., Warmerdam, L., Barkham, M., Bilich, L., Lovell, K. and Liu, E. T. 2013. Influence of initial severity of depression on effectiveness of low intensity interventions: meta-analysis of individual patient data. *British Medical Journal,* 346: f540.

Bowling, A. 2005. *Measuring Health: A Review of Quality of Life Measurement Scales.* Maidenhead: McGraw-Hill Education.

Brailsford, S. C., Lattimer, V. A., Tarnaras, P. and Turnbull, J. C. 2004. Emergency and on-demand health care: modelling a large complex system. *Journal of the Operational Research Society,* 55: 34–42.

Brailsford, S. C., Harper, P. R., Patel, B. and Pitt, M. 2009. An analysis of the academic literature on simulation and modelling in healthcare. *Journal of Simulation,* 3: 130–40.

Brailsford, S. C., Harper, P. R. and Sykes, J. 2012. Incorporating human behaviour in simulation models of screening for breast cancer. *European Journal of Operational Research,* 219: 491–507.

Brazier, J., McCabe, C. and Edlin, R. 2005. Health economics and cost consequences analysis: a step back in time. *British Medical Journal,* 329: 1233.

Brazier, J., Ratcliffe, J., Salomon, J. A. and Tsuchiya, A. 2007. *Measuring and Valuing Health Benefits for Economic Evaluation.* Oxford: Oxford University Press.

Brettschneider, C., Luhmann, D. and Raspe, H. 2011. Informative value of Patient Reported Outcomes (PRO) in Health Technology Assessment (HTA). *GMS Health Technology Assessment,* 7: Doc. 01.

Briggs, A. H. and O'Brien, B. J. 2001. The death of cost-minimization analysis? *Health Economics,* 10: 179–84.

Briggs, A. H., Claxton, K. and Sculpher, M. 2006. *Decision Modelling for Health Economic Evaluation.* Oxford: Oxford University Press.

Brouwer, W. B. and Koopmanschap, M. A. 2000. On the economic foundations of CEA: ladies and gentlemen, take your positions! *Journal of Health Economics,* 19: 439–59.

Brouwer, W. B., Culyer, A. J., van Exel, N. J., Job, A. and Rutten, F., 2008. Welfarism vs extra welfarism. *Journal of Health Economics,* 27: 325–38.

Brown, C. A. and Lilford, R. J. 2006. The stepped wedge trial design: a systematic review. *BMC Medical Research Methodology,* 6: 54–62.

Brown, C. E., Wickline, M. A., Ecoff, L. and Glaser, D. 2008. Nursing practice, knowledge, attitudes and perceived barriers to evidence-based practice at an academic medical center. *Journal of Advanced Nursing,* 65: 371–81.

Brown, D. and McCormack, B. 2006. Determining factors that impact upon effective evidence based pain management with older people, following colorectal surgery: an ethnographic study. *Journal of Clinical Nursing,* 15: 1287–98.

——2011. Developing the practice context to enable more effective pain management with older people: an action research approach. *Implementation Science,* 6: 1–14.

Brown, L. D., Cai, T. T., DasGupta, A., Agresti, A., Coull, B. A., Casella, G., Corcoran, C., Mehta, C., Ghosh, M. and Santner, T. J. 2001. Interval estimation for a binomial proportion. *Statistical Science,* 16: 101–33.

Browne, R. H. 1995. On the use of a pilot sample for sample size determination. *Statistics in Medicine,* 14: 1933–40.

Brownson, R. C., Colditz, G. A. and Proctor, E. K. 2012. *Dissemination and Implementation Research in Health: Translating Science to Practice.* Oxford: Oxford University Press.

Brueton, V. C., Tierney, J., Stenning, S., Harding, S., Meredith, S., Nazareth, I. and Rait, G. 2013. Strategies to improve retention in randomised trials. *Cochrane Database of Systematic Reviews*, 12: MR000032. doi: 10.1002/14651858.MR000032.pub2.

Bryant, J., Boyes, A., Jones, K., Sanson-Fisher, R., Carey, M. and Fry, R. 2014. Examining and addressing evidence-practice gaps in cancer care: a systematic review. *Implementation Science,* 9: 37.

Bryson, J. M., Patton, M. Q. and Bowman, R. A. 2011. Working with evaluation stakeholders: a rationale, step-wise approach and toolkit. *Evaluation and Program Planning,* 34: 1–12.

Byford, S., Sharac, J., Lloyd-Evans, B., Gilburt, H., Osborn, D. P. J., Leese, M., Johnson, S. and Slade, M. 2010. Alternatives to standard acute in-patient care in England: readmissions, service use and cost after discharge. *British Journal of Psychiatry,* 197: S20–5.

Cabana, M. D., Rand, C. S., Powe, N. R., Wu, A. W., Wilson, M. H., Abboud, P. A. and Rubin, H. R. 1999. Why don't physicians follow clinical practice guidelines? A framework for improvement. *JAMA: Journal of the American Medical Association,* 282: 1458–65.

Caldwell, P. H. Y., Hamilton, S., Tan, A. and Craig, J. C. 2010. Strategies for increasing recruitment to randomised controlled trials: systematic review. *PLoS Medicine,* 7: e1000368.

Cameron, I., Gillespie, L., Robertson, M., Murray, G., Hill, K., Cumming, R. and Kerse, N. 2012. Interventions for preventing falls in older people in care facilities and hospitals. *Cochrane Database of Systematic Reviews,* 12: CD005465.

Campbell, M., Fitzpatrick, R., Haines, A., Kinmonth, A. L., Sandercock, P., Spiegelhalter, D. and Tyrer, P. 2000. Framework for design and evaluation of complex interventions to improve health. *British Medical Journal,* 321: 694–6.

Campbell, N. C., Murray, E., Darbyshire, J., Emery, J., Farmer, A., Griffiths, F., Guthrie, B., Lester, H., Wilson, P. and Kinmonth, A. L. 2007. Designing and evaluating complex interventions to improve health care. *British Medical Journal,* 334: 455–9.

Campbell, R., Quilty, B. and Dieppe, P. 2003. Discrepancies between patients' assessments of outcome: qualitative studies nested within randomised controlled trials. *British Medical Journal*, 326: 252–3.

Campbell, R., Peters, T., Grant, C., Quilty, B. and Dieppe, P. 2005. Adapting the randomized consent (Zelen) design for trials of behavioural interventions for chronic disease: feasibility study. *Journal of Health Services Research and Policy,* 10: 220–5.

Cane, J., O'Connor, D. and Michie, S. 2012. Validation of the theoretical domains framework for use in behaviour change and implementation research. *Implementation Science,* 7: 37.

Carfoot, S., Williamson, P. R. and Dickson, R. 2004. The value of a pilot study in breastfeeding research. *Midwifery*, 20: 188–93.

Carr, E. 2000. Exploring the effect of postoperative pain on patient outcome following surgery. *Acute Pain*, 3: 183–93.

Carroll, C., Patterson, M., Wood, S., Booth, A., Rick, J. and Balain, S. 2007. A conceptual framework for implementation fidelity. *Implementation Science,* 2: 40.

Cartwright, N., Goldfinch, A. and Howick, J. 2007. *Evidence-Based Policy: Where is Our Theory of Evidence?* Technical Report 07/07. Contingency and Dissent in Science Project, Centre for Philosophy of Natural and Social Science, London School of Economics and Political Science.

Castro, F. G., Barrera, M. and Martinez, C. R. 2004. The cultural adaptation of prevention interventions: resolving tensions between fidelity and fit. *Prevention Science,* 5: 41–5.

Centre for Reviews and Dissemination. 2007. *NHS Economic Evaluation Database Handbook.* Centre for Reviews and Dissemination, University of York.

Centre for Reviews and Dissemination. 2009. *Systematic Reviews: CRD's Guidance for Undertaking Reviews in Health Care.* University of York, Centre for Reviews and Dissemination. http://www.york.ac.uk/inst/crd/pdf/Systematic_Reviews.pdf.

Chalmers, I. and Glasziou, P. 2009. Avoidable waste in the production and reporting of research evidence. *The Lancet,* 374: 86–9.

Chalmers, I., Bracken, M. B., Djulbegovic, B., Garattini, S., Grant, J., Gulmezoglu, A. M., Howells, D. W., Ioannidis, J. P. A. and Oliver, S. 2014. How to increase value and reduce waste when research priorities are set. *The Lancet,* 383: 156–65.

Chan, A. W., Tetzlaff, J., Gøtzsche, P. C., Altman, D. G., Mann, H., Berlin, J. A., Dickersin, K., Hróbjartsson, A., Schulz, K. F., Parulekar, W. R., Krleža-Jerić, K., Laupacis, A. and Moher, D. 2013. SPIRIT 2013 explanation and elaboration: guidance for protocols of clinical trials. *British Medical Journal,* 346: e7586.

Chan, A. W., Song, F. J., Vickers, A., Jefferson, T., Dickersin, K., Gotzsche, P. C., Krumholz, H. M., Ghersi, D. and Van Der Worp, H. B. 2014. Increasing value and reducing waste: addressing inaccessible research. *The Lancet,* 383: 257–66.

Charchalis, M., Cossette, S. and Frasure-Smith, N. 2013. Feasibility and acceptability of an individualized nursing intervention aimed at increasing adaptation among patients with newly implanted cardiac defibrillators: a pilot randomized clinical trial. *Canadian Journal of Cardiology,* 28: S433.

Charnes, A., Cooper, W. and Rhodes, E. 1978. Measuring the efficiency of decision-making units. *European Journal of Operational Research,* 2: 429–44.

Cheater, F., Baker, R., Gillies, C., Hearnshaw, H., Flottorp, S., Robertson, N., Shaw, E. J. and Oxman, A. D. 2005. Tailored interventions to overcome identified barriers to change: effects on professional practice and health care outcomes. *Cochrane Database of Systematic Reviews,* 3: CD005470.

Checkland, P. and Poulter, J. 2006. *Learning for Action: A Short Definitive Account of Soft Systems Methodology, and Its Use for Practitioners, Teachers and Students.* Chichester: John Wiley.

Cheng, S. K., Dietrich, M. S. and Dilts, M. 2010. A sense of urgency: evaluating the link between clinical trial development time and the accrual performance of cancer therapy evaluation program (NCI-CTEP) sponsored studies. *Clinical Cancer Research,* 16: 5557–63.

Ciliberto, M. A., Sandige, H. and Ndekha, M. J. 2005. Comparison of home-based therapy with ready-to-use therapeutic food with standard therapy in the treatment of malnourished Malawian children: a controlled, clinical effectiveness trial. *American Journal of Clinical Nutrition,* 81: 864–70.

Clarke, M., Hopewell, S. and Chalmers, I. 2010. Clinical trials should begin and end with systematic reviews of relevant evidence: 12 years and waiting. *The Lancet,* 376: 20–1.

Claxton, K. 2008. Exploring uncertainty in cost-effectiveness analysis. *PharmacoEconomics,* 26: 781–98.

Claxton, K., Ginnelly, L., Sculpher, M., Philips, Z. and Palmer, S. 2004. A pilot study on the use of decision theory and value of information analysis as part of the NHS Health Technology Assessment programme. *Health Technology Assessment,* 8: 1–103.

Claxton, K. P., Sculpher, M. J. and Ades, T. 2005. Cost consequences: implicit, opaque and anti-scientific. *British Medical Journal,* 329: 1233.

Coast, J. 2004. Is economic evaluation in touch with society's health values? *British Medical Journal,* 329: 1233–6.

Coast, J., Smith, R. and Lorgelly, P. 2008a. Welfarism, extra-welfarism and capability: the spread of ideas in health economics. *Social Science & Medicine*, 67: 1190–8.

——. 2008b. Should the capability approach be applied in health economics? *Health Economics*, 17: 667–70.

Cochrane Collaboration. 2005. *Glossary of terms in the Cochrane Collaboration, version 4.2.5.*

Cochrane Effective Practice and Organisation of Care Review Group. 2002. *Data Collection Checklist.* http://epoc.cochrane.org/sites/epoc.cochrane.org/files/uploads/data collectionchecklist.pdf [accessed 27 February 2014].

Cochrane Effective Practice and Organisation of Care Group. 2012. *Welcome to the EPOC Website.* http://epoc.cochrane.org/ [accessed 27 February 2014].

Collins, K. M. T. and O'Cathain, A. 2009. Ten points about mixed methods research to be considered by the novice researcher. *International Journal of Multiple Research Approaches,* 3: 2–7.

Collins, L. M., Murphy, S. A., Nair, V. N. and Strecher, V. J. 2005. A strategy for optimizing and evaluating behavioral interventions. *Annals of Behavioral Medicine*, 30: 65–73.

Collins, L. M., Murphy, S. A. and Strecher, V. 2007. The multiphase optimization strategy (MOST) and the sequential multiple assignment randomized trial (SMART): new methods for more potent eHealth interventions. *American Journal of Preventive Medicine,* 32: S112–18.

Colquhoun, H. L., Brehaut, J. C., Sales, A., Ivers, N., Grimshaw, J., Michie, S., Carroll, K., Chalifoux, M. and Eva, K. W. 2013. A systematic review of the use of theory in randomized controlled trials of audit and feedback. *Implementation Science*, 8: 66.

CONSORT (Consolidated Standards of Reporting Trials). http://www.consort-statement. org.

Cook, T. D. and Campbell, D. T. 1979. *Quasi-Experimentation: Design & Analysis Issues for Field Settings.* Boston: Houghton Mifflin.

Cooper, C. L., Hind, D., Parry, G. D., Isaac, C. L., Dimairo, M., O'Cathain, A., Rose, A., Freeman, J. V., Martin, L., Kaltenthaler, E. C., Thake, A. and Sharrack, B. 2011. Computerised cognitive behavioural therapy for the treatment of depression in people with multiple sclerosis: external pilot trial. *Trials,* 12: 259.

Corry, M., Clarke, M., While, A. E. and Lalor, J. 2013. Developing complex interventions for nursing: a critical review of key guidelines. *Journal of Clinical Nursing,* 22: 2366–86.

Cortés-Jofré, M., Rueda, J. R., Corsini-Muñoz, G., Fonseca-Cortes, C., Caraballoso, M. and Bonfill Cosp, X. 2012. Drugs for preventing lung cancer in healthy people. *Cochrane Database of Systematic Reviews,* 10: CD002141.

Cossette, S., D'Aoust, L.-X., Morin, M., Heppell, S. and Frasure-Smith, N. 2009. The systematic development of a nursing intervention aimed at increasing enrollment in cardiac rehabilitation for acute coronary syndrome patients. *Progress in Cardiovascular Nursing,* 24: 71–9.

Cossette, S., Frasure-Smith, N., Dupuis, J., Juneau, M. and Guertin, M.-C. 2012. Randomized controlled trial of tailored nursing interventions to improve cardiac rehabilitation enrollment. *Nursing Research*, 61: 119–28.

Cossette, S., Vadeboncoeur, A., Frasure-Smith, N., McCusker, J., Perreault, D. and Guertin, M.-C. 2013. Randomized controlled trial of a nursing intervention to reduce emergency department revisits. *Canadian Journal of Emergency Medicine*, 15: 1–8.

Côté, J., Rouleau, G., Godin, G., Ramirez-Garcia, P., Gueheneuc, Y. G., Nahas, G., Tremblay, C., Otis, J. and Hernandez, A. 2012. Acceptability and feasibility of a virtual intervention to help people living with HIV manage their daily therapies. *Journal of Telemedicine & Telecare*, 18: 409–12.

Craig, L. E., Bernhardt, J., Langhorne, P. and Wu, O. 2010. Early mobilization after stroke: an example of an individual patient data meta-analysis of a complex intervention. *Stroke,* 41: 2632–6.

Craig, P. and Petticrew, M. 2013. Developing and evaluating complex interventions: reflections on the 2008 MRC guidance. *International Journal of Nursing Studies,* 50: 585–92.

Craig, P., Dieppe, P., Macintyre, S., Michie, S., Nazareth, I. and Petticrew, M. 2008. Developing and evaluating complex interventions: the new Medical Research Council guidance. *British Medical Journal,* 337: a1655.

Craig, P., Cooper, C., Gunnell, D., Haw, S., Lawson, K., Macintyre, S., Ogilvie, D., Petticrew, M., Reeves, B., Sutton, M. and Thompson, S. 2012. Using natural experiments to evaluate population health interventions: new Medical Research Council guidance. *Journal of Epidemiology and Community Health,* 66: 1182–6.

Craigie, A. M., Caswell, S., Paterson, C., Treweek, S., Belch, J. J. F., Daly, F., Rodger, J., Thompson, J., Kirk, A., Ludbrook, A., Stead, M., Wardle, J., Steele, R. J. C. and Anderson, A. S. 2011. Study protocol for BeWEL: the impact of a BodyWEight and physicaL activity intervention on adults at risk of developing colorectal adenomas. *BMC Public Health,* 11: 184.

Creswell, J. W. 2003. *Research Design: Qualitative, Quantitative, and Mixed Methods Approaches.* Thousand Oaks, CA: Sage.

Creswell, J. W. 2007. *Qualitative Inquiry & Research Design: Choosing among Five Approaches,* 2nd edn. London: Sage.

Creswell, J. W. and Miller, D. L. 2000. Determining validity in qualitative inquiry. *Theory into Practice,* 39: 124–30.

Creswell, J. W. and Plano Clark, V. L. 2007. *Designing and Conducting Mixed Methods Research.* Thousand Oaks, CA: Sage.

——2011. *Designing and Conducting Mixed Methods Research,* 2nd edn. Thousand Oaks, CA: Sage.

Culyer, A. J. 1991. The normative economics of health care finance and provision. In: A. McGuire, P. Fenn and K. Mayhew (eds), *Providing Health Care: The Economics of Alternative Systems of Finance and Delivery.* Oxford: Oxford University Press, pp. 65–98.

Dal-Ré, R., Moher, D., Gluud, C., Treweek, S., Demotes-Mainard, J. and Carné, X. 2011. Disclosure of investigators' recruitment performance in multicenter clinical trials: a further step for research transparency. *PLoS Medicine,* 8: e1001149.

Damschroder, L. J., Aron, D. C., Keith, R. E., Kirsh, S. R., Alexander, J. A. and Lowery, J. C. 2009. Fostering implementation of health services research findings into practice: a consolidated framework for advancing implementation science. *Implementation Science,* 4: 50.

Dancet, E. A., D'Hooghe, T. M., Spiessens, C., Sermeus, W., De Neubourg, D., Karel, N., Kremer, J. A. and Nelen, W. L. 2013. Quality indicators for all dimensions of infertility care quality: consensus between professionals and patients. *Human Reproduction,* 28: 1584–97.

Dane, A. V. and Schneider, B. H. 1998. Program integrity in primary and early secondary prevention: are implementation effects out of control? *Clinical Psychology Review,* 18: 23–45.

Dangerfield, B. C. 1999. System dynamics application to European health care issues. *Journal of the Operational Research Society,* 50: 345–53.

Daskin, M. S. 2008. What you should know about location modeling. *Naval Research Logistics,* 55: 283–94.

Database of Instruments for Resource Use Measurement. http://www.dirum.org/about [accessed 28 February 2014].

Datta, J. and Petticrew, M. 2013. Challenges to evaluating complex interventions: a content analysis of published papers. *BMC Public Health,* 13: 568.

Davenport, A., Gura, V., Ronco, C., Beizai, M., Ezon, C. and Rambod, E. 2008. A wearable haemodialysis device for patients with end-stage renal failure: a pilot study. *The Lancet,* 370: 2005–10.

Davis, D. and Taylor-Vaisey, A. 1997. Translating guidelines into practice: a systematic review of theoretic concepts, practical experience and research evidence in the adoption of clinical practice guidelines. *Canadian Medical Association Journal,* 157: 408–16.

de Bruin, M., Viechtbauer, W., Hospers, H., Schaalma, H. and Kok, G. 2009. Standard care quality determines treatment outcomes in control groups of HAART-adherence intervention studies: implications for the interpretation and comparison of intervention effects. *Health Psychology,* 28: 668–74.

de Bruin, M., Viechtbauer, W., Schaalma, H. P., Kok, H., Abraham, C. and Hospers, H. J. 2010. Standard care impact on effects of highly active antiretroviral therapy adherence interventions: a meta-analysis of randomized controlled trials. *Annals of Internal Medicine,* 170: 240–50.

DeBar, L. L., Elder, C., Ritenbaugh, C., Aickin, M., Deyo, M., Meenan, R., Dickerson, J., Webster, J. A. and Yarborough, B. J. 2011. Acupuncture and chiropractice care for chronic pain in an integrated health plan: a mixed methods study. *BMC Complementary & Alternative Medicine,* 11: 118. http://www.biomedcentral.com/1472–6882/11/118.

Deeks, J., Higgins, J. and Altman, D. on behalf of the CSMG. 2011. Analysing data and undertaking meta-analyses. In: J. P. T. Higgins and S. Green (eds), *Cochrane Handbook for Systematic Reviews of Interventions Version 5.1.0,* chapter 9. http://www.cochrane-handbook.org [accessed 8 May 2014].

Denton, B., Viapiano, J. and Vogl, A. 2007 Optimization of surgery sequencing and scheduling decisions under uncertainty. *Health Care Management Science,* 10: 13–24.

Denzin, N. and Lincoln, Y. 2000. *Sage Handbook of Qualitative Research,* 3rd edn. Thousand Oaks, CA: Sage.

Ding, Y., Hu, Y. and Rahm Hallberg, I. 2013. Health-related quality of life and associated factors in Chinese women with cervical cancer: a 9-month follow up. *Cancer Nursing,* 36: 18–26.

Dobson, D. and Cook, T. J. 1980. Avoiding type III error in program evaluation: results from a field experiment. *Evaluation and Program Planning,* 3: 269–76.

Doctor Foster. 2004. *Adult Chronic Pain Management Services in Primary Care.* In association with Long-term Medical Conditions Alliance and the Patients Association. London.

Dolan, P. 2008. Developing methods that really do value the 'Q' in the QALY. *Health Economics, Policy and Law,* 3: 69–77.

Dolan, P., Gudex, C., Kind, P. and Williams, A. 1995. *A Social Tariff for EuroQol: Results from a UK General Population Survey.* York: University of York Discussion Paper 138.

Domholdt, E. 2000. *Physical Therapy Research: Principles and Applications.* Philadelphia: W. B. Saunders.

Donnell, A., Nicholl, J. and Read, S. M. 2003. Acute pain teams in England: current provision and their role in postoperative pain management. *Journal of Clinical Nursing,* 12: 387–93.

Donner, A. and Klar, N. S. 2000. *Design and Analysis of Cluster Randomisation Trials.* London: Arnold.

Donovan, J. L., Paramasivan, S., de Salis, I. and Toerien, M. 2014. Clear obstacles and hidden challenges: understanding recruiter perspectives in six pragmatic randomised controlled trials. *Trials,* 15: 5.

Drummond, M. F., Sculpher, M. J., Torrance, G. W., O'Brien, B. J. and Stoddart, G. L. 2005. *Methods for the Economic Evaluation of Health Care Programmes.* New York: Oxford University Press.

Dumville, J. C., Soares, M. O., O'Meara, S. and Cullum, N. 2012. Systematic review and mixed treatment comparison: dressings to heal diabetic foot ulcers. *Diabetologia*, 55: 1902–10.

Dumville, J. C., Deshpande, S., O'Meara, S. and Speak, K. 2013a. Hydrocolloid dressings for healing diabetic foot ulcers. *Cochrane Database of Systematic Reviews*, 8: CD009099.

——2013b. Foam dressings for healing diabetic foot ulcers. *Cochrane Database of Systematic Reviews*, 6: CD009111.

Dumville, J. C., O'Meara, S., Deshpande, S. and Speak, K. 2013c. Hydrogel dressings for healing diabetic foot ulcers. *Cochrane Database of Systematic Reviews*, 7: CD009101.

——2013d. Alginate dressings for healing diabetic foot ulcers. *Cochrane Database of Systematic Reviews*, 6: CD009110.

Durst, C., Viol, J. and Wickramasinghe, N. 2013. Online social networks, social capital and health-related behaviours: a state-of-the-art analysis. *Communications of the Association for Information Systems*, 32: 134–58.

Dusenbury, L., Brannigan, R., Falco, M. and Hansen, W. B. 2003. A review of research on fidelity of implementation: implications for drug abuse prevention in school settings. *Health Education Research*, 18: 237–56.

Eccles, M., Grimshaw, J., Walker, A., Johnston, M. and Pitts, N. 2005. Changing the behavior of healthcare professionals: the use of theory in promoting the uptake of research findings. *Journal of Clinical Epidemiology*, 58: 107–12.

Egger, M., Davey Smith, G. and Altman, D. G. (eds). 2001. *Systematic Reviews in Health Care: Meta-Analysis in Context*. London: British Medical Journal Books.

Ekwall, A. K and, Rahm Hallberg, I. 2007. The association between caregiving satisfaction, difficulties and coping among elderly family caregivers. *Journal of Clinical Nursing*, 16: 832–44.

Eldridge, S. and Kerry, S. 2012. *A Practical Guide to Cluster Randomised Trials in Health Services Research*. Chichester: John Wiley.

Eldridge, S. M., Ukoumunne, O. C. and Carlin, J. B. 2009. The intra-cluster correlation coefficient in cluster randomized trials: a review of definitions. *International Statistical Review*, 77: 378–94.

Elliott, J. 2011. *Reconstructing Teacher Education*. Abingdon: Routledge.

Elliott, R. A. and Payne, K. 2005. *Essentials of Economic Evaluation in Healthcare*. London: The Pharmaceutical Press.

Elliott, R. A., Putman, K., Franklin, M., Annemans, L., Verhaeghe, N., Eden, M., Hayre, J., Rodgers, S., Sheikh, A. and Avery, A. J. 2014a. Cost effectiveness of a pharmacist-led IT-based intervention with simple feedback in reducing rates of clinically important errors in medicines management in general practices (PINCER) *PharmacoEconomics*, 32: 573–90.

Elliott, R. A., Putman, K., Davies, J. and Annemans, L. 2014b. A review of the methodological challenges in assessing the cost effectiveness of pharmacist interventions. *PharmacoEconomics*, 32: 1185–99.

Elliott, W. J. and Meyer, P. M. 2007. Incident diabetes in clinical trials of antihypertensive drugs: a network meta-analysis. *The Lancet*, 369: 201–7.

Ennis, L. and Wykes, T. 2013. Impact of patient involvement in mental health research: longitudinal study. *British Journal of Psychiatry*, 203: 381–6.

Entwistle, V. A., Renfrew, M. J., Yearley, S., Forrester, J. and Lamont, T. 1998. Lay perspectives: advantages for health research. *British Medical Journal*, 316: 463–6.

Ernst, A. T., Jiang, H., Krishnamoorthy, M. and Sier, D. 2004. Staff scheduling and rostering: a review of applications, methods and models. *European Journal of Operational Research*, 153: 3–27.

Estabrooks, C. A., Scott, S., Squires, J. E., Stevens, B., O'Brien-Pallas, L., Watt-Watson, J., Profetto-McGrath, J., McGilton, K., Golden-Biddle, K., Lander, J., Donner, G., Boschma, G., Humphrey, C. K. and Williams, J. 2008. Patterns of research utilization on patient care units. *Implementation Science,* 3: 31.

Estabrooks, C. A., Squires, J. E., Cummings, G. G., Birdsell, J. M. and Norton, P. G. 2009. Development and assessment of the Alberta Context Tool. *BMC Health Services Research,* 9: 234.

Estabrooks, C. A., Squires, J. E., Hayduk, L. A., Cummings, G. G. and Norton, P. G. 2011. Advancing the argument for validity of the Alberta Context Tool with healthcare aides in residential long-term care. *BMC Medical Research Methodology,* 11: 107.

Ethgen, M., Boutron, I., Baron, G., Giraudeau, B., Sibilia, J. and Ravaud, P. 2005. Reporting of harm in randomized, controlled trials of nonpharmacologic treatment for rheumatic disease. *Annals of Internal Medicine,* 143: 20–5.

European Medicines Agency (EMA). 2008. Guideline on the evaluation of medicinal products for cardiovascular disease prevention. Doc. Ref. EMEA/CHMP/EWP/3118902007.

European Science Foundation (ESF). 2011. *Implementation of Medical Research in Clinical Practice.* ESF Science Policy Briefing, September. http://www.esf.org/index.php?eID=tx_nawsecuredl&u=0&file=fileadmin/be_user/research_areas/emrc/FL/FLIP/SPB45_2012_ImplMedRes_ClinPract.pdf&t=1402481174&hash=48aa7cb92f358a587794ce45c351255fd2e76ed5.

Euroqol. 2014. The EQ-5D. http://www.euroqol.org/ [accessed 28 February 2014].

Everitt, B. 2006. *Medical Statistics from A to Z: A Guide for Clinicians and Medical Students.* Cambridge: Cambridge University Press.

Farmer, A., Légaré, F., Turcot, L., Grimshaw, J., Harvey, E., McGowan, J. and Wolf, F. 2008. Printed educational materials: effects on professional practice and health care outcomes. *Cochrane Database of Systematic Reviews,* 16: CD004398.

Fay, B. 1987. *Critical Social Science.* Cambridge: Polity Press.

Feeley, N., Zelkowitz, P., Charbonneau, L., Cormier, C., Lacroix, A., Papageorgiou, A. and Ste Marie, C. 2008. Promoting mothers' ability to interact sensitively with their very-low birthweight infant: a pilot study. *Advances in Neonatal Care,* 8: 276–84.

Feeley, N., Cossette, S., Côté, J., Héon, M., Stremler, R., Martorella, G. and Purden, M. 2009. The importance of piloting an RCT intervention. *Canadian Journal of Nursing Research,* 41: 84–99.

Feldt, K. S., Ryden, M. B. and Miles, S. 1998. Treatment of pain in cognitively impaired compared with cognitively intact older patients with hip fracture. *Journal of the American Geriatrics Society,* 46: 1079–85.

Fenwick, E., Claxton, K. and Sculpher, M. 2008. The value of implementation and the value of information: combined and uneven development. *Medical Decision Making,* 28: 21–32.

Fetter, R. B. and Thompson, J. D. 1965. The simulation of hospital systems. *Operations Research,* 13: 689–711.

Finch, T., Mair, F., O'Donnell, C., Murray, E. and May, C. 2012. From theory to 'measurement' in complex interventions: methodological lessons from the development of an e-health normalisation instrument. *BMC Medical Research Methodology,* 12: 69.

Finch, T. L., Rapley, T., Girling, M., Mair, F. S., Murray, E., Treweek, S., McColl, E., Steen, I. N. and May, C. R. 2013. Improving the normalization of complex interventions: measure development based on normalization process theory (NoMAD): study protocol. *Implementation Science,* 8: 43.

Fineout-Overholt, E. and Johnston, L. 2005. Teaching EBP: asking searchable, answerable clinical questions. *Worldviews on Evidence-Based Nursing,* 2: 157–60.

Fishbein, M., Triandis, H. C., Kanfer, F. H., Becker M., Middlestadt, S. E. and Eichler, A. 2001. Factors influencing behavior and behavior change. In: A. Baum, T. A. Revenson and J. E. Singer (eds), *Handbook of Health Psychology*. Mahwah, NJ: Lawrence Erlbaum Associates, pp. 3–17.

Fisher, J. D. and Fisher, W. A. 1992. Changing AIDS-risk behavior. *Psychological Bulletin*, 111: 455–71.

Fixsen, D. L., Naoom, S. F., Blase, K. A., Friedman, R. M. and Wallace, F. 2005. *Implementation Research: A Synthesis of the Literature*. Tampa, FL: University of South Florida, Louis de la Parte Florida Mental Health Institute, The National Implementation Research Network (FMHI publication 231).

Fletcher, B., Gheorghe, A., Moore, D., Wilson, S. and Damery, S. 2012. Improving the recruitment activity of clinicians in randomised controlled trials: a systematic review. *British Medical Journal Open*, 2: e000496-6.

Flick, U. 2007. *The Sage Qualitative Research Kit*. Thousand Oaks, CA: Sage.

Flodgren, G., Eccles, M. P., Shepperd, S., Scott, A., Parmelli, E. and Beyer, F. R. 2011. An overview of reviews evaluating the effectiveness of financial incentives in changing healthcare professional behaviours and patient outcomes. *Cochrane Database of Systematic Reviews*, 7: CD009255.

Foresight. 2007. *Tackling Obesities: Future Choices-Project Report*. London: The Stationery Office.

Forsetlund, L., Bjørndal, A., Rashidian, A., Jamtvedt, G., O'Brien, M., Wolf, F., Davis, D., Odgaard-Jensen, J. and Oxman, A. 2009. Continuing education meetings and workshops: effects on professional practice and health care outcomes. *Cochrane Database of Systematic Reviews*, 15: CD003030.

Foy, R., Parry, J., Duggan, A., Delaney, B., Wilson, S., Lewin-Van Den Broek, N. T., Lassen, A., Vickers, L. and Myres, P. 2003. How evidence based are recruitment strategies to randomized controlled trials in primary care? Experience from seven studies. *Family Practice*, 20: 83–92.

Francis, J. J., O'Connor, D. and Curran, J. 2012. Theories of behaviour change synthesised into a set of theoretical groupings: introducing a thematic series on the theoretical domains framework. *Implementation Science*, 7: 35.

Fraser, M. W., Richman, J. M. and Galinsky, M. J. 2009. *Intervention Research: Developing Social Programs*. New York: Oxford University Press.

Freire, P. 1987. *Pedagogy of the Oppressed, trans*. Myra Bergman Ramos. New York: Continuum.

French, S. D., Green, S. E., O'Connor, D. A., McKenzie, J. E., Francis, J. J., Michie, S., Buchbinder, R., Schattner, P., Spike, N. and Grimshaw, J. M. 2012. Developing theory-informed behaviour change interventions to implement evidence into practice: a systematic approach using the Theoretical Domains Framework. *Implementation Science*, 7: 38.

Frost, J., Anderson, R., Argyle, C., Daly, M., Harris-Golesworthy, F., Harris, J., Gibson, A., Ingram, W., Pinkney, J., Ukoumunne, O. C., Vaidya, B., Vickery, J. and Britten, N. 2013. A pilot randomised controlled trial of a preconsultation web-based intervention to improve the care quality and clinical outcomes of diabetes patients (DIAT). *British Medical Journal Open*, 3: e003396.

Fu, R., Gartlehner, G., Grant, M., Shamliyan, T., Sedrakyan, A., Wilt, T. J., Griffith, L., Oremus, M., Raina, P., Ismaila, A., Santaguida, P., Lau, J. and Trikalinos, T. A. 2008. Conducting quantitative synthesis when comparing medical interventions: AHRQ and the effective health care program. In: *Methods Guide for Effectiveness and Comparative Effectiveness Reviews*. Rockville, MD: Agency for Healthcare Research and Quality (USA). http://www.ncbi.nlm.nih.gov/books/NBK49407/ [accessed 22 July 2013].

Fuller, C., Michie, S., Savage, J., McAteer, J., Besser, S., Charlett, A., Hayward, A., Cookson, B. D., Cooper, B. S., Duckworth, G., Jeanes, A., Roberts, J., Teare, L. and Stone, S. 2012. The Feedback Intervention Trial (FIT) – improving hand-hygiene compliance in UK healthcare workers: a stepped wedge cluster randomised controlled trial. *PloS One,* 7: e41617.

Funk, S. G., Champagne, M. T., Wiese, R. A. and Tornquist, E. M. 1991. BARRIERS: the barriers to research utilization scale. *Applied Nursing Research,* 4: 39–45.

Gabbay, J. and le May, A. 2004. Evidence based guidelines or collectively constructed "mindlines"? Ethnographic study of knowledge management in primary care. *British Medical Journal,* 329: 1013.

Georgakellos, D. A. and Macris, A. M. 2009. Application of the semantic learning approach in the feasibility studies preparation training process. *Information Systems Management,* 26: 231–40.

Gibson, A., Britten, N. and Lynch, J. 2012. Theoretical directions for an emancipatory concept of patient and public involvement. *Health (London),* 16: 531–47.

Gillespie, L. D., Robertson, M. C., Gillespie, W. J., Sherrington, C., Gates, S., Clemson, L. M. and Lamb, S. E. 2012. Interventions for preventing falls in older people living in the community. *Cochrane Database of Systematic Reviews,* 9: CD007146.

Glasgow, R. E., Vogt, T. M. and Boles, S. M. 1999. Evaluating the public health impact of health promotion interventions: the RE-AIM framework. *American Journal of Public Health,* 89: 1322–7.

Glasziou, P., Meats, E., Heneghan, C. and Shepperd, S. 2008. What is missing from descriptions of treatment in trials and reviews? *British Medical Journal,* 336: 1472–4.

Glasziou, P., Chalmers, I., Altman, D. G., Bastian, H., Boutron, I., Brice, A., Jamtvedt, G., Farmer, A., Ghersi, D., Groves, T., Heneghan, C., Hill, S., Lewin, S., Michie, S., Perera, R., Pomeroy, V., Tilson, J., Shepperd, S. and Williams, J. W. 2010. Taking healthcare interventions from trial to practice. *British Medical Journal,* 341: c3852.

Glasziou, P., Altman, D. G., Bossuyt, P., Boutron, I., Clarke, M., Julious, S., Michie, S., Moher, D. and Wager, E. 2014. Reducing waste from incomplete or unusable reports of biomedical research. *The Lancet,* 383: 267–76.

Glenton, C., Lewin, S. and Scheel, I. 2011. Still too little qualitative research to shed light on results from reviews of effectiveness trials: a case study of a Cochrane review on the use of lay health workers. *Implementation Science,* 6: 53.

Glenton, C., Colvin, C. J., Carlsen, B., Swartz, A., Lewin, S., Noyes, J. and Rashidian, A. 2013. Barriers and facilitators to the implementation of lay health worker programmes to improve access to maternal and child health: qualitative evidence synthesis. *Cochrane Database of Systematic Reviews,* 10: CD010414.

Godin, G., Bélanger-Gravel, A., Eccles, M. and Grimshaw, J. 2008. Healthcare professionals' intentions and behaviours: a systematic review of studies based on social cognitive theories. *Implementation Science,* 3: 36.

Gollwitzer, P. M. and Sheeran, P. 2006. Implementation intentions and goal achievement: a meta-analysis of effects and processes. *Advances in Experimental Social Psychology,* 38: 249–68.

Gonnella C. 1989. Single subject experimental paradigm as a clinical decision tool. *Physical Therapy,* 69: 601–9.

Gough, D., Oliver, S. and Thomas, J. 2012. *An Introduction to Systematic Reviews.* Thousand Oaks, CA, Sage.

GRADE working group. The grading of Recommendations, Assessments, Development and Evaluation. www.gradeworkinggroup.org

Graffy, J., Bower, P., Ward, E., Wallace, P., Delaney, B., Kinmonth, A.-L., Collier, D. and Miller, J. 2010. Trials within trials? Researcher, funder and ethical perspectives on the practicality and acceptability of nesting trials of recruitment methods in existing primary care trials. *BMC Medical Research Methodology*, 10: 38.

Graham, J. E., Karmarkar, A. M. and Ottenbach, K. J. 2012. Small sample research designs for evidence based rahabilitaion: issues and methods. *Archives of Physical Medicine and Rehabilitation,* 93: S111–16.

Graneheim, U. H. and Lundman, B. 2004. Qualitative content analysis in nursing research: concepts, procedures and measures to achieve trustworthiness. *Nurse Education Today*, 24: 105–12.

Grant, A., Treweek, S., Dreischulte, T., Foy, R. and Guthrie, B. 2013. Process evaluations for cluster-randomised trials of complex interventions: a proposed framework for design and reporting. *Trials,* 14: 15.

Green, J. and Thorogood, N. 2004. *Qualitative Methods for Health Research.* London: Sage.

Greenhalgh, T. and Peacock, R. 2005. Effectiveness and efficiency of search methods in systematic reviews of complex evidence: audit of primary sources. *British Medical Journal,* 331: 1064–5.

Greenhalgh, T., Robert, G., Macfarlane, F., Bate, P. and Kyriakidou, O. 2004. Diffusion of innovations in service organizations: systematic review and recommendations. *Milbank Quarterly,* 82: 581–629.

Greenhalgh, T., Robert, G., Bate, P., Macfarlane, F. and Kyriakidou, O. 2005. *Diffusion of Innovations in Health Service Organisations: A Systematic Literature Review.* Malden, MA: Blackwell.

Greenhalgh, T., Kristjansson, E. and Robinson, V. 2007. Realist review to understand the efficacy of school feeding programmes. *British Medical Journal*, 335: 858–61.

Griffiths, P. 2012. Qualitative or quantitative? Developing and evaluating complex interventions: time to end the paradigm wars. *International Journal of Nursing Studies*, 50: 583–4.

Grimshaw, J. M. and Hutchinson, A. 1995. Clinical practice guidelines: do they enhance value for money in health care? *British Medical Bulletin,* 51: 927–40.

Grimshaw, J. M., Shirran, L., Thomas, R., Mowatt, G., Fraser, C., Bero, L., Grilli, R., Harvey, E., Oxman, A. and O'Brien, M. A. 2001. Changing provider behavior: an overview of systematic reviews of interventions. *Medical Care,* 39, Suppl. 2: 2–45.

Grimshaw, J. M., Eccles, M. P., Walker, A. E. and Thomas, R. E. 2002. Changing physicians' behavior: what works and thoughts on getting more things to work. *Journal of Continuing Education in the Health Professions,* 22: 237–43.

Grimshaw, J.M., Alderson, P., Bero, L., Grilli, R., Oxman, A. and Zwarenstein, M. 2003. Study designs accepted for inclusion in EPOC reviews. *EPOC Newsletter*, March. Cochrane Effective Practice and Organization of Care Review Group. http://epoc.cochrane.org/newsletters.

Grimshaw, J. M., Thomas, R. E., MacLennan, G., Fraser, C., Ramsay, C. R., Vale, L., Whitty, P., Eccles, M. P., Matowe, L., Shirran, L., Wensing, M., Dijkstra, R. and Donaldson, C. 2004. Effectiveness and efficiency of guideline dissemination and implementation strategies. *Health Technology Assessment,* 8: 6.

Grol, R. and Wensing, M. 2013. Implementation of change in healthcare: a complex problem. In: R. Grol, M. Wensing, M. Eccles and D. Davis (eds), *Improving Patient Care: The Implementation of Change in Healthcare.* Chichester: John Wiley, pp. 3–17.

Grol, R., Wensing, M. and Eccles, M. (eds). 2005. *Improving Patient Care: The Implementation of Change in Clinical Practice.* London: Elsevier.

Grol, R., Wensing, M., Eccles, M. and Davis, D. (eds). 2013 *Improving Patient Care: The Implementation of Change in Healthcare*, 2nd edn. Chichester: John Wiley.

Guise, J, Chang, C., Viswanathan, M., Glick, S., Treadwell, J., Umscheid, C., Whitlock, E., Fu, R., Berliner, E., Paynter, R., Anderson, J., Motu'apuaka, M. and Trikalinos, T. 2014. Systematic reviews of complex multicomponent health care interventions. Research White Paper. AHRQ Publication No. 14-EHC003-EF. Rockville, MD: Agency for Healthcare Research and Quality.

Gunal, M. and Pidd, M. 2010. Discrete event simulation for performance modelling in health care: a review of the literature. *Journal of Simulation*, 41: 42–51.

Gunn, J. M., Palmer, V. J., Dowrick, C. F., Herrman, H. E., Griffiths, F. E., Kokanovic, R., Blashki, G. A., Hegarty, K. L., Johnson, C. L., Potiriadis, M. and May, C. R. 2010. Embedding effective depression care: using theory for primary care organisational and systems change. *Implementation Science*, 5: 62.

Gupta, D. and Denton, B. 2008. Appointment scheduling in health care: challenges and opportunities. *IIE Transactions*, 40: 800–19.

Gustafsson, J. and Nilsson-Wikmar, L. 2008. Influence of specific muscle training on pain, activity limitation and kinesiophobia in women with back pain post-partum: a 'single-subject research design'. *Physiotherapy Research International*, 13: 18–30.

Guyatt, G., Oxman, A., Akl, E., Kunz, R., Vist, G., Brozek, J., Norris, S., Falck-Ytter, Y., Glasziou, P., deBeer, H., Jaeschke, R., Rind, D., Meerpohl, J., Dahm, P. and Schünemann, H. J. 2011. GRADE guidelines: 1. Introduction – GRADE evidence profiles and summary of findings tables. *Journal of Clinical Epidemiology*, 64: 383–94.

Habermas, J. 1981. *The Theory of Communicative Action*, trans. Thomas McCarthy. Cambridge: Polity Press.

Hansen, W. B., Graham, J. W., Wolkenstein, B. H. and Rohrbach, L. A. 1991. Program integrity as a moderator of prevention program effectiveness: results for fifth-grade students in the adolescent alcohol prevention trial. *Journal of Studies on Alcohol*, 52: 568–79.

Harden, A. and Thomas, J. 2005. Methodological issues in combining diverse study types in systematic reviews. *International Journal of Social Research Methodology*, 8: 257–71.

Harper, P. R. and Pitt, M. A. 2004. On the challenges of healthcare modelling and a proposed project life-cycle for successful implementation. *Journal of the Operational Research Society*, 55: 657–61.

Harris, J. 2011. Using qualitative research to develop robust effectiveness questions and protocols for Cochrane systematic reviews. In: J. Noyes, A. Booth, K. Hannes, A. Harden, J. Harris, S. Lewin and C. Lockwood (eds), *Supplementary Guidance for Inclusion of Qualitative Research in Cochrane Systematic Reviews of Interventions Version 1* (updated August 2011), chapter 2. http://cqrmg.cochrane.org/supplemental-handbook-guidance.

Hasson, H. 2010. Study protocol: systematic evaluation of implementation fidelity of complex interventions in health and social care. *Implementation Science*, 5: 67.

Hasson, H. and Topo, P. 2014. Implementation of a complex improvement program in aged care. In: A. K. Leist, J. Kulmala and F. Nyqvist (eds), *Health and Cognition in Old Age*. New York: Springer, pp. 219–32.

Hasson, H., Andersson, M. and Bejerholm, U. 2011. Barriers in implementation of evidence-based practice: supported employment in Swedish context. *Journal of Health Organization and Management*, 25: 332–45.

Hasson, H., Blomberg, S. and Dunér, A. 2012. Fidelity and moderating factors in complex interventions: a case study of a continuum of care program for frail elderly people in health and social care. *Implementation Science*, 7: 23.

Hausner, E., Waffenschmidt, S., Kaiser, T. and Simon, M. 2012. Routine development of objectively derived search strategies. *Systematic Reviews*, 1: 19.

Haynes, R. B., Sackett, D. L., Guyatt, G. H. and Tugwell, P. (eds). 2006. *Clinical Epidemiology: How to Do Clinical Practice Research*, 3rd edn. Philadelphia: Lippincott Williams and Wilkins.

Helfrich, C. D., Li, Y. F., Sharp, N. D. and Sales, A. E. 2009. Organizational readiness to change assessment (ORCA): development of an instrument based on the Promoting Action on Research in Health Services (PARIHS) framework. *Implementation Science,* 4: 38.

Herdman, M., Gudex, C., Lloyd, A., Janssden, M. F., Kind, P., Parkin, D., Bonsel, G. and Badia, X. 2011. Development and preliminary testing of the new five-level version of EQ-5D (EQ-5D-5L). *Quality of Life Research,* 20: 1727–36.

Hermens, M. L., Muntingh, A., Franx, G., van Splunteren, P. T. and Nuyen, J. 2014. Stepped care for depression is easy to recommend, but harder to implement: results of an explorative study within primary care in the Netherlands. *BMC Family Practice,* 15: 5.

Hewitt, C. E., Kumaravel, B., Dumville, J. C. and Torgerson, D. J. (Trial Attrition Study Group). 2010. Assessing the impact of attrition in randomized controlled trials. *Journal of Clinical Epidemiology,* 63: 1264–70.

Heyvaert, M., Maes, B. and Onghena, P. 2013. Mixed methods research synthesis: definition, framework, and potential. *Quality and Quantity,* 47: 659–76.

Heyvaert, M., Saenen, L., Maes, B. and Onghena, P. 2014a. Systematic review of restraint interventions for challenging behaviour among persons with intellectual disabilities: focus on experiences. *Journal of Applied Research in Intellectual Disabilities.* doi: 10.1111/jar.12095.

——2014b. Systematic review of restraint interventions for challenging behaviour among persons with intellectual disabilities: focus on effectiveness in single-case experiments. *Journal of Applied Research in Intellectual Disabilities.* doi: 10.1111/jar.12094.

Higgins, J. P. T. and Green, S. (eds). 2009. *Cochrane Handbook for Systematic Reviews of Interventions Version 5.0.2.* http://www.cochrane-handbook.org.

——2011. *Cochrane Handbook for Systematic Reviews of Interventions Version 5.1.0.* http://www.cochrane-handbook.org [accessed 8 May 2014].

Higgins, J. P. T., Thompson, S., Deeks, J. and Altman, D. 2003. Measuring inconsistency in meta-analyses. *British Medical Journal,* 327: 557–60.

Higgins, J. P. T., Altman, D. and Sterne, J. on behalf of the CSMG and the CBMG. 2011a. Assessing risk of bias in included studies. In: J. P. T. Higgins and S. Green (eds), *Cochrane Handbook for Systematic Reviews of Interventions Version 5.1.0,* chapter 8. http://www.cochrane-handbook.org [accessed 8 May 2014].

Higgins, J. P. T., Altman, D. G., Gøtzsche, P. C., Jüni, P., Moher, D., Oxman, A. D., Savović, J., Schulz, K. F., Weeks, L. and Sterne, J. A. C. (Cochrane Bias Methods Group, Cochrane Statistical Methods Group). 2011b. The Cochrane Collaboration's tool for assessing risk of bias in randomised trials. *British Medical Journal,* 343: d5928.

Hill, A. B. 1965. The environment and disease: association or causation? *Proceedings of the Royal Society of Medicine,* 58: 295–300.

Hoben, M., Bär, M., Mahler, C., Berger, S., Squires, J. E., Estabrooks, C. A., Kruse, A. and Behrens, J. 2014. Linguistic validation of the Alberta Context Tool and two measures of research use, for German residential long term care. *BMC Research Notes,* 7: 67.

Hoddinott, P., Britten, J. and Pill, R. 2010. Why do interventions work in some places and not others? A breastfeeding support group trial. *Social Science & Medicine,* 70: 769–78.

Hodnett, E. D., Kaufman, K., O'Brien-Pallas, L., Chipman, M., Watson-MacDonell, J. and Hunsburger, W. 1996. A strategy to promote research-based nursing care: effects on childbirth outcomes. *Research in Nursing & Health,* 19: 13–20.

Hoffmann, T. C., Glasziou, P. P., Boutron, I., Milne, R., Perera, R., Moher, D., Altman, D. G., Barbour, V., Macdonald, H., Johnston, M., Lamb, S. E., Dixon-Woods, M., McCulloch, P.,

Wyatt, J. C., Chan, A. W. and Michie, S. 2014. Better reporting of interventions: template for intervention description and replication (TIDieR) checklist and guide. *British Medical Journal,* 348: g1687.

Holleman, G., Eliens, A., van Vliet, M. and van Achterberg, T. 2006. Promotion of evidence-based practice by professional nursing associations: literature review. *Journal of Advanced Nursing*, 53: 702–9.

Howard, L. and Thornicroft, G. 2006. Patient preference randomized controlled trials in mental health research. *British Journal of Psychiatry*, 188: 303–4.

Howell, E. M. and Yemane, A. 2006. An assessment of evaluation designs: case studies of 12 large federal evaluations. *American Journal of Evaluation,* 27(2): 219–36.

Howes, C. 1988. Peer interaction of young children. *Monographs of the Society for Research in Child Development*, 53: 1–88.

Howick, J., Glasziou, P. and Aronson, J. K. 2009. The evolution of evidence hierarchies: what can Bradford Hill's 'guidelines for causation' contribute? *Journal of the Royal Society of Medicine,* 102: 186–94.

Hróbjartsson, A., Thomsen, A. S. S., Emanuelsson, F., Tendal, B., Hilden, J., Boutron, I., Ravaud, P. and Brorson, S. 2012. Observer bias in randomised clinical trials with binary outcomes: systematic review of trials with both blinded and non-blinded outcome assessors. *British Medical Journal,* 344: e1119.

Huijg, J. M., Gebhardt, W. A., Crone, M. R., Dusseldorp, E. and Presseau, J. 2014. Discriminant content validity of a theoretical domains framework questionnaire for use in implementation research. *Implementation Science,* 9: 11.

Huis, A., Schoonhoven, L., Grol, R., Borm, G., Adang, E., Hulscher, M. and van Achterberg, T. 2011. Helping hands: a cluster randomised trial to evaluate the effectiveness of two different strategies for promoting hand hygiene in hospital nurses. *Implementation Science,* 6: 101.

Huis, A., Holleman, G., van Achterberg, T., Grol, R., Schoonhoven, L. and Hulscher, M. 2013a. Explaining the effects of two different strategies for promoting hand hygiene in hospital nurses: a process evaluation alongside a cluster randomised controlled trial. *Implementation Science,* 8: 1.

Huis, A., Schoonhoven, L., Grol, R., Donders, R., Hulscher, M. and van Achterberg, T. 2013b. Impact of a team and leaders-directed strategy to improve nurses' adherence to hand hygiene guidelines: a cluster randomised trial. *International Journal of Nursing Studies,* 50: 464–74.

Hurley, M., Dickson, K., Walsh, N., Hauari, H., Grant, R., Cumming, J. and Oliver, S. 2013. Exercise interventions and patient beliefs for people with chronic hip and knee pain: a mixed methods review. *Cochrane Database of Systematic Reviews*, 12. http://onlinelibrary.wiley.com/doi/10.1002/14651858.CD010842/abstract;jsessionid=8B00557A93AC003E0BFBEAA211258C17.f01t04.

Husereau, D., Petrou, S., Carwell, C., Moher, D., Greenberg, D., Augustovski, F., Briggs, A. H., Lindsay, W. R., Mauskopf, J. and Loder, E. 2013. Consolidated Health Economic Evaluation Reporting Standards (CHEERS) statement. *British Medical Journal,* 346: f1049.

Hussey, M. A. and Hughes, J. P. 2007. Design and analysis of stepped wedge cluster randomized trials. *Contemporary Clinical Trials*, 28: 182–91.

Hutchinson, A. M. and Johnston, L. 2006. Beyond the BARRIERS scale: commonly reported barriers to research use. *Journal of Nursing Administration,* 36: 189–99.

ICECAP. 2014. Measures of capability. http://www.birmingham.ac.uk/research/activity/mds/projects/HaPS/HE/ICECAP/index.aspx [accessed 28 February 2014].

ICMJE; International Committee of Medical Journal editors. www.icmje.org

Ingolfsson, A., Budge, S. and Erkut, E. 2008. Optimal ambulance location with random delays and travel times. *Health Care Management Science*, 113: 262–74.

Institute of Medicine (IOM). 2002. *Crossing the Quality Chasm: A New Health System for the 21st Century*. Washington, DC: National Academy Press.

Ioannidis, J. P. 2005. Why most published research findings are false. *PLoS Medicine*, 2: 0696–07001.

Ioannidis, J. P. A., Patsopoulos, N. A. and Rothstein, H. R. 2008. Reasons or excuses for avoiding meta-analysis in forest plots. *British Medical Journal,* 336: 1413–15.

Ioannidis, J. P. A., Greenland, S., Hlatky, M. A., Khoury, M. J., Macleod, M. R., Moher, D., Schulz, K. F. and Tibshirani, R. 2014. Increasing value and reducing waste in research design, conduct, and analysis. *The Lancet,* 383: 166–75.

ISPOR. 2006. Guidelines for pharmacoeconomic research, updated version. http://www.ispor.org/PEguidelines/source/HTAGuidelinesNLupdated2006.pdf [accessed 28 February 2014].

ISPOR. 2014. Pharmacoeconomic Guidelines Around the World. http://www.ispor.org/PEguidelines/index.asp [accessed 28 February 2014].

Ivers, N. M., Sales, A., Colquhoun, H., Michie, S., Foy, R., Francis, J. J. and Grimshaw, J. M. 2014. No more 'business as usual' with audit and feedback interventions: towards an agenda for a reinvigorated intervention. *Implementation Science,* 9: 14.

Jacobs, S. R., Weiner, B. J. and Bunger, A. C. 2014. Context matters: measuring implementation climate among individuals and groups, *Implementation Science*, 9: 46. http://www.implementationscience.com/content/pdf/1748–5908–9-46.pdf.

Jaeschke, R., Singer, J. and Guyatt, G. H. 1989. Measurement of health status: ascertaining the minimal clinically important difference. *Controlled Clinical Trials,* 10: 407–15.

Jamtvedt, G., Young. J., Kristoffersen, D., O'Brien, M. and Oxman, A. 2006. Does telling people what they have been doing change what they do? A systematic review of the effects of audit and feedback. *Quality and Safety in Health Care*, 15: 433–6.

Janevic, M. R., Janz, N. K., Dodge, J. A., Lin, X., Pan, W., Sinco, B. R. and Clark, N. M. 2003. The role of choice in health education intervention trials: a review and case study. *Social Science & Medicine,* 56: 1581–94.

Johnson, R. B. and Onwuegbuzie, A. J. 2004. Mixed methods research: a research paradigm whose time has come. *Educational Researcher*, 33: 14–26.

Johnson, R. B., Onwuegbuzie, A. J. and Turner, L. A. 2007. Toward a definition of mixed methods research. *Journal of Mixed Methods Research*, 1: 112–33.

Jun, T. and Clarkson, J. E. 2008. *Modelling and Simulation Techniques for Supporting Healthcare Decision Making: A Selection Framework*. Cambridge: Engineering Design Centre.

Katsaliaki, K. and Mustafee, N. 2011. Applications of simulation wthin the healthcare context. *Journal of the Operational Research Society,* 62: 1431–51.

Kazdin, A. E. 1982. *Single-Case Research Designs: Methods for Clinical and Applied Settings*. Oxford: Oxford University Press.

Kehlet, H. and Dahl, J. 2003. Anaesthesia, surgery, and challenges in postoperative recovery. *The Lancet*, 362: 1921–8.

Keith, R. E., Hopp, F. P., Subramanian, U., Wiitala, W. and Lowery, J. C. 2010. Fidelity of implementation: development and testing of a measure. *Implementation Science,* 5: 99.

Kellogg Foundation. 2004. *Logic Model Development Guide*. Battle Creek, MI: W. K. Kellogg Foundation.

Kemmis, S. and McTaggart, R. 2005. Participatory action research: communicative action and the public sphere. In: N. K. Denzin and Y. S. Lincoln (eds), *Handbook of Qualitative Research,* 3rd edn. Beverley Hills, CA: Sage, pp. 559–604.

Kemmis, S., McTaggart, R. and Nixon, R. 2014. *The Action Research Planner: Doing Critical Participatory Action Research.* Dordrecht: Springer.

Kennedy, A., Rogers, A., Bowen, R., Lee, V., Blakeman, T., Gardner, C., Morris, R., Protheroe, J. and Chew-Graham, C. 2013. Implementing, embedding and integrating self-management support tools for people with long-term conditions in primary care nursing: a qualitative study. *International Journal of Nursing Studies*, 51: 1103–13.

Kerry, R., Eriksen, T. E., Lie, S. A. N., Mumford, S. D. and Anjum, R. L. 2012. Causation and evidence-based practice: an ontological review. *Journal of Evaluation in Clinical Practice*, 18: 1006–12.

Kettles, A. M., Creswell, J. W. and Zhang, W. 2011. Mixed methods research in mental health nursing. *Journal of Psychiatric and Mental Health Nursing*, 18: 535–42.

Kilbourne, A. M., Neumann, M. S., Pincus, H. A., Bauer, M. S. and Stall, R. 2007. Implementing evidence-based interventions in health care: application of the replicating effective programs framework. *Implementation Science*, 2: 42.

King, M., Nazareth, I., Lampe, F., Bower, P., Chandler, M., Morou, M., Sibbald, B. and Lai, R. 2005. Impact of participant and physician intervention preferences on randomized trials: a systematic review. *JAMA: Journal of the American Medical Association,* 293: 1089–99.

Kirkham, J. J., Dwan, K. M., Altman, D. G., Gamble, C., Dodd, S., Smyth, R. and Williamson, P. R. 2010. The impact of outcome reporting bias in randomised controlled trials on a cohort of systematic reviews. *British Medical Journal,* 340: c365.

Kirkwood, B. R. and Sterne, J. A. C. 2003. *Essential Medical Statistics.* Oxford: Blackwell Science.

Kitson, A. 1995. The multi-professional agenda and clinical effectiveness. In: M. Deighan and S. Hitch (eds), *Clinical Effectiveness from Guidelines to Cost Effective Practice.* London: Department of Health.

Kitson, A., Harvey, G. and McCormack, B. 1998. Enabling the implementation of evidence based practice: a conceptual framework. *Quality in Health Care*, 7: 149–58.

Kitson, A. L., Rycroft-Malone, J., Harvey, G., McCormack, B., Seers, K. and Titchen, A. 2008. Evaluating the successful implementation of evidence into practice using the PARiHS framework: theoretical and practical challenges, *Implementation Science*, 3: 1. http://www.implementationscience.com/content/3/1/1.

Knol, M. J., Groenwold, R. H. and Grobbee, D. E. 2012. P-values in baseline tables of randomised controlled trials are inappropriate but still common in high impact journals. *European Journal of Preventive Cardiology,* 19: 231–2.

Knox, C. R., Lall, R., Hansen, Z. and Lamb, S. E. 2014. Treatment compliance and effectiveness of a cognitive behavioural intervention for low back pain: a complier average causal effect approach to the BeST data set. *BMC Musculoskeletal Disorders,* 15: 17.

Koehn, M. L. and Lehman, K. 2008. Nurses' perceptions of evidence-based nursing practice. *Journal of Advanced Nursing,* 62: 209–15.

Kraemer, H. C., Mintz, J., Noda, A., Tinklenberg, J. and Yesavage, J. A. 2006. Caution regarding the use of pilot studies to guide power calculations for study proposals. *Archives of General Psychiatry,* 63: 484–9.

Kroenke, K., Spitzer, R. L. and Williams, J. B. 2001. The PHQ-9: validity of a brief depression severity measure. *Journal of General Internal Medicine,* 16: 606–13.

Lachin, J. M. 2000. Statistical considerations in the intent-to-treat principle. *Controlled Clinical Trials,* 21: 167–9.

Lancaster, G. A., Dodd, S. and Williamson, P. R. 2004. Design and analysis of pilot studies: recommendations for good practice. *Journal of Evaluation in Clinical Practice,* 10: 307–12.

Langendam, M. W., Akl, E. A., Dahm, P., Glasziou, P., Guyatt, G. and Schünemann, H. J. 2013. Assessing and presenting summaries of evidence in Cochrane reviews. *Systematic Reviews,* 2: 81.

Langhorne, P. and Pollock, A. 2002. What are the components of effective stroke unit care? *Age and Ageing,* 31: 365–71.

Langhorne, P., Stott, D., Knight, A., Bernhardt, J., Barer, D. and Watkins, C. 2010. Very early rehabilitation or intensive telemetry after stroke: a pilot randomised trial. *Cerebrovascular Diseases* (Basel, Switzerland), 29: 352–60.

Last, J. M. (ed.). 2001. *A Dictionary of Epidemiology.* Oxford: Oxford University Press.

Law, A. 2006. *Simulation Modelling and Analysis,* 4th edn. New York: McGraw-Hill.

Leal, J., Wordsworth, S., Legood, R. and Blair, E. 2007. Eliciting expert opinion for economic models: an applied example. *Value in Health,* 10: 195–203.

LeBlanc, A., Légaré, F., Labrecque, M., Godin, G., Thivierge, R., Laurier, C., Côté, L., O'Connor, A. M. and Rousseau, M. 2011. Feasibility of a randomised trial of a continuing medical education program in shared decision-making on the use of antibiotics for acute respiratory infections in primary care: the DECISION+ pilot trial. *Implementation Science,* 6: 5.

Lefebvre, C., Manheimer, E. and Glanville, J. on behalf of the CIRMG. 2011. Searching for studies. In: J. P. T. Higgins and S. Green (eds), *Cochrane Handbook for Systematic Reviews of Interventions Version 5.1.0,* chapter 6. http://www.cochrane-handbook.org [accessed 8 May 2014].

Légaré, F. and Zhang, P. 2013. Barriers and facilitators-strategies for identification and measurement. In: S. E. Straus, J. Tetroe and I. D. Graham (eds), *Knowledge Translation in Health Care: Moving from Evidence to Practice,* 2nd edn. Chichester: John Wiley and Sons, Ltd., pp. 121–36.

Légaré, F., Ratté, S., Gravel, K. and Graham, I. D. 2008. Barriers and facilitators to implementing shared decision-making in clinical practice: update of a systematic review of health professionals' perceptions. *Patient Education and Counseling,* 73: 526–35.

Leighl, N. B., Shepherd, F. A., Zawisza, D., Burkes, R. L., Feld, R., Waldron, J., Sun, A., Payne, D., Bezjak, A. and Tattersall, M. H. N. 2008. Enhancing treatment decision-making: pilot study of a treatment decision aid in stage IV non-small cell lung cancer. *British Journal of Cancer,* 98: 1769–73.

Leiva-Fernández, F., Leiva-Fernández, J., Zubeldia-Santoyo, F., García-Ruiz, A., Prados-Torres, D. and Barnstein-Fonseca, P. 2012. Efficacy of two educational interventions about inhalation techniques in patients with chronic obstructive pulmonary disease (COPD). TECEPOC: study protocol for a partially randomized controlled trial (preference trial). *Trials,* 13: 64.

Lenz, M., Steckelberg, A., Richter, B. and Mühlhauser, I. 2007. Meta-analysis does not allow appraisal of complex interventions in diabetes and hypertension self-management: a methodological review. *Diabetologia,* 50: 1375–83.

Leon, A. C., Davis, L. L. and Kraemer, H. C. 2011. The role and interpretation of pilot studies in clinical research. *Journal of Psychiatric Research,* 45: 626–9.

Leon, N., Lewin, S. and Mathews, C. 2013. Implementing a provider-initiated testing and counselling (PITC) intervention in Cape Town, South Africa: a process evaluation using the normalisation process model. *Implementation Science,* 8: 97.

Lewin, K. 1946. Action research and minority problems. *Journal of Social Issues,* 2: 34–46.

Lewin, S., Glenton, C. and Oxman, A. 2009. Use of qualitative methods alongside randomised controlled trials of complex healthcare interventions: methodological study. *British Medical Journal,* 339: b3496.

Lewis, R. A., Williams, N. H., Sutton, A. J., Burton, K., Din, N. U., Matar, H. E., Hendry, M., Phillips, C. J., Nafees, S., Fitzsimmons, D., Rickard, I. and Wilkinson, C. 2013. Comparative clinical effectiveness of management strategies for sciatica: systematic review and network meta-analyses. *Spine Journal*, pii:S1529–9430(13)01497–6.

Liberati, A., Altman, D., Tetzlaff, J., Mulrow, C., Gøtzsche, P., Ioannidis, J., Apte, M., Devereaux, P., Kleijnen, J. and Moher, D. 2009. The PRISMA statement for reporting systematic reviews and meta-analyses of studies that evaluate health care interventions: explanation and elaboration. *PLoS Medicine,* 6: e1000100.

Lieberson, S. and Lynn, F. B. 2002. Barking up the wrong branch: scientific alternatives to the current model of sociological science. *Annual Review of Sociology,* 28: 1–19.

Lindemann, E. 1944. Symptomatology and management of acute grief. *American Journal of Psychiatry*, 101: 141–8.

Lipworth, W. L., Davey, H. M., Carter, S. M., Hooker, C. and Hu, W. 2010. Beliefs and beyond: what can we learn from qualitative studies of lay people's understandings of cancer risk? *Health Expectations,* 13: 113–24.

Little, R. J., D'Agostino, R., Cohen, M. L., Dickersin, K., Emerson, S. S., Farrar, J. T., Frangakis, C., Hogan, J. W., Molenberghs, G., Murphy, S. A., Neaton, J. D., Rotnitzky, A., Scharfstein, D., Shih, W. J., Siegel, J. P. and Stern, H. 2012. The prevention and treatment of missing data in clinical trials. *New England Journal of Medicine,* 367: 1355–60.

Lloyd, J. J., Logan, S., Greaves, C. J. and Wyatt, K. M. 2011. Evidence, theory and context: using intervention mapping to develop a school-based intervention to prevent obesity in children. *International Journal of Behavioral Nutrition and Physical Activity*, 8: 73.

Lloyd, J. J., Wyatt, K. M. and Creanor, S. 2012. Behavioural and weight status outcomes from an exploratory trial of the Healthy Lifestyles Programme (HeLP): a novel school-based obesity prevention programme. *BMJ Open*, 2: e000390.

Lodewijckx, C., Decramer, M., Sermeus, W., Panella, M., Deneckere, S. and Vanhaecht, K. 2012. Eight-step method to build the clinical content of an evidence-based care pathway: the case for COPD exacerbation. *Trials*, 13: 229.

Loeb, M. 2002. Application of the development stages of a cluster randomized trial to a framework for evaluating complex health interventions. *BMC Health Services Research*, 2: 13.

Lohr, K. N. and Steinwachs, D. M. 2002. Health service research: an evolving definition of the field. *Health Service Research*, 37: 15–17.

Luszczynska, A., Sobczyk, A. and Abraham, C. 2007. Planning to lose weight: randomized controlled trial of an implementation intention prompt to enhance weight reduction among overweight and obese women. *Health Psychology*, 26: 507–12.

Lutge, E., Lewin, S., Volmink, J., Friedman, I. and Lombard, C. 2013. Economic support to improve tuberculosis treatment outcomes in South Africa: a pragmatic cluster-randomized controlled trial. *Trials*, 14: 154.

McCaffery, K. J., Turner, R., Macaskill, P., Walter, S. D., Chan, S. F. and Irwig, L. 2011. Determining the impact of informed choice: separating treatment effects from the effects of choice and selection in randomized trials. *Medical Decision Making,* 31: 229–36.

McCann, S. K. 2007. Patients' perspectives on participation in randomised controlled trials. PhD dissertation, University of Aberdeen.

McCann, S. K., Campbell, M. K. and Entwistle, V. A. 2010. Reasons for participating in randomised controlled trials: conditional altruism and considerations for self. *Trials*, 11: 31.

McCormack, B. and Titchen, A. 2006. Critical creativity: melding, exploding, blending. *Educational Action Research: An International Journal*, 14: 239–66.

McCormack, B., Kitson, A., Harvey, G., Rycroft-Malone, J., Titchen, A. and Seers, K. 2002. Getting evidence into practice: the meaning of 'context'. *Journal of Advanced Nursing*, 38: 94–104.

McCormack, B., McCarthy, G., Wright, J., Slater, P. and Coffey, A. 2009a. Development and testing of the Context Assessment Index (CAI). *Worldviews on Evidence-Based Nursing*, 6: 27–35.

McCormack, B., Henderson, E., Wilson, V. and Wright, J. 2009b. The Workplace Culture Critical Analysis Tool. *Practice Development in Healthcare*, 8: 28–43.

McCormack, B., Rycroft-Malone, J., DeCorby, K., Hutchinson, A., Bucknall, T., Kent, B., Schultz, A., Snelgrove-Clarke, E., Stetler, C., Titler, M., Wallin, L. and Wilson, V. 2013. A realist review of interventions and strategies to promote evidence-informed healthcare: a focus on change agency. *Implementation Science*, 8: 107. http://www.implementation-science.com/content/pdf/1748–5908-8-107.pdf.

McCormack, B., Manley, K. and Titchen, A. (eds). 2014. *Practice Development in Nursing and Healthcare*. Oxford: Wiley-Blackwell.

McDonald, A. M., Knight, R. C., Campbell, M. K., Entwistle, V. A., Grant, A. M., Cook, J. A., Elbourne, D. R., Francis, D., Garcia, J., Roberts, I. and Snowdon, C. 2006. What influences recruitment to randomised controlled trials? A review of trials funded by two UK funding agencies. *Trials*, 7: 9.

McEvoy, R., Ballini, L., Maltoni, S., O'Donnell, C., Mair, F. and MacFarlane, A. 2014. A qualitative systematic review of studies using the normalization process theory to research implementation processes. *Implementation Science*, 9: 2.

McGlynn, E. A., Asch, S. M., Adams, J., Keesey, J., Hicks, J., DeCristofaro, A. and Kerr, E. A. 2003. The quality of health care delivered to adults in the United States. *New England Journal of Medicine*, 348: 2635–45.

McGrew, J. H. and Griss, M. E. 2005. Concurrent and predictive validity of two scales to assess the fidelity of implementation of supported employment. *Psychiatric Rehabilitation Journal*, 29: 41–7.

McGuire, T., Wells, K. B., Bruce, M. L., Miranda, J., Scheffler, R., Durham, M., Ford, D. E. and Lewis, L. 2002. Burden of illness. *Mental Health Services Research*, 4: 179–85.

McInnes, E., Jammali-Blasi, A., Bell-Syer, S. E. M., Dumville, J. C. and Cullum, N. 2011. Support surfaces for pressure ulcer prevention. *Cochrane Database of Systematic Reviews*, 4: CD001735.Machta, B. B., Chachra, R., Transtrum, M. K. and Sethna, J. P. 2013. Parameter space compression underlies emergent theories and predictive models. *Science*, 342: 604–7.

Macleod, M. R., Michie, S., Roberts, I., Dirnagl, U., Chalmers, I., Ioannidis, J. P. A., Salman, R. A., Chan, A. W. and Glasziou, P. 2014. Biomedical research: increasing value, reducing waste. *The Lancet*, 383: 101–4.

Mailhot, T., Cossette, S., Bourbonnais, A., Cote, J., Denault, A., Cote, M. C., Lamarche, Y. & Guertin, M. C. 2014. Evaluation of a nurse mentoring intervention to family caregivers in the management of delirium after cardiac surgery (MENTOR_D): a study protocol for a randomized controlled pilot trial. *Trials*, 15: 306.

Mangiapane, S. and Velasco Garrido, M. 2009. Use of surrogate end points in HTA. *GMS Health Technology Assessment*, 5: Doc. 12.

Mantzoukas, S. 2009. The research evidence published in high impact nursing journals between 2000 and 2006: a quantitative content analysis. *International Journal of Nursing Studies*, 46: 479–89.

Marklund, I. and Klässbo, M. 2006. Effects of lower limb intensive mass practice in post-stroke patients: single-subject experimental design with long-term follow-up. *Clinical Rehabilitation*, 20: 568–76.

Marteau, T. M., Dormandy, E. and Michie, S. 2001. A measure of informed choice. *Health Expectations,* 4: 99–108.

MASHnet. 2014. *MASHnet – The UK Network of Modelling and Simulation in Healthcare.* http://www.mashnet.info [accessed 12 June 2014].

Matthews, J. N. S. 2000. *An Introduction to Randomized Trials.* London: Arnold.

May, C. 2006. A rational model for assessing and evaluating complex interventions in health care. *BMC Health Services Research,* 6: 1–11.

May, C. 2013. Towards a general theory of implementation. *Implementation Science,* 8: 18. http://www.implementationscience.com/content/pdf/1748–5908–8-18.pdf.

May, C. and Finch, T. 2009. Implementing, embedding, and integrating practices: an outline of normalization process theory. *Sociology: Journal of the British Sociological Association,* 43: 535–54.

May, C., Mair, F. S., Finch, T., MacFarlane, A., Dowrick, C., Treweek, S., Rapley, T., Ballini, L., Ong, B. N., Rogers, A., Murray, E., Elwyn, G., Legare, F., Gunn, J. and Montori, V. M. 2009. Development of a theory of implementation and integration: Normalization Process Theory. *Implementation Science,* 4: 29.

May, C., Sibley, A. and Hunt, K. 2014. The nursing work of hospital-based clinical practice guideline implementation: an explanatory systematic review using Normalisation Process Theory. *International Journal of Nursing Studies,* 51: 289–99.

May, G. S., DeMets, D. L., Friedman, L., Furberg, C. and Passamani, E. 1981. The randomised clinical trial: bias in analysis. *Circulation,* 64: 669–73.

Mayoh, J., Bond, C. S. and Todres, L. 2012. An innovative mixed methods approach to studying the online health information seeking experience of adults with chronic health conditions. *Journal of Mixed Methods Research,* 6: 21–33.

Mayo-Wilson, E., Grant, S., Hopewell, S., Macdonald, G., Moher, D. and Montgomery, P. 2013. Developing a reporting guideline for social and psychological intervention trials. *Trials,* 14: 242.

Medical Research Council. 2000. *A Framework for Development and Evaluation of RCTs for Complex Interventions to Improve Health.* London: Medical Research Council.

Medical Research Council. 2008. *Developing and Evaluating Complex Interventions: New Guidance.* London: Medical Research Council.

Meleis, A. I. 2004. *Theoretical Nursing: Development and Progress,* 3rd revised edn. Philadelphia: Lippincott.

Melnyk, M. B. 2012. The role of technology in enhancing evidence-based practice, education, heathcare quality, and patient outcomes: a call for randomized controlled trials and comparative effectiveness research. *Worldviews on Evidence-Based Nursing,* 9: 63–5.

Meyer, G. and Mühlhauser, I. 2006. Hip protectors in the elderly: lack of effectiveness or just suboptimal implementation? *European Review of Aging and Physical Activity,* 3: 85–90.

Micevski, V., Sarkissian, S., Byrne, J. and Smirnis, J. 2004. Identification of barriers and facilitators to utilizing research in nursing practice. *Worldviews on Evidence-Based Nursing,* 1: 229.

Michie, S., Johnston, M., Abraham, C., Lawton, R., Parker, D. and Walker, A. 2005. Making psychological theory useful for implementing evidence based practice: a consensus approach. *Quality and Safety in Health Care,* 14: 26–33.

Michie, S., Johnston, M., Francis, J., Hardeman, W. and Eccles, M. 2008. From theory to intervention: mapping theoretically derived behavioural determinants to behaviour change techniques. *Applied Psychology: An International Review/Psychologie Appliquée: Revue Internationale,* 57: 660–80.

Michie, S., Fixsen, D., Grimshaw, J. M. and Eccles, M. P. 2009. Specifying and reporting complex behaviour change interventions: the need for a scientific method. *Implementation Science,* 4, 40.

Michie, S., Abraham, C., Eccles, M. P., Francis, J. J., Hardeman, W. and Johnston, M. 2011. Strengthening evaluation and implementation by specifying components of behaviour change interventions: a study protocol. *Implementation Science,* 6: 10.

Michie, S., Richardson, M., Johnston, M., Abraham, C., Francis, J., Hardeman, W., Eccles, M. P., Cane, J. and Wood, C. E. 2013. The behavior change technique taxonomy (v1) of 93 hierarchically clustered techniques: building an international consensus for the reporting of behavior change interventions. *Annals of Behavioral Medicine,* 46: 81–95.

Mihalic, S. 2004. The importance of implementation fidelity. *Emotional & Behavioral Disorders in Youth,* 4: 83–6.

Mihaylova, B., Briggs, A., O'Hagan, A. and Thompson, S. G. 2011. Review of statistical methods for analysing healthcare resources and costs. *Health Economics,* 20: 897–916.

Mitchell, N., Hewitt, C. E., Lenaghan, E., Platt, E., Shepstone, L. and Torgerson, D. J. 2012. Prior notification of trial participants by newsletter increased response rates: a randomized controlled trial. *Journal of Clinical Epidemiology,* 65: 1348–52.

Moffatt, S., White, M., Macintosh, J. and Howel, D. 2006. Using quantitative and qualitative data in health services research: what happens when mixed method findings conflict? *BMC Health Service Research,* 6: 28. http://www.biomedcentral.com/1472–6963/6/28.

Moher, D., Hopewell, S., Schulz, K. F., Montori, V., Gøtzsche, P. C., Devereaux, P. J., Elbourne, D., Egger, M. and Altman, D. G. 2010. CONSORT 2010 explanation and elaboration: updated guidelines for reporting parallel group randomised trials. *British Medical Journal,* 340: c869.

Möhler, R., Bartoszek, G., Köpke, S. and Meyer, G. 2012. Proposed criteria for reporting the development and evaluation of complex interventions in healthcare (CReDECI): guideline development. *International Journal of Nursing Studies,* 49: 40–6.

Monks, T., Pitt, M. A., Stein, K. and Ma, J. 2012. Maximising the population benefit from thrombolysis in acute ischemic stroke: a modeling study of in-hospital delays. *Stroke,* 43: 2706–11.

Montgomery, P., Grant, S., Hopewell, S., Macdonald, G., Moher, D. and Michie, S. 2013. Protocol for CONSORT-SPI: an extension for social and psychological interventions. *Implementation Science,* 8: 99.

Moore, G. F., Raisanen, L., Moore, L., Din, N. U. and Murphy, S. 2013. Mixed-method process evaluation of the Welsh National Exercise Referral Scheme. *Health Education,* 113: 476–501.

Moore, G., Audrey, S., Barker, M., Bond, L., Bonell, C., Cooper, C., Hardeman, W., Moore, L., O'Cathain, A., Tinati, T., Wight, D. and Baird, J. 2014. Process evaluation in complex public health intervention studies: the need for guidance. *Journal of Epidemiology and Community Health,* 68: 101–2.

Morgan, D. L. 1998. Practical strategies combining qualitative and quantitative methods: applications to health research. *Qualitative Health Research,* 8: 362–76.

Morgan, M. S. 2013. Nature's experiments and natural experiments in the social sciences. *Philosophy of the Social Sciences,* 43: 341–57.

Moulding, N. T., Silagy, C. A. and Weller, D. P. 1999. A framework for effective management of change in clinical practice: dissemination and implementation of clinical practice guidelines. *Quality in Health Care,* 8: 177–83.

Mowbray, C. T., Holter, M. C., Teague, G. B. and Bybee, D. 2003. Fidelity criteria: development, measurement, and validation. *American Journal of Evaluation,* 24: 315.

Mühlhauser, I., Lenz, M. and Meyer, G. 2011. Entwicklung, Bewertung und Synthese von komplexen Interventionen: eine methodische Herausforderung [Development, appraisal and synthesis of complex interventions: a methodological challenge, in German]. *Zeitschrift für Evidenz, Fortbildung und Qualität im Gesundheitswesen,* 105: 751–61.

Munro, A. and Bloor, M. 2010. Process evaluation: the new miracle ingredient in public health research? *Qualitative Research,* 10: 699–713.

Munro, S., Lewin, S., Swart, T. and Volmink, J. 2007. A review of health behavior theories: how useful are these for developing interventions for long-term medication adherence for HIV/AIDS? *BMC Public Health,* 7: 104.

Murray, E., Treweek, S., Pope, C., MacFarlane, A., Ballini, L., Dowrick, C., Finch, T., Kennedy, A., Mair, F., O'Donnell, C., Ong, B. N., Rapley, T., Rogers, A. and May, C. 2010. Normalisation process theory: a framework for developing, evaluating and implementing complex interventions. *BMC Medicine,* 8: 63.

Nabitz, U., Schramade, M. and Schippers, G. 2006. Evaluating treatment process redesign by applying the EFQM Excellence Model. *International Journal for Quality in Health Care,* 18: 336–45.

National Institute of Clinical Studies. 2006. *Identifying Barriers to Evidence Uptake.* https://www.nhmrc.gov.au/_files_nhmrc/file/nics/material_resources/Identifying%20Barriers%20to%20Evidence%20Uptake.pdf [accessed 27 February 2014].

Ng, Y. 1983. *Welfare Economics: Introduction and Basic Concepts.* London: Macmillan.

NICE. 2012. *Methods for the Development of NICE Public Health Guidance.* London: National Institute for Health and Care Excellence.

NICE. 2013a. *Social Care Guidance Manual.* London: National Institute for Health and Care Excellence.

NICE. 2013b. *Guide to the Methods of Technology Appraisal.* London: National Institute for Health and Care Excellence.

Nieminen, T., Prättälä, R., Martelin, T., Härkänen, T., Hyyppä, M. T., Alanen, E. and Koskinen, S. 2013. Social capital, health behaviours and health: a population-based associational study. *BMC Public Health,* 13: 613.

Nilsson Kajermo, K., Nordström, G., Krusebrant, Å. and Björvell, H. 1998. Barriers to and facilitators of research utilization, as perceived by a group of registered nurses in Sweden. *Journal of Advanced Nursing,* 27: 798–807.

Nilsson Kajermo, K., Boström, A. M., Thompson, D. S., Hutchinson, A. M., Estabrooks, C. A. and Wallin, L. 2010. The BARRIERS scale – the barriers to research utilization scale: a systematic review. *Implementation Science,* 5: 32.

Nolan, T. and Berwick, D. M. 2006. All-or-none measurement raises the bar in performance. *JAMA: Journal of the American Medical Association,* 295: 1168–70.

Norberg, A., Melin, E. and Asplund, K. 1986. Reactions to music, touch and object presentation in the final stage of dementia: An exploratory study. *International Journal of Nursing Studies,* 23: 315–23.

Noyes, J. and Lewin, S. 2011. Supplemental guidance on selecting a method of qualitative evidence synthesis, and integrating qualitative evidence with Cochrane Intervention Reviews. In: J. Noyes, A. Booth, K. Hannes, A. Harden, J. Harris, S. Lewin and C. Lockwood (eds), *Supplementary Guidance for Inclusion of Qualitative Research in Cochrane Systematic Reviews of Interventions Version 1* (updated August 2011), chapter 6. http://cqrmg.cochrane.org/supplemental-handbook-guidance.

Noyes, J., Popay, J., Pearson, A., Hannes, K. and Booth, A. 2008. Qualitative research and Cochrane reviews. In: J. P. T. Higgins and S. Green (eds), *Cochrane Handbook for Systematic Reviews of Interventions Version 5.0.1* (updated September 2008), chapter 20. http://www.cochrane-handbook.org.

O'Cathain, A. 2009. Mixed methods research in the health sciences: a quiet revolution. *Journal of Mixed Methods Research,* 3: 3–6.

O'Cathain, A., Murphy, E. and Nicholl, J. 2007. The quality of mixed methods studies in health service research. *Journal of Health Service Research & Policy,* 13: 92–8.

O'Cathain, A., Murphy, E. and Nicholl, J. 2008. Multidisciplinary, interdisciplinary, or dysfunctional? Team working in mixed-methods research. *Qualitative Health Research,* 18: 1574–85.

O'Cathain, A., Murphy, E. and Nicholl, J. 2010. Three techniques for integrating data in mixed methods studies. *British Medical Journal*, 341: c4587.

O'Meara, S., Tierney, J., Cullum, N., Bland, J. M., Franks, P. J., Mole, T. and Scriven, M. 2009. Four layer bandage compared with short stretch bandage for venous leg ulcers: systematic review and meta-analysis of randomised controlled trials with data from individual patients. *British Medical Journal,* 338: 1054–7.

Oakley, A., Strange, V., Bonell, C., Allen, E., Stephenson, J. and RIPPLE Study Team. 2006. Process evaluation in randomised controlled trials of complex interventions. *British Medical Journal*, 332: 413–16.

Odendaal, W., Marais, S., Munro, S. and Van Niekerk, A. 2008. When the trivial becomes meaningful: reflections on a process evaluation of a home visitation programme in South Africa. *Evaluation and Program Planning,* 31: 209–16.

Oliver, S., Clarke-Jones, L., Rees, R., Milne, R., Buchanan, P., Gabbay, J., Gyte, G., Oakley, A. and Stein, K. 2004. Involving consumers in research and development agenda setting for the NHS: developing an evidence-based approach. *Health Technology Assessment,* 8: 1–148.

Oliver, S. R., Rees, R. W., Clarke-Jones, L., Milne, R., Oakley, A. R., Gabbay, J., Stein, K., Buchanan, P. and Gyte, G. 2008. A multidimensional conceptual framework for analysing public involvement in health services research. *Health Expectations,* 11: 72–84.

Olschewski, M. and Scheurlen, H. 1985. Comprehensive cohort study: an alternative to randomized consent design in a breast preservation trial. *Methods of Information in Medicine,* 24: 131–4.

Onwuegbuzie, A. J. and Collins, K. 2007. A typology of mixed methods sampling designs in social science research. *The Qualitative Report*, 12: 281–316.

Onwuegbuzie, A. J. and Leech, N. L. 2006. Linking research questions to mixed methods data analysis procedures. *The Qualitative Report*, 11: 474–98.

Onwuegbuzie, A. J. and Teddlie, C. 2003. A framework for analyzing data in mixed methods research. In: A. Tashakkori and C. Teddlie (eds), *Handbook of Mixed Methods in Social & Behavioral Research*. Thousand Oaks, CA: Sage, pp. 351–83.

Östlund, U., Kidd, L., Wengström, Y. and Rowa-Dewar, N. 2011. Combining qualitative and quantitative research within mixed method research designs: a methodological review. *International Journal of Nursing Studies*, 48: 369–83.

Ottenbacher, K. J. 1986. *Evaluating Clinical Change: Strategies for Occupational and Physical Therapists.* Baltimore, MD: Williams & Wilkins.

Owen, R. R., Drummond, K. L., Viverito, K. M., Marchant, K., Pope, S. K., Smith, J. L. and Landes, R. D. 2013. Monitoring and managing metabolic effects of antipsychotics: a cluster randomized trial of an intervention combining evidence-based quality improvement and external facilitation. *Implementation Science,* 8: 120.

Oxman, A. D., Thomson, M. A., Davis, D. A. and Haynes, R. B. 1995. No magic bullets: a systematic review of 102 trials of interventions to improve professional practice. *Canadian Medical Association Journal,* 153: 1423–31.

Parahoo, K. and McCaughan, E. M. 2001. Research utilization among medical and surgical nurses: a comparison of their self reports and perceptions of barriers and facilitators. *Journal of Nursing Management,* 9: 21–30.

Parker, M., Gillespie, W. and Gillespie, L. 2006. Effectiveness of hip protectors for preventing hip fractures in elderly people: systematic review. *British Medical Journal,* 332: 571–4.

Partridge, N. and Scadding, J. 2004. The James Lind Alliance: patients and clinicians should jointly identify their priorities for clinical trials. *The Lancet,* 364: 1923–4.

Patton, M. Q. 2012. *Essentials of Utilization-Focused Evaluation.* Thousand Oaks, CA: Sage.

Pawson, R. and Tilley, N. 1997. *Realistic Evaluation.* London: Sage.

——2001. Realistic evaluation bloodlines. *American Journal of Evaluation,* 22: 317–24.

Pearson, A., Wiechula, R., Court, A. and Lockwood, C. 2005. The JBI model of evidence-based healthcare. *International Journal of Evidence-Based Healthcare,* 2: 207–15.

Pearson, M., Monks, T., Gibson, A., Allen, M., Komashie, A., Fordyce, A., Harris-Golesworthy, F., Pitt, M. A., Brailsford, S., Stein, K. and Al, E. 2013. Involving patients and the public in healthcare operational research: the challenges and opportunities. *Operations Research for Health Care,* 2: 86–9.

Petticrew, M. 2011. When are complex interventions 'complex'? When are simple interventions 'simple'? *European Journal of Public Health,* 21: 397–8.

Petticrew, M., Anderson, L., Elder, R., Grimshaw, J., Hopkins, D., Hahn, R., Krause, L., Kristjansson, E., Mercer, S., Sipe, T., Tugwell, P., Ueffing, E., Waters, E. and Welch, V. 2013a. Complex interventions and their implications for systematic reviews: a pragmatic approach. *Journal of Clinical Epidemiology,* 66: 1209–14.

Petticrew, M., Rehfuess, E., Noyes, J., Higgins, J. P. T., Mayhew, A., Pantoja, T., Shemilt, I. and Sowden, A. 2013b. Synthesizing evidence on complex interventions: how meta-analytical, qualitative, and mixed-method approaches can contribute. *Journal of Clinical Epidemiology,* 66: 1230–43.

Philips, Z., Bojke, L., Sculpher, M., Claxton, K. and Golder, S. 2006. Good practice guidelines for decision-analytic modelling in health technology assessment: a review and consolidation of quality assessment. *PharmacoEconomics,* 24: 355–71.

Pigott, T. and Shepperd, S. 2013. Identifying, documenting, and examining heterogeneity in systematic reviews of complex interventions. *Journal of Clinical Epidemiology,* 66: 1244–50.

Ploeg, J., Davies, B., Edwards, N., Gifford, W. and Miller, P. E. 2007. Factors influencing best-practice guideline implementation: lessons learned from administrators, nursing staff, and project leaders. *Worldviews on Evidence-Based Nursing,* 4: 210–19.

Pocock, S. 1983. *Clinical Trials: A Practical Approach.* Chichester: John Wiley.

Polit, D. F. and Tatano Beck, C. 2012. *Nursing Research: Generating and Assessing Evidence for Nursing Practice,* 9th edn. Philadelphia, PA: Wolters Kluwer Health/Lippincott Williams & Wilkins.

Pope, C. and Mays, N (eds). 2006. *Qualitative Research in Healthcare.* Oxford: Blackwell.

Pope, C., Ziebland, S. and Mays, N. 2000. Analysing qualitative data. *British Medical Journal,* 320: 114–16.

Pound, P., Britten, N., Morgan, M., Yardley, L., Pope, C., Daker-White, G. and Campbell, R. 2005. Resisting medicines: a synthesis of qualitative studies of medicine taking. *Social Science & Medicine,* 61: 133–55.

Prescott, R. J., Counsell, C. E., Gillespie, W. J., Grant, A. M., Russell, I. T., Kiauka, S., Colthart, I. R., Ross, S., Shepherd, S. M. and Russell, D. 1999. Factors that limit the quality, number and progress of randomised controlled trials. *Health Technology Assessment,* 3: 1–143.

Putland, C., Baum. F., Ziersch, A., Arthurson, K. and Pomagalska, D. 2013. Enabling pathways to health equity: developing a framework for implementing social capital in practice. *BMC Public Health,* 13: 517.

Raftery, J. and Powell, J. 2013. Health technology assessment in the UK. *The Lancet,* 382: 1278–85.

Rahm Hallberg, I. 2006. Challenges for future nursing research: providing evidence for health-care practice. *International Journal of Nursing Studies,* 43: 923–7.

——2009. Moving nursing research forward towards a stronger impact on health care practice. *International Journal of Nursing Studies,* 46: 407–12.

Rapport, F., Storey, M., Porter, A., Snooks, H., Jones, K., Peconi, J., Sanches, A., Siebert, S., Thorne, K., Clement, C. and Russell, I. 2013. Qualitative research within trials: creating a standard operating procedure for a clinical trials unit. *Trials,* 14: 54.

Rawat, R., Nguyen, P. H., Ali, D., Saha, K., Alayon, S., Kim, S. S., Ruel, M. and Menon, P. 2013. Learning how programs achieve their impact: embedding theory-driven process evaluation and other program learning mechanisms in Alive & Thrive. *Food and Nutrition Bulletin,* 34: S212–25.

Reason, P. and Bradbury-Huang, H. 2013. *The Sage Handbook of Action Research: Participative Inquiry and Practice,* 2nd edn. London: Sage.

Reason, P. and Rowan, J. 1981. *Human Inquiry: A Sourcebook of New Paradigm Research.* Chichester: John Wiley.

Reeves, S., Albert, M., Kuper, A. and Hodges, B. D. 2008. Why use theories in qualitative research? *British Medical Journal,* 337: a949.

Reeves, S., Lewin, S., Espin, S. and Zwarenstein, M. 2010. *Interprofessional teamwork for health and social care.* Oxford: Wiley-Blackwell.

Relton, C., Torgerson, D., O'Cathain, A. and Nicholl, J. 2010. Rethinking pragmatic randomized controlled trials: introducing the 'cohort multiple randomized controlled trial' design. *British Medical Journal,* 340: c1066.

Relton, C., O'Cathain, A. and Nicholl, J. 2012. A pilot 'cohort multiple randomized controlled trial' of treatment by a homeopath for women with menopausal hot flushes. *Contemporary Clinical Trials,* 33: 853–9.

Rennick, J.E., Constantin, E., Stremler, R., Horwood, L., Antonacci, M., Aita, M., Majnemer, A. 2014. Abstract 24: acceptability and feasibility of an intervention to promote child comfort and psychological well-being during and following PICU hospitalization. *Pediatric Critical Care Medicine,* 15: (4); suppl p9

Richards, D. A. and Borglin, G. 2011. Complex interventions and nursing: looking through a new lens at nursing research. *International Journal of Nursing Studies,* 48: 531–3.

Richards, D. A. and Hamers, J. P. 2009. RCTs in complex nursing interventions and laboratory experimental studies. *International Journal of Nursing Studies,* 46: 588–92.

Richards, D.A., Meakins, J., Tawfik, J., Dutton, E., Richardson, G. and Russel, D. 2002. Nurse telephone triage for same day appointments in general practice: multiple interrupted time series trial of effect on workload and costs. *British Medical Journal,* 325: 1214–20.

Richards, D. A., Lankshear, A. J., Fletcher, J., Rogers, A., Barkham, M., Bower, P., Gask, L., Gilbody, S. and Lovell, K. 2006. Developing a UK protocol for collaborative care: a qualitative study. *General Hospital Psychiatry,* 28: 296–305.

Richards, D.A., Lovell, K., Gilbody, S., Gask, L., Torgerson, D., Barkham, M., Bland, M., Bower, P., Lankshear, A. J., Simpson, A., Fletcher, J., Escott, D., Hennessy, S. and Richardson, R. 2008. Collaborative care for depression in UK primary care: a randomized controlled trial. *Psychological Medicine,* 38: 279–87.

Richards, D. A., Hughes-Morley, A., Hayes, R. A., Araya, R., Barkham, M., Bland, J. M., Bower, P., Cape, J., Chew-Graham, C. A., Gask, L., Gilbody, S., Green, C., Kessler, D., Lewis, G., Lovell, K., Manning, C. and Pilling, S. 2009. Collaborative Depression Trial (CADET): multi-centre randomised controlled trial of collaborative care for depression – study protocol. *BMC Health Services Research,* 9: 188.

Richards, D. A., Hill, J. J., Gask, L., Lovell, K., Chew-Graham, C., Bower, P., Cape, J., Pilling, S., Araya, R., Kessler, D., Bland, J. M., Green, C., Gilbody, S., Lewis, G., Manning, C.,

Hughes-Morley, A. and Barkham, M. 2013. Clinical effectiveness of collaborative care for depression in UK primary care (CADET): cluster randomized controlled trial. *British Medical Journal*, 347: f4913.

Richards, D. A., Coultard, V. and Borglin, G. 2014. The state of European nursing research: dead, alive or chronically diseased? A systematic literature review. *Worldviews on Evidence-Based Nursing*, 11: 147–55.

Richie, J. and Spencer, L. 1994. Qualitative data analysis for applied policy research. In: A. Bryman and R. G. Burgess (eds), *Analysing Qualitative Data*. London: Routledge, pp. 173–94.

Riley, R. D., Lambert, P. C. and Abo-Zaid, G. 2010. Meta-analysis of individual participant data: rationale, conduct, and reporting. *British Medical Journal*, 340: c221.

Riley, R. D., Higgins, J. P. T. and Deeks, J. J. 2011. Interpretation of random effects meta-analyses. *British Medical Journal*, 342: d549.

Ritchie, J., & Spencer, L. 1994. Qualitative data analysis for applied policy research. In A. Bryman & R. G. Burgess (Eds.), *Analyzing qualitative data*. Oxford: Routledge.

Robert, G. and Fulop, N. 2014. The role of context in successful improvement. In: Health Foundation, *Perspectives on Context: A Selection of Essays Considering the Role of Context in Successful Quality Improvement*. London: Health Foundation, pp. 31–58.

Roberts, K., Dixon-Woods, M., Fitzpatrick, R., Abrams, K. and Jones, D. R. 2002. Factors affecting uptake of childhood immunisation: an example of Bayesian synthesis of qualitative and quantitative evidence. *The Lancet*, 360: 1596–9.

Rogers, P. J. 2008. Using programme theory to evaluate complicated and complex aspects of interventions. *Evaluation*, 14(1): 29–48.

Rohrbach, L. A., Graham, J. W. and Hansen, W. B. 1993. Diffusion of a school-based substance abuse prevention program: predictors of program implementation. *Preventive Medicine*, 22: 237–60.

Rosenhead, J. 1996. What's the problem? An introduction to problem structuring methods. *Interfaces*, 266: 117–31.

Rosenhead, J. and Mingers, J. 2001. *Rational Analysis for a Problematic World Revisited: Problem Structuring Methods for Complexity, Uncertainty and Conflict*, 2nd edn. Chichester: John Wiley.

Rossi, P. H., Lipsey, M. W. and Freeman, H. E. 2004. *Evaluation: A Systematic Approach*, 7th edn. Thousand Oaks, CA: Sage.

Rossouw, J. E., Anderson, G. L., Prentice, R. L., Lacroix, A. Z., Kooperberg, C., Stefanick, M. L., Jackson, R. D., Beresford, S. A., Howard, B. V., Johnson, K. C., Kotchen, J. M. and Ockene, J. 2002. Risks and benefits of estrogen plus progestin in healthy postmenopausal women: principal results from the Women's Health Initiative randomized controlled trial. *Journal of the American Medical Association*, 288: 321–33.

Rothwell, P. M. 2005. External validity of randomised controlled trials: 'to whom do the results of this trial apply?' *The Lancet*, 365: 82–93.

Rottingen, J. A., Regmi, S., Eide, M., Young, A. J., Viergever, R. F., Ardal, C., Guzman, J., Edwards, D., Matlin, S. A. and Terry, R. F. 2013. Mapping of available health research and development data: what's there, what's missing, and what role is there for a global observatory? *The Lancet*, 382: 1286–307.

Rücker, G. 1989. A two-stage trial design for testing treatment, self-selection and treatment preference effects. *Statistics in Medicine*, 8: 477–85.

Ryan, R., Santesso, N., Hill, S., Lowe, D., Kaufman, C. and Grimshaw, J. 2011. Consumer-oriented interventions for evidence-based prescribing and medicines use: an overview of systematic reviews. *Cochrane Database of Systematic Reviews*, 5: CD007768.

Rycroft-Malone, J., Harvey, G., Seers, K., Kitson, A., McCormack, B. and Titchen, A. 2004. An exploration of the factors that influence the implementation of evidence into practice. *Journal of Clinical Nursing,* 13: 913–24.

Rycroft-Malone, J., McCormack, B., Hutchinson, A. M., DeCorby, K., Bucknall, T. K., Kent, B., Schultz, A., Snelgrove-Clarke, E., Stetler, C. B., Titler, M., Wallin, L. and Wilson, V. 2012. Realist synthesis: illustrating the method for implementation research. *Implementation Science,* 7: 33.

Sackett, D. L., Rosenberg, W. M., Gray, J. A., Haynes, R. B. and Richardson, W. S. 1996. Evidence based medicine: what it is and what it isn't. *British Medical Journal,* 312: 71–2.

Saini, M. and Schlonsky, A. 2012. *Systematic Synthesis of Qualitative Research.* New York: Oxford University Press.

Salanti, G. 2012. Indirect and mixed-treatment comparison, network, or multiple-treatments meta-analysis: many names, many benefits, many concerns for the next generation evidence synthesis tool. *Research Synthesis Methods,* 3: 80–97.

Salanti, G., Ades, A. E. and Ioannidis, J. P. A. 2011. Graphical methods and numerical summaries for presenting results from multiple-treatment meta-analysis: an overview and tutorial. *Journal of Clinical Epidemiology,* 64: 163–71.

Sales, A. E. and Helfrich, C. D. 2006. Value in development of complex interventions *American Journal of Managed Care,* 12: 253–4.

Sales, A., Smith, J., Curran, G. and Kochevar, L. 2006. Models, strategies, and tools: theory in implementing evidence-based findings into health care practice. *Journal of General Internal Medicine,* 21, Suppl. 2: S43–9.

Salman, R. A., Beller, E., Kagan, J., Hemminki, E., Phillips, R. S., Savulescu, J., Macleod, M., Wisely, J. and Chalmers, I. 2014. Increasing value and reducing waste in biomedical research regulation and management. *The Lancet,* 383: 176–85.

Sandelowski, M., Voils, C. I. and Barroso, J. 2006. Defining and designing mixed research synthesis studies. *Research in the Schools,* 13: 29–40.

Santesso, N., Carrasco-Labra, A. and Brignardello-Petersen, R. 2014. Hip protectors for preventing hip fractures in older people. *Cochrane Database Systematic Reviews,* 31: CD001255.

Schulz, K. F. and Grimes, D. A. 2002. Sample size slippages in randomised trials: exclusions and the lost and wayward. *The Lancet,* 359: 781–5.

Sculpher, M., Drummond, M. and Buxton, M. 1997. The iterative use of economic evaluation as part of the process of health technology assessment. *Journal of Health Services & Research Policy,* 2: 26–30.

Sculpher, M. J., Claxton, K., Drummond, M. J. and McCabe, C. 2006. Whither trial-based economic evaluation for health care decision making? *Health Economics,* 15: 677–87.

Seers, K., Cox, K., Crichton, N. J., Edwards, R. T., Eldh, A. C., Estabrooks, C. A., Harvey, G., Hawkes, C., Kitson, A., Linck, P., McCarthy, G., McCormack, B., Mockford, C., Rycroft-Malone, J., Titchen, A. and Wallin, L. 2012. FIRE (Facilitating Implementation of Research Evidence): a study protocol. *Implementation Science,* 7: 25.

Shadish, W., Cook, T. and Campbell, D. 2002. *Experimental and Quasi-Experimental Designs for Generalized Causal Inference.* Boston: Houghton Mifflin.

Shanyinde, M., Pickering, R. M. and Weatherall, M. 2011. Questions asked and answered in pilot and feasibility randomized controlled trials. *BMC Medical Research Methodology,* 11: 117.

Shepperd, S., Lewin, S., Straus, S., Clarke, M., Eccles, M., Fitzpatrick, R., Wong, G. and Sheikh, A. 2009. Can we systematically review studies that evaluate complex interventions? *PLoS Medicine,* 6: e1000086.

Shieh, G. 2013. On using a pilot sample variance for sample size determination in the detection of differences between two means: power consideration. *Psicologica*, 34: 125–43.

Sidani, S. and Braden, C. J. 2011. *Design, Evaluation, and Translation of Nursing Interventions.* Chichester: Wiley-Blackwell.

Sleikeu, K. A. 1990. *Crisis Intervention: A Handbook for Practice and Research.* Boston: Pearson Education.

Smith, C. T., Hickey, H., Clarke, M., Blazeby, J., & Williamson, P. 2014. The trials methodological research agenda: Results from a priority setting exercise. *Trials*, 15: 32

Smith, H. K., Laporte, G. and Harper, P. R. 2009. Locational analysis: highlights of growth to maturity. *Journal of the Operational Research Society*, 60: 140–8.

Smith, J. R. and Donze, A. 2010. Assessing environmental readiness: first steps in developing an evidence-based practice implementation culture. *Journal of Perinatal & Neonatal Nursing*, 24: 61–71.

Smith, R. D. 2003. Construction of the contingent valuation market in health care: a critical assessment. *Health Economics*, 12: 609–28.

Smith, R. D. and Sach, T. H. 2009. Contingent valuation: (still) on the road to nowhere? *Health Economics*, 18: 863–6.

——. 2010. Contingent valuation: what needs to be done? *Health Economics Policy and Law*, 5: 91–111.

Social Care Institute for Excellence (SCIE). 2011. *SCIE's Approach to Economic Evaluation in Social Care.* http://www.scie.org.uk/publications/reports/report52.pdf [accessed 28 February 2014].

Somekh, B. 2005. *Action Research: A Methodology for Change and Development.* Maidenhead: Open University Pres/McGraw-Hill Education.

Spangaro, J., Poulos, R. G. and Zwi, A. B. 2011. Pandora doesn't live here anymore: normalization of screening for intimate partner violence in australian antenatal, mental health, and substance abuse services. *Violence and Victims*, 26: 130–44.

Squires, J. E., Estabrooks, C. A., Gustavsson, P. and Wallin, L. 2011. Individual determinants of research utilization by nurses: a systematic review update. *Implementation Science*, 6: 1.

Squires, J. E., Suh, K. N., Linklater, S., Bruce, N., Gartke, K., Graham, I. D., Karovitch, A., Read, J., Roth, V., Stockton, K., Tibbo, E., Woodhall, K., Worthington, J. and Grimshaw, J. M. 2013a. Improving physician hand hygiene compliance using behavioural theories: a study protocol. *Implementation Science*, 8: 16.

Squires, J. E., Valentine, J. C. and Grimshaw, J. M. 2013b. Systematic reviews of complex interventions: framing the review question. *Journal of Clinical Epidemiology*, 66: 1215–22.

Steckler, A. and Linnan, L. (eds). 2002. *Process Evaluation for Public Health Interventions and Research.* San Francisco, CA: Jossey-Bass.

Stein, K. F., Sargent, J. T. and Rafaels, N. 2007. Intervention research: establishing fidelity of the independent variable in nursing clinical trials. *Nursing Research*, 56: 54–62.

Sterman, J. D. 2000. *Business Dynamics: Systems Thinking and Modeling for a Complex World.* New York: Irwin/McGraw-Hill.

Sterne, J. A., White, I. R., Carlin, J. B., Spratt, M., Royston, P., Kenward, M. G., Wood, A. M. and Carpenter, J. R. 2009. Multiple imputation for missing data in epidemiological and clinical research: potential and pitfalls. *British Medical Journal*, 338: b2393.

Stetler, C. B., Ritchie, J. A., Rycroft-Malone, J., Schultz, A. A. and Charns, M. P. 2009. Institutionalizing evidence-based practice: an organizational case study using a model of strategic change. *Implementation Science*, 4: 78.

Stewart, L. A., Tierney, J. F. and Clarke, M. 2011. Reviews of individual patient data. In: J. P. T. Higgins and S. Green (eds), *Cochrane Handbook for Systematic Reviews of Interventions Version 5.1.0*. http://www.cochrane-handbook.org.

Stirling, C., Andrews, S., Croft, T., Vickers, J., Turner, P. and Robinson, A. 2010. Measuring dementia carers' unmet need for services: an exploratory mixed method study. *BMC Health Service Research,* 10: 122. http://www.biomedcentral.com/1472–6963/10/122.

Stoller, E. P., Webster, N. J., Blixen, C. E., McCormick, R. A., Hund, A. J., Kanuch, S. W., Thomas, C. L., Kercher, K. and Dawson, N. V. 2009. Alcohol consumption decision among nonabusing drinkers diagnosed with hepatitis C: an exploratory sequential mixed methods study. *Journal of Mixed Method Research,* 3: 65–86.

Stroke Unit Trialists' Collaboration. 2013. Organised inpatient (stroke unit) care for stroke [Systematic Review]. *Cochrane Database of Systematic Reviews,* 9: CD000197.

Sullivan, F. M., Swan, I. R. C., Donnan, P. T., Morrison, J. M., Smith, B. H., McKinstry, B., Davenport, R. J., Vale, L. D., Clarkson, J. E., Hayavi, S., McAteer, A., Stewart, K. and Daly, F. 2007. Early treatment with prednisolone or acyclovir in Bell's palsy. *New England Journal of Medicine,* 357:1598–607.

Sullivan, P. W., Slejko, J. F., Sculpher, M. J. and Ghushchyan, V. 2011. Catalogue of EQ-5D scores for the United Kingdom. *Medical Decision Making,* 31: 800–4.

Sullivan, S. D., Mauskopf, J. A., Augustovski, F., Caro, J., Lee, K. M., Minchin, M., Orlewska, E., Penna, P., Rodriguez Barrios, J. M. and Shau, W. Y. 2014. Budget impact analysis – principles of good practice: report of the ISPOR 2012 Budget Impact Analysis Good Practice II Task Force. *Value in Health,* 17: 5–14.

Sullivan, W. N. and Payne, K. 2011. The appropriate elicitation of expert opinion in economic models: making expert data fit for purpose. *PharmacoEconomics,* 29: 455–9.

Sully, B. G. O, Julious, S. A. and Nicholl, J. 2013. A reinvestigation of recruitment to randomised, controlled, multicenter trials: a review of trials funded by two UK funding agencies. *Trials,* 14: 1.

Tabak, R. G., Khoong, E. C., Chambers, D. A. and Brownson, R. C. 2012. Bridging research and practice: models for dissemination and implementation research. *American Journal of Preventive Medicine,* 43: 337–50.

Tallon, D., Chard, J. & Dieppe, P. 2000a. Consumer involvement in research is essential. *British Medical Journal,* 320: 380–1.

Tallon, D., Chard, J. and Dieppe, P. 2000b. Relation between agendas of the research community and the research consumer. *The Lancet,* 355: 2037–40.

Tansella, M. and Thornicroft, G. 2009. Implementation science: understanding the translation of evidence into practice. *British Journal of Psychiatry,* 195: 283–5.

Tashakkori, A. and Creswell, J. 2007. The new era of mixed methods. *Journal of Mixed Methods Research,* 1: 3–7.

Taylor, N., Lawton, R., Slater, B. and Foy, R. 2013. The demonstration of a theory-based approach to the design of localized patient safety interventions. *Implementation Science,* 8: 123.

Teddlie, C. and Tashakkori, A. 2009. *Foundations of Mixed Methods Research: Integrating Quantitative and Qualitative Approaches in the Social and Behavioral Sciences.* Thousand Oaks, CA: Sage.

Thabane, L., Ma, J., Chu, R., Cheng, J., Ismaila, A., Rios, L. P., Robson, R., Thabane, M., Giangregorio, L. and Goldsmith, C. H. 2010. A tutorial on pilot studies: the what, why and how. *BMC Medical Research Methodology,* 10: 1. http://www.ncbi.nlm.nih.gov/pmc/articles/PMC2824145/.

Thomas, F. 2007. Eliciting emotions in HIV/AIDS research: a diary-based approach. *Area,* 39: 74–82.

Thompson, A. R., Newman, W. G., Elliott, R. A., Tricker, K. and Payne, K. 2014. The cost-effectiveness of a pharmacogenetic test: a trial-based evaluation of TPMT testing for azathioprine. *Value in Health*, 17: 22–33.

Thompson, D. R. and Clark, A. M. 2012. Addressing the complexity conundrum in and of nursing. *International Journal of Nursing Studies*, 49: 247–8.

Thompson, S. G. and Higgins, J. P. T. 2002. How should meta-regression analyses be undertaken and interpreted? *Statistics in Medicine*, 21: 1559–73.

Tickle-Degnen, L. 2013. Nuts and bolts of conducting feasibility studies. *American Journal of Occupational Therapy*, 67: 171–6. http://www.ncbi.nlm.nih.gov/pmc/articles/PMC3722658/

Titchen, A. and Armstrong, H. 2007. Re-directing the vision: dancing with light and shadows. In: J. Higgs. A. Titchen, D. Horsfall and H. B. Armstrong (eds), *Being Critical and Creative in Qualitative Research*. Sydney: Hampden Press, pp. 151–63.

Tong, A., Flemming, K., Mcinnes, E., Oliver, S. and Craig, J. 2012. Enhancing transparency in reporting the synthesis of qualitative research: ENTREQ. *BMC Medical Research Methodology*, 12: 181.

Torgerson, D. and Roland, M. 1998. Understanding controlled trials: what is Zelen's design? *British Medical Journal*, 316: 606.

Treweek, S., Mitchell, E., Pitkethly, M., Cook, J., Kjeldstrøm, M., Johansen, M., Taskila, T. K., Sullivan, F., Wilson, S., Jackson, C., Jones, R. and Lockhart, P. 2010. Strategies to improve recruitment to randomised controlled trials. *Cochrane Database of Systematic Reviews*, 4: MR000013. doi: 10.1002/14651858.MR000013.pub5.

Treweek, S., Barnett, K., MacLennan, G., Bonetti, D., Eccles, M. P., Francis, J. J., Jones, C., Pitts, N. B., Ricketts, I. W., Weal, M. and Sullivan, F. 2012. E-mail invitations to general practitioners were as effective as postal invitations and were more efficient. *Journal of Clinical Epidemiology*, 65: 793–7.

Treweek, S., Lockhart, P., Pitkethly, M., Cook, J. A., Kjeldstrøm, M., Johansen, M., Taskila, T. K., Sullivan, F., Wilson, S., Jackson, C., Jones, R. and Mitchell, E. 2013. Methods to improve recruitment to randomised controlled trials: Cochrane systematic review and meta-analysis. *British Medical Journal Open*, 3: e002360.

Treweek, S., Wilkie, E., Craigie, A., Caswell, S., Thompson, J., Steele, R. and Anderson, A. 2014. Meeting the challenges of recruitment to multicentre, community-based, lifestyle-change trials: a case study of the BeWEL trial. *Trials*, 14: 436.

Tritter, J. Q. 2009. Revolution or evolution: the challenges of conceptualizing patient and public involvement in a consumerist world. *Health Expectations*, 12: 275–87.

Tritter, J. Q. and Lutfey, K. 2009. Bridging divides: patient and public involvement on both sides of the Atlantic. *Health Expectations*, 12: 221–5.

Turley, R., Saith, R., Bhan, N., Doyle, J., Jones, K. and Waters, E. 2013a. Slum upgrading review: methodological challenges that arise in systematic reviews of complex interventions. *Journal of Public Health*, 35: 171–5.

Turley, R., Saith, R., Bhan, N., Rehfuess, E. and Carter, B. 2013b. Slum upgrading strategies involving physical environment and infrastructure interventions and their effects on health and socio-economic outcomes. *Cochrane Database of Systematic Reviews*, 1. doi: 10.1002/14651858.CD010067.pub2.

Turner, R. M., Thompson, S. G. and Spiegelhalter, D. J. 2005. Prior distributions for the intra-cluster correlation coefficient, based on multiple previous estimates, and their application in cluster randomized trials. *Clinical Trials*, 2: 108–18.

United Kingdom Back Pain Exercise and Manipulation (UK BEAM) randomised trial. 2004. Effectiveness of physical treatments for back pain in primary care. *British Medical Journal*, 329: 1377–81.

US Department of Health and Human Services: Food and Drug Administration (FDA). 2007. Guidance for industry: clinical trial endpoints for the approval of cancer drugs and biologics. http://www.fda.gov/downloads/Drugs/GuidanceComplianceRegulatoryInformation/Guidances/ucm071590.pdf.

US Department of Health and Human Services: Food and Drug Administration (FDA). 2009. Guidance for industry: patient-reported outcome measures – use in medical product development to support labeling claims. http://www.fda.gov/downloads/Drugs/Guidances/UCM193282.pdf.

US Department of Veterans Affairs. 2013. *VA HSR&D QUERI Implementation Guide*. http://www.queri.research.va.gov/implementation/.

van der Wouden, J. C., Blankenstein, A. H., Huibers, M. J. H., van der Windt, D. A. W. M., Stalman, W. A. B. and Verhagen, A. P. 2007. Survey among 78 studies showed that Lasagna's law holds in Dutch primary care research. *Journal of Clinical Epidemiology*, 60: 819–24.

van Hout, B., Janssen, M. F., Feng, Y. S., Kohlmann, T., Busschbach, J., Golicki, D., Lloyd, A., Scalone, L., Kind, P. and Pickard, A. S. 2012. Interim scoring for the EQ-5D-5L: mapping the EQ-5D-5L to EQ-5D-3L value sets. *Value in Health*, 15: 708–15.

Van Vliet, E. J., Sermeus, W., van Gaalen, C. M., Sol, J. C. and Vissers, J. M. 2010. Efficacy and efficiency of a lean cataract pathway: a comparative study. *Quality & Safety in Health Care*, 19: e13.

van Woerkom, C. 1990. 'Education as a policy instrument'. Inaugural address, Wageningen University, Wageningen, The Netherlands.

Vanhaecht, K., Van Gerven, E., Deneckere, S., Lodewijckx, C., Janssen, I., van Zelm, R., Boto, P, Mendes, R., Panella, M., Eva Biringer, E. and Sermeus, W. 2012. The 7-phase method to design, implement and evaluate care pathways, *International Journal of Person Centered Medicine*, 2: 341–51.

Vickers, A. J. and Altman, D. G. 2001. Analysing controlled trials with baseline and follow up measurements. *British Medical Journal*, 323: 1123.

Vickers, A. J., Cronin, A. M., Maschino, A. C., Lewith, G., MacPherson, H., Foster, N. E., Sherman, K. J., Witt, C. M., Linde, K. and Acupuncture Trialists' Collaboration. 2012. Acupuncture for chronic pain: individual patient data meta-analysis. *Archives of Internal Medicine*, 172: 1444–53.

Virtue, A., Chaussalet, T. and Kelly, J. 2013. Healthcare planning and its potential role increasing operational efficiency in the health sector: a viewpoint. *Journal of Enterprise Information Management*, 26: 8–20.

Voils, C. I., Hasselblad, V., Chang, Y., Crandell, J. L., Lee, E. J. and Sandelowski, M. 2009. A Bayesian method for the synthesis of evidence from qualitative and quantitative reports: an example from the literature on antiretroviral medication adherence. *Journal of Health Services Research and Policy*, 14: 226–33.

von Thiele Schwarz, U., Hasson, H. and Lindfors, P. 2013. Using a fidelity framework to balance adaptation and adherence: examples from a physical exercise intervention. Submitted.

Walker, A. E., Grimshaw, J., Johnston, M., Pitts, N., Steen, N. and Eccles, M. 2003. PRIME–PRocess modelling in ImpleMEntation research: selecting a theoretical basis for interventions to change clinical practice. *BMC Health Services Research*, 3: 22.

Walker, M. F., Leonardi-Bee, J., Bath, P., Langhorne, P., Dewey, M., Corr, S., Drummond, A., Gilbertson, L., Gladman, J. R. F., Jongbloed, L., Logan, P. and Parker, C. 2004. Individual patient data meta-analysis of randomized controlled trials of community occupational therapy for stroke patients. *Stroke*, 35: 2226–32.

Walsh, M., Srinathan, S.K., McAuley, D.F., Mrkobrada, M., Levine, O., Ribic, C., Molnar, A. O., Dattani, N. D., Burke, A., Guyatt, G., Thabane, L., Walter, S. D., Pogue, J. & Devereaux,

P. J., Devereaux, P.J. 2014. The statistical significance of randomized controlled trial results is frequently fragile: A case for a fragility index. *Journal of Clinical Epidemiology*, 67: (6); 622–628.

Wand, T., White, K. and Patching, J. 2010. Applying a realist(ic) framework to the evaluation of a new model of emergency department based mental health nursing practice. *Nursing Inquiry*, 17: 231–9.

Wang, D. and Bakhai, A. (eds). 2006. *Clinical Trials: A Practical Guide to Design, Analysis, and Reporting*. London: Remedica.

Warden, D., Trivedi, M. H., Greer, T. L., Nunes, E., Grannemann, B. D., Horigian, V. E., Somoza, E., Ring, K., Kyle, T. and Szapocznik, J. 2012. Rationale and methods for site selection for a trial using a novel intervention to treat stimulant abuse. *Contemporary Clinical Trials*, 33: 29–37.

Warren, F. C., Stych, K., Thorogood, M., Sharp, D. J., Murphy, M., Turner, K. M., Holt, T. A., Searle, A., Bryant, S., Huxley, C., Taylor, R. S., Campbell, J. L. and Hillsdon, M. 2014. Evaluation of different recruitment and randomisation methods in a trial of general practitioner-led interventions to increase physical activity: a randomised controlled feasibility study with factorial design. *Trials*, 15: 134.

Waters, E., Hall, B. J., Armstrong, R., Doyle, J., Pettman, T. L. and de Silva-Sanigorski, A. 2011. Essential components of public health evidence reviews: capturing intervention complexity, implementation, economics and equity. *Journal of Public Health*, 33: 462–5.

Watson, J. M. and Torgerson, D. J. 2006. Increasing recruitment to randomised trials: a review of randomised controlled trials. *BMC Medical Research Methodology*, 6: 34.

Webster, F. and Robins, K. 1989. Plan and control: towards a cultural history of the information-society. *Theory and Society*, 18: 323–51.

Weiner, B. 2009. A theory of organizational readiness for change. *Implementation Science*, 4: 67.

Welton, N. J., Caldwell, D. M., Adamopoulos, E. and Vedhara, K. 2009. Mixed treatment comparison meta-analysis of complex interventions: psychological interventions in coronary heart disease. *American Journal of Epidemiology*, 169: 1158–65.

Wennberg, J. E., Barry, M. J., Fowler, F. J. and Mulley, A. 1993. Outcomes research, PORTS, and health care reform. *Annals of the New York Academy of Sciences*, 703: 52–62.

Whynes, D. K., Frew, E. J. and Wolstenholme, J. L. 2003. A comparison of two methods for eliciting contingent valuations of colorectal cancer screening. *Journal of Health Economics*, 22: 555–74.

Wilhelmson, K., Duner, A., Eklund, K., Gosman-Hedstrom, G., Blomberg, S., Hasson, H., Gustafsson, H., Landahl, S. and Dahlin-Ivanoff, S. 2011. Continuum of care for frail elderly people: design of a randomized controlled study of a multi-professional and multidimensional intervention targeting frail elderly people. *BMC Geriatrics*, 11: 24.

Wisdom, J. P., Cavaleri, M. A., Onwuegbuzie, A. J. and Green, C. A. 2012. Methodological reporting in qualitative, quantitative and mixed methods health service research articles. *Health Service Research*, 47: 721–45.

Wittes, J. and Brittain, E. 1990. The role of internal pilot studies in increasing the efficiency of clinical trials. *Statistics in Medicine*, 9: 65–71 (discussion 71–2).

WMA Declaration of Helsinki – Ethical principles for medical research involving human subjects. Last updated 2013. http://www.wma.net/en/30publications/10policies/b3/.

Wong, G., Pawson, R. and Owen, L. 2011. Policy guidance on threats to legislative interventions in public health: a realist synthesis. *BMC Public Health*, 11: 222.

Wong, G., Greenhalgh, T., Westhorp, G., Buckingham, J. and Pawson, R. 2013a. RAMESES publication standards: meta-narrative reviews. *BMC Medicine*, 11: 20.

——2013b. RAMESES publication standards: realist syntheses. *BMC Medicine*, 11: 21.

World Health Organization (WHO). 2006. *Quality of Care: A Process for Making Strategic Choices in Health Systems.* Geneva: World Health Organization. http://www.who.int/management/quality/assurance/QualityCare_B.Def.pdf.

World Health Organization (WHO). 2010. WHO's role and responsibilities in health research. Sixty-third World Health Assembly Document A63/21 approved on 21 May 2010. http://apps.who.int/gb/ebwha/pdf_files/WHA63/A63_R21-en.pdf.

Worrall, J. 2002. *What Evidence in Evidence-Based Medicine?* Technical Report 01/03. Centre for Philosophy of Natural and Social Science Causality: Metaphysics and Methods. London School of Economics.

——2010. Evidence: philosophy of science meets medicine. *Journal of Evaluation in Clinical Practice,* 16: 356–62.

Wyatt, K. M., Lloyd, J. J., Creanor, S. and Logan, S. 2011. The development, feasibility and acceptability of a school-based obesity prevention programme: results from three phases of piloting. *BMJ Open,* 1: 1.

Wyatt, K. M., Lloyd, J., Abraham, C., Creanor, S., Dean, S., Densham, E., Daurge, W., Green, C., Hillsdon, M., Pearson, V., Taylor, R., Tomlinson, R. and Logan, S. 2013. The Healthy Lifestyles Programme (HeLP), a novel school-based intervention to prevent obesity in school children: study protocol for a randomised controlled trial. *Trials,* 14: 95. http://www.trialsjournal.com/content/14/1/95.

Yarcheski, A., Mahon, N. E. and Yarcheski, T. J. 2012. A descriptive study of research published in scientific nursing journals from 1985 to 2010. *International Journal of Nursing Studies,* 49: 1112–21.

Young, T., Brailsford, S., Connell, C., Davies, R., Harper, P. and Klein, J. H. 2004. Using industrial processes to improve patient care. *British Medical Journal,* 328: 162–4.

Yu, S. C., Hao, Y. T., Zhang, J., Xiao, G. X., Liu, Z., Zhu, Q., Ma, J. Q. and Wang, Y. 2012. Using interrupted time series design to analyze changes in hand, foot, and mouth disease incidence during the declining incidence periods of 2008–2010 in China. *Biomedicine Environmental Science,* 25: 645–52.

Yu, X. and Zhang, J. 2007. Factor analysis and psychometric evaluation of the Connor-Davidson resilience scale (CD-RISC) with Chinese people. *Social Behavior and Personality,* 35: 19–30.

Zelen, M. 1979. A new design for randomized clinical trials. *New England Journal of Medicine,* 300: 1242–5.

——1990. Randomized consent designs for clinical trials: an update. *Statistics in Medicine,* 9: 645–56.

INDEX

References to tables are in *italics* and diagrams in **bold**.

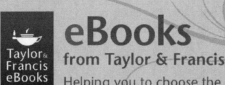